The Thinking Person's

Guide to

PERFECT HEALTH

The Transformation of Medicine

by

Ron Kennedy, M.D.

Context Publications

About the author...

Dr. Kennedy received his Bachelor of Science degree in chemistry and zoology from Texas A. and M. University in 1965. He attended medical school at the University of Texas Medical Branch in Galveston and received his M.D. degree in 1969. Dr. Kennedy interned at Hennepin County General Hospital and did his residency training in neurology and psychiatry at the University of Texas Medical Branch in Galveston. He was board certified in 1975. At present, he practices nutritional family medicine in Santa Rosa, California.

Library of Congress Cataloging in Publication Data
Main entry under title:

The Thinking Person's Guide to Perfect Health, The Transformation of Medicine

Includes index.

Library of Congress catalogue card number: 96-83373

ISBN: 0-932654-13-4

Printed in the United States of America

Editing by Necia Dixon Liles and Suzanne Stasa

Cover design by Ron Kennedy and Necia Dixon Liles

Consultant: Bob Warden

Context Publications
P.O. Box 2909
Rohnert Park, California 94927
(707) 576-1700

Ron Kennedy, M.D.
Santa Rosa, California

Table of Contents

What leaders of the nutritional medicine movement in America have to say about this book...

"This extremely insightful, thought-provoking guide covers the gamut of natural therapies. It will serve as a valuable reference tool for physician and patient alike."

Julian Whitaker, M.D.
President of The American Preventive Medicine Association

"*The Thinking Person's Guide to Perfect Health* details many of the approaches, treatments and major issues of 'alternative' health care in an in-depth and highly readable way. This book is highly recommended for anyone taking responsibility for his or her own health."

Jonathan Wright, M.D.
Vice President of The American Preventive Medicine Association

"*The Thinking Person's Guide to Perfect Health* is a great summary of alternatives in medicine. Patients who are better informed are highly motivated. Having several copies around the office makes my job easier."

L. Terry Chappell, M.D.
President of The American College for Advancement in Medicine

"What an interesting text! I particularly found the chapters 'Chelation Therapy,' 'Dental Amalgam Mercury Poisoning,' and 'Human Growth Hormone,' to be of considerable interest."

H. Richard Casdorph, M.D., Ph.D., F.A.C.P.
Past President of The American College for Advancement in Medicine

INTRODUCTION

INTRODUCTION

The word *doctor*, in Latin, means "teacher." The Latin word *docere* translates: "to teach." When you go to your doctor, you should expect not only to get well but to learn about health and healing also. If you want to learn and your "doctor" doesn't want to teach you, I suggest you get a real doctor.

A good teacher also is a student — otherwise there is soon nothing to teach. Is the ordinary doctor a serious student? To give you an idea of the answer to this question, let me tell you this: most state medical boards require that each doctor have at least thirty hours of "continuing medical education" each year to maintain his or her license. To really keep up with developments, about 300 hours of study per year are required for a fast learner. The fact that medical boards must require thirty documented hours per year reveals how little continued learning is valued by most doctors compared to such things as, for example, managing their business interests.

Most doctors study thousands of hours to make it through each year of medical training, and after that, they feel entitled to believe whatever they did not learn is not worth learning. "If I didn't hear about it in medical school, it must not be any good." That is the unfortunate, unspoken — and sometimes spoken — attitude.

This book is about "progressive" medicine. All good teachers think for themselves. However, most doctors believe what they are told to believe by their teachers in medical school, and this uniformity in beliefs results in "community standards" of medical practice. This term, "community standards," is a semi-legal term used to harass doctors who dare to think for themselves about medical care and who realize "community standards" is merely another term for institutionalized mediocrity.

The Allopathic Paradigm

A paradigm is a model for how things are. It is so deeply believed as to be unexaminable by the person who holds to that paradigm. A paradigm is an unconscious belief that organizes the perception of reality. For example, the paradigm for war is conflict. When you hear the word "war," you assume conflict. A paradigm is not examined or questioned and almost all of what we know to be "true" is paradigm derived. It is not possible to think for yourself until you become aware of the nature of paradigms and conscious of your own particular paradigms. Very few people ever attempt this, and fewer still master it.

Standard medical care is based on the allopathic paradigm. An "allopath" is a standard mainstream doctor following "community standards." These folks assume the body to be basically a machine that functions normally until attacked by a specific disease with a single cause. Find the cause, kill it (usually with a synthetic drug, radiation or a scalpel) and pronounce a cure, if the patient does not die from the treatment, of course.

This paradigm — this unquestioned assumption — is the foundation stone of standardized medical care. From the point of view of a holistic doctor (a "teacher of the whole person") this is a woefully inadequate and mediocre paradigm from which to render medical care.

The Holistic Paradigm

A holistic doctor is necessarily one who has overcome medical school dogma and thinks for him/herself. He/she thinks from a different model of illness and health: the holistic paradigm. This kind of doctor believes illness is almost always multifactorial in cause, and that an important factor in causation of overt illness is the condition of the patient when in the "healthy" state, that is to say, an apparently healthy person may be ill without yet showing symptoms. The holistic doctor believes it is best to treat the patient before symptoms appear because of the difficulty involved in treating after symptoms appear. This is called "preventive medicine."
The holistic doctor believes correction of illness before it is apparent also is the best way to contain health costs. And finally, the holistic doctor sees his or her role as that of an expert advisor with the goal to create an informed patient more able to prevent disease on his own. (This book is meant to assist that process.)

This is the paradigm, or model, with which the holistic doctor approaches the patient. However, the allopathic model with its single cause, doctor-as-God approach is still the predominant medical model in North America. It is popular, because it gives over responsibility for health matters to the doctor.

All professions practice their skills in a socioeconomic context. There are great political pressures on holistic doctors to conform to "community standards" of medical practice. Therefore, your holistic doctor is, by nature, a person willing to think and act in your best interests, despite pressure from his allopathic peers. Your holistic doctor also is termed an "alternative" physician, meaning that because she/he is not of the allopathic paradigm, he/she provides an alternative to that approach.

Perhaps the state of medicine can best be made clear by making what Albert Einstein (a real doctor, a teacher) called a "thought experiment." In this case, our experiment is a social-political-economic-medical thought experiment. Imagine for a moment a plant is discovered having the following characteristics: the seeds are readily available; it is easily grown in any climate; eating this plant instantly cures all of the diseases of aging including arterial occlusion, spinal problems, and also cancer. In addition, this plant works to prevent all other diseases.

What do you suppose would be the reaction of the medical establishment to such a plant? By the term "medical establishment" I am not referring to individual doctors, rather to the advertising/propaganda machines created by the various trade unions associated with medicine: the American Medical Association, the American Pharmaceutical Association, the American Dental Association, etc. I also refer to the FDA, which is staffed by former members of the medical establishment and thus has the same mentality, even though it is supposed to impartially regulate the rest of the medical establishment. The medical establishment is a state of mind created by propaganda machines.

Individual doctors listen to these propaganda machines just as does the rest of the public. Doctors believe most of what they believe about medicine because these trade unions have told them to believe it and have overwhelmed them with propaganda to support their point of view.

To get the answer to the question about the plant that cures all disease, you have to remember this plant, if properly understood by the public, will replace most of modern medicine, putting doctors, pharmaceutical companies, hospitals, medical insurance companies, the professional trade unions (AMA, APA, ADA, etc.) and almost all related industries out of business overnight.

Trauma surgeons, emergency rooms, cosmetic surgeons, obstetricians and a few others still would be in business, everyone else would be scanning the "help wanted" column of the newspaper along with the multi billion dollar pharmaceutical industry and the manufacturers of most medical equipment. An entire industry would be rendered obsolete.

The reaction of the medical establishment to this plant would, of course, be more than negative. Given any chance whatsoever, the medical community would mount a propaganda campaign to discredit this new discovery. This propaganda campaign would be unmatched by any the world has ever seen. Powerful vested interests would not yield easily to this simple plant.

If such a plant were discovered, you probably would never hear of it, or if you did, it would be in the form of the medical establishment's denouncement of this plant as a hoax.

Pure medical science and capitalism do not mix in the same pot. All medical advances occur in a political/economic context. If there is no great profit to be made from an advance in medicine, that advance is downplayed, ignored, or attracts a powerful negative reaction that brands it a hoax.

The fact is, as far as I know, such a plant has not been discovered. However, if you take a handful of relatively obscure medical treatments, that currently are in use, you will have something close to the equivalent of such a magical plant. Probably, you have never heard of them, because they have been downplayed, ignored, or (if that failed) outright attacked by the medical establishment.

In this book I will be telling you about this handful of therapies. The claims that can be made by these therapies are truly astounding and hard to believe. "Why hasn't my doctor told me?" you will ask. "Why haven't I read about these therapies in the paper?" you will want to know. Your doctor hasn't told you, because probably your doctor is also unaware. Doctors listen to the medical establishment, as does the general public, and doctors believe what they are told by the medical establishment, which they trust.

You haven't read about these therapies in the paper, because the media print only that which has general medical agreement. Therefore, the therapies that I will describe in this book are not for everyone.

Most people are hypnotized by the advice to "Listen to your doctor, and do exactly what your doctor tells you!" This is good advice, if you have not informed yourself in such a way that you can become a partner in your own health care rather than merely the passive recipient. Most people should listen to their doctors, and do what those doctors tell them. I am not writing this book for "most people." This book is for the exceptional person, the person who has the intellect and will to question authority, not to be rebellious, simply in recognition of the fact authority is not always correct. This book is for the person who can, and will, think for him/herself.

Let me tell you about the revolution underway in American medicine and in medicine worldwide. On one side is the old order: the medical establishment, espousing allopathic medicine — one disease, one cure — supported by the pharmaceutical industry, churning out one laboratory-made drug after another, providing short-term benefits with significant risks and sacrificing long-term health. Also, lined up with the old order is the Federal Drug Administration (FDA) which collects over 200 million dollars for its participation in the approval process of each new drug, drugs which, after they are approved, are estimated to cause 25,000 deaths outright every year in the U. S. alone and contribute to another 115,000 deaths each year.

On the other side of this war are people who believe in healing by natural means, people who know synthetic drugs are universally toxic and who also know there is no job done by a synthetic drug that cannot be done better by natural agents — vitamins, herbs, botanicals (plant derived), homeopathic preparation, or some other agent derivative from nature. These doctors also know that many times diet and lifestyle changes alone will effect a cure much better than any synthetic drug.

The pharmaceutical industry also is aware of this last fact and is extremely anxious to prevent the public from learning about these superior preparations. Above all, they are terrified doctors will come to appreciate these facts and cease handing out synthetic drugs as if they were candy and begin practicing medicine in a more sensible way. When doctors make this change the pharmaceutical industry is history, and they know it. For this reason they provide a never-ending stream of propaganda aimed at doctors and medical schools (future doctors). They buy large amounts of advertising space in the major medical journals, effectively coercing these journals not to publish research on botanicals, vitamins, and minerals, etc. that would undermine their profits.

The FDA is heavily allied with the pharmaceutical industry with a high priority on protecting drug company profits (and thus their own 200-plus million dollars per drug approval). They have proclaimed regulations to shut the mouths of the manufacturers of vitamins, botanicals, etc. These companies are prohibited from printing the truth on bottles of vitamins, minerals, botanicals, etc. regarding their health benefits and uses. They are forbidden from distributing books and brochures proclaiming these truths. For this reason only people who have taken the time to educated themselves in these matters are aware of the situation.

When these dictatorial regulations are breached, the FDA has no problem putting on their flack jackets, loading their guns, busting into doctors' offices, vitamin stores, vitamin and botanical companies etc., roughing people up, stealing patient and research records, stock, property, and pat-searching personnel, including women. (I can back these assertions up with data.)

The FDA would like to ban the sale of books proclaiming these truths. They would like to regulate vitamins as if they were dangerous synthetic drugs and, if not ban them, at least put them on prescription or, failing that, at least permit only the sale of greatly reduced dosages. These things have actually happened in many countries and if we are not eternally vigilant, they also will happen in the U.S.

All doctors participate in this monumental struggle for the future of your right to be informed and to make informed decisions regarding your health care. Unfortunately, most doctors are participating by doing nothing, by staying locked into the "system," practicing medicine as it was taught to them in medical school and as they are encouraged by the American Medical Association (AMA), the FDA, their state medical boards and other organizations such as the American Cancer Society (ACS) and the National Cancer Institute (NCI).

By the way, if you think these assertions are outrageous and hard to believe, let me invite you to educate yourself. All of these assertions, and many more, are documented in a book entitled *The Assault on Medical Freedom* by P. Joseph Lisa. You can order this book by dialing (800) 357-2211. The cost is $14.95 plus shipping. You will be amazed. I especially encourage other doctors to order this book. So many of us are not informed.

The Transformation of Medicine

There exists a network of doctors in America and throughout the world, among whom I include myself, who are not satisfied to live out their lives practicing the kind of medicine they were taught to practice in medical school, regardless of how obscene the income it can generate. These people understand time marches on, things change, and advances are made. They understand the medical monopoly and choose not to participate in it. Indeed, these doctors want to break the medical monopoly and create a condition some have called "freedom of health care." These doctors think for themselves, practice their art with integrity and courage, and are open-minded to the newest advances in the healing arts whether or not these advances were taught in medical school—and even if these advances do not further line the pockets of the medical establishment.

The latest advances, even if they favor the generation of large incomes for doctors, hospitals, and medical insurance companies, take ten years to make it from the research labs to teaching centers, and at least another ten years to make it to the medical practice of typical doctors. This twenty year lag period makes it too late for many people. Those advances which are not patentable — which reveal the power of vitamins, nutrients, natural human hormones, and other natural substances to heal — would never make it to the consumer except for dedicated practitioners of progressive medicine and their colleagues in research labs and compounding pharmacies.

The network of doctors of which I speak believes in bypassing this pyramid of medical authority and bringing these advances directly to the public. This was the way medicine was designed to be practiced before it became big business. We commit ourselves to a renewal, a renaissance, a transformation of medicine.

This transformation seems to be provoking an inquisiton as doctors are harrassed, persecuted and even prosecuted by the FDA and state medical boards for nothing more than beating the timetable by twenty years and offering therapies which actually work. But, never mind, we can handle the inquisition.

Ron Kennedy, M.D.

Ron Kennedy, M.D.

This book is not intended to replace your relationship with a doctor. If you are ill, do two things: inform yourself about your illness, and find a good doctor. Do not try to treat yourself. Choose your doctor on a rational, informed basis. This book is intended solely as an educational device. It will help you inform yourself and thus be able to choose your doctor on a rational basis, then function as a partner in your own health care.

Ron Kennedy, M.D.

PROGRESSIVE

MEDICAL

THERAPIES

CHELATION THERAPY

Chelation (pronounced key-lay-shun) is a chemical reaction that results in a bond being formed between a metal ion and an organic (i.e., carbon-based—made mostly of carbon) molecule. The resulting complex, metal bound to molecule, is called a "chelate" and contains one or more rings of atoms in which the metal ion is so firmly bound it cannot escape. This allows the metal ion to be transported in the same manner as a prisoner, first handcuffed, then moved from one location to another.

In the presence of aging and disease, the cells' ability to move metal ions through the system and eliminate them when they are in excess becomes progressively impaired. This is especially true for calcium.

Calcium has vital functions in the human body. Without calcium, teeth and bones could not exist. Nevertheless, as the body ages, lipid peroxidation damages the walls of the arterial tree which is repaired leaving a scar. Then calcium and oxidized cholesterol are incorporated into the resulting scar tissue.

There are several known, and easily avoided, risk factors at work in the creation of atherosclerosis. Lipid peroxidation begins the inflammatory process in the wall of the artery and is facilitated by the presence of: (1) polyunsaturated fatty acids (present in many "junk-foods"), (2) oxidized cholesterol (from cooked, i.e., pasteurized, milk and other animal foods cooked in open air), (3) the relative absence of antioxidants, such as vitamins A, C and E, and (4) high levels of homocysteine (a condition easily prevented with vitamins B_6, B_{12} and folate). Tobacco smoke drains the body's resources of antioxidants, particularly vitamin C, and further accelerates atherosclerosis. If you know and apply these facts from an early age, there is no reason for atherosclerosis to develop in your body. To know and apply these facts, you have to be willing to think for yourself and ah, there is the reason atherosclerosis will continue to kill people. Maybe the good do die young but so do the uninformed and dogmatic.

"Hardening of the arteries," or *arterio*sclerosis, on the other hand, is apparently an inevitable change of aging. The walls of blood vessels become stiffer as time passes, as does all connective tissue of the body. This is caused by cross-linkage of collagen, the protein which makes up the connective tissue of artery walls. This cross-linkage results in loss of elasticity and flexability. We believe the process can be slowed, but not entirely prevented, by the liberal intake of antioxidants, especially vitamin C.

With *athero*sclerosis, as the years pass, calcium deposits build up, and calcified atherosclerotic plaques form, lining the walls of the arterial vessels. This plaque is composed of various lipids, so-called foam cells, scar tissue, and overgrown smooth muscles cells from the artery wall. In many people, this process begins in early childhood.

With *arterio*sclerosis, calcium also builds up and becomes many times more concentrated in the wall of the normal artery than it was in childhood. Calcium content is what atherosclerosis and arteriosclerosis have in common. Aging can be thought of as a progressive dysfunction of calcium metabolism.

The exact content of the plaques is determined by the individual's diet, antioxidant intake and duration of the process. Regardless of where on the atherosclerotic continuum any particular individual falls, the result is the same: less and less fresh oxygen delivered to the tissues of the body.

It once was thought this process began in middle or old age. It is now known to begin in childhood in many people. The severity of this life-long process is determined by genetics, level of exercise and dietary habits. By age 21, many individuals have arterial disease, easily recognized at surgery or autopsy.

This is a disease of modern civilization. Never before have people so young had atherosclerosis. As recently as the year 1900, heart disease was very rare. It may be that airborne industrial pollutants, as well as herbicides, pesticides and preservatives in our food, have something to do with the development of atherosclerosis.

The cholesterol content of these plaques can be handled by shifting to a no-fat, high-fiber diet. Plaques actually decrease in size, and the cholesterol content can eventually disappear. Lipid peroxidation itself can be halted by the liberal intake of antioxidants such as Beta-carotene (the precursor of vitamin A), mixed tocopherols (vitamin E) and vitamin C, so no further damage is caused to the arterial tree.

The calcium content of the scar-plaques already present is another matter. Diet and pure water have little effect on it. Therefore, if you want to restore your health to a completely youthful condition, you are facing a real challenge.

The list of problems that can be caused by artery disease is truly impressive, but it should not be surprising that it is so extensive given that a fresh supply of oxygenated blood is absolutely necessary for proper functioning in any organ. Even diseases that are more complicated, in that they have causes other than decreased blood flow, are made worse by arterial disease.

A prime example is Alzheimer's Disease. True Alzheimer's Disease is mimicked by simple aterio-/athero-sclerosis of the arteries and arterioles supplying the brain. Diabetes is known to be made worse by poor blood flow to the pancreas, and poor blood supply also can cause decreased output of digestive enzymes from the exocrine part of the pancreas, causing incomplete digestion.

Decreased blood supply to the kidneys results in the inappropriate release of angiotensin by the kidneys, inducing hypertension throughout the vascular tree. The joints, particularly the joints of the low back, react with inflammation and pain to decreasing blood flow and this, along with the degeneration of ligament tissue and disc disease, is responsible for the so-called "low back syndrome."

Atherosclerosis plays a big part in the cause of arthritis throughout the body due to poor blood supply to the joints. The effect of this process on the heart is angina (chest pain originating in the heart) and eventually infarction and death. Poor blood supply to the stomach and small intestines results in poor digestion. Poor blood supply to the colon causes slowing of the colon with resulting colon disease.

The effect on the extremities is cold hands and feet, and in an advanced case, gangrene of the extremities can result. Impotence can be caused by decreased blood flow to the penis due to clogged arterioles. Frigidity can be caused by decreased blood flow to the pelvis. Cancer is known to be accelerated by decreased blood flow to the affected tissues. When blood flow is decreased to the immunocompetent cells in the bone marrow and spleen, the immune system itself is weakened.

The list of pains, aches, discomforts and diseases caused, or made worse by, Atherosclerosis goes on and on. The above discussion is not complete and could not be made complete unless expanded to book size. Fortunately, there is a way to deal with atherosclerosis. The answer is chelation.

Prevention of Atherosclerosis: Antioxidants

An ounce of prevention certainly is worth a pound of cure. The oral antioxidants (sometimes misnamed as "oral chelating agents") serve admirably to prevent or halt the progression of atherosclerosis, but do little to reverse the disease once it is present. You probably already are taking one of the oral antioxidants, vitamin C. This is an excellent oral chelating agent and also easily available. Also, fresh vegetables are loaded with other natural and effective chelating agents.

Exercise-generated Chelation

Lactic acid, produced from exercise, is an excellent chelating agent. It is the metabolic byproduct of sustained, vigorous muscle contraction. To get this chelating agent, you must exercise regularly. Exercise also increases your body's ability to reduce, and thus neutralize, free radicals, which are at the heart of degenerative diseases.

There is a host of more exotic substances (Anginin, Unithol, Vaso Elastin, DMS, NTA, Hexopal Forte, Syntrival) that I think you should ignore, since they are not readily available, they are expensive, and the agents already easily available to you are excellent.

Reversal of the Effects of Atherosclerosis by Intravenous Chelation

In distinction to the oral chelating agents that serve to prevent atherosclerosis, intravenous chelation has been shown to actually reverse the effects of the disease. The agent used is Ethylene-diamine-tetra-acetic Acid, also known as "EDTA," sold commercially as Sodium Edetate.

EDTA is a synthetic amino acid. The usual dose is 2000-3000 mg. (adjusted to body weight, age, and kidney function) added to 500 ml. of "carrier solution" — sterile water with a mixture of vitamins and minerals. Most chelation doctors add vitamin C along with B vitamins, bicarbonate and magnesium.

The solution is infused slowly, one drop per second, and one treatment requires about three hours. The prisoner (calcium) is moved out of the body using thesheriff's handcuffs (EDTA). The half life of EDTA in the body is one hour; i.e., one-half is removed (filtered into the urine) after one hour, another half of what is left is removed after one more hour, etc. Within 24 hours 99% of the EDTA is gone from the body, and you are left with only the therapeutic benefit.

In addition, to the transitory transport of calcium, many other metal ions are transported and rearranged, which brings up the subject of how EDTA works. In the early days of EDTA therapy, physicians had no idea how it worked. As physicians do, they reached for the nearest reasonable explanation. They said it decalcified the walls of arteries clogged with atherosclerotic plaque, a kind of chemical ROTO-ROOTERTM. This is now known not to be the only benefit of EDTA, even though decalcification of plaques does occur. The action of EDTA is more complex than the simple-minded comparison with a ROTO-ROOTER can reflect.

To be sure, the action of EDTA is to increase blood flow throughout the body. One of the hallmarks of aging is decreased blood flow to all the organs. It has been shown conclusively: EDTA restores this lost blood flow. How can this happen, if EDTA is not a "ROTO-ROOTER?"

Delivery of oxygen to cells is not explainable by merely comparing the circulatory system to a set of pipes. Blood vessels are living organs, not pipes. Once oxygen is delivered to a cell there is still the matter of how efficiently it can be used. EDTA, as it turns out, operates at all these levels. Here are the effects of EDTA, the final manifestation of which is the healing of degenerative diseases of many kinds.

1. EDTA lowers blood calcium and thus stimulates the production of parathormone from the parathyroid glands. This mild pulse of parathormone is responsible for the removal of calcium from abnormal locations (such as arteries) and the deposition of calcium in

locations (such as bones) where it should be. This accounts for the mild recalcification of osteoporotic bones seen with EDTA.

2. EDTA stimulates the enlargement of small vessels, so that they serve the purpose of collateral circulation around a blockage, rendering the blockage irrelevant.

3. EDTA controls free radical damage due to lipid peroxidation by serving as a powerful antioxidant.

4. EDTA removes abnormally located metal ions, such as copper and iron, that accumulate with age.

5. EDTA removes lead, cadmium, aluminum, mercury and other metals, restoring enzyme systems to their proper functions.

6. EDTA enhances the integrity of cellular and mitochondrial membranes.

7. EDTA helps reestablish prostaglandin hormone balance. Prostaglandins, among other things, are responsible for the balancing act between contraction and relaxation of arterial walls and between clotting and the free flow of blood. Prostaglandins are produced from fatty acids, therefore lipid peroxidation upsets the balance of these vital hormones. EDTA chelates out the catalyzing metallic co-enzymes and thus inhibits lipid peroxidation, also serving the same function as an antioxidant.

8. EDTA reduces the tendency of platelets to cause coagulation too readily. This tends to prevent inappropriate thrombosis, which blocks coronary arteries during a heart attack.

9. EDTA increases tissue flexibility by uncoupling age-related cross-linkages that are responsible for loss of skin tone and for wrinkling.

I recommend any individual over the age of forty to have a series of twenty EDTA treatments, followed by six to twelve per year for maintenance after that, simply to restore youthful vitality lost due to aging and atherosclerosis. A person who is already symptomatic with a cardiovascular disease will require more than twenty treatments. We look for the end of troublesome symptoms such as chest pain, leg pain, transient dizziness, intellectual impairment, and fatigue — all attributable to loss of blood flow to vital organs — to know when there have been enough treatments. A good rule of thumb to estimate the maximum number of treatments needed is one treatment for every year of your age, minus 20, but this is only a rough estimate.

You should expect to pay $90-120 per treatment, which admittedly is a nice piece of change. Most people would spend more money on a new car than on their health, so you have to ask yourself how much your health is worth. In the long run, the money you spend on chelation should more than repay itself in health, vitality and the absence of illness. If this were not so, I would not recommend it to you, and I would not be a chelation therapist.

The number of physicians who carry out this procedure is relatively small, but growing rapidly—a few hundred in the U.S. at present. This relative unavailability is surprising, given the great benefits available through this relatively inexpensive, extremely safe treatment.

A Short History of EDTA

EDTA was developed in Germany in the early 1930s as a substitute for citric acid. Citric acid was produced in England and used by Germany for binding mordant dyes. The development of EDTA was part of Germany's effort to become independent of other countries. No one dreamed at the time that it would ever have a medical use. It has been available in the U.S. for medical purposes since 1948. The controversy has been raging since then, and it is not going away, much to the chagrin of the medical/pharmaceutical complex.

Background Information

Many physicians who administer EDTA are people who have benefited from it themselves, many of whom have been brought back from death's door, most commonly from heart disease. As I write this, I am experiencing the absence of a severe low back pain condition, which had been with me for thirteen years, relief I attribute to EDTA! Also my hearing, which was beginning to fail, has cleared up dramatically, and my kids are now puzzled that I can hear them from the other room.

I was introduced to EDTA by an 84-year-old former surgeon, Martin Weiss, M.D., who had been given a death sentence by a cardiovascular surgeon at age 67 unless he would immediately undergo coronary bypass. He knew the dangers of surgery and looked around for an alternative. He learned of EDTA and through treatment became free of heart disease without the risk of anesthesia or surgery. He then decided to offer EDTA to his patients.

Many physicians are closet chelators who perform chelations on themselves and their loved ones and relatives, but do not offer it to the general public because of the threat of condemnation by the medical community. These physicians are severely constrained by their need to be accepted by their peers. The freedoms we enjoy in America were not won by such people.

Medical Politics

One can speculate about why this treatment is not more well-known and commonly administered in modern medicine in the U.S. It is interesting to observe, the patent on EDTA ran out in 1948, and it is therefore very inexpensive, because it can be produced by any drug company and must therefore face free market competition. It hardly matters how effective any drug is, when the patent expires, you probably will not hear much more about it. Drug companies have no fortune to make and thus no motivation to advertise EDTA to doctors. This kind of advertisement, believe it or not, is the most important factor determining which drugs many doctors prescribe, because it is this advertising doctors rely on for the bulk of their "continuing education."

Also, if EDTA became commonly used, there would be a lot of cardiovascular surgeons looking for something else to do, as EDTA is a reasonably priced (cost: $2,000-4000), *safe*, nonsurgical alternative to balloon angioplasty (cost: around $20,000), and coronary bypass operations (cost: in the range of $50,000!). Many of these surgeons make over two million dollars per year doing drastic procedures for illnesses which could have been prevented with oral chelation, and many — even most — of which can still be treated successfully with EDTA. If these surgeons go out of business so does a section of hospital surgery suites and with those, many hospitals. The economic phalanx lined up against chelation therapy is solid and deep.

It is interesting to note a recent study in a publication called *Medical Care* (1995;33(7):715-728). This study reports that coronary bypass surgery is 96% more likely to be recommended when the patient is covered by private insurance versus Medicare (which pays less), and 117% more likely to be recommended versus the noninsured (which pays even less).

I recently attended the thirty year reunion at the university where I took my premed training. There I met an old friend who had become a vascular surgeon. This man was a wonderful student who never made less than an "A" on any test. I thought that, of all people, Ed would have looked over the relevant studies and would have a well-thought-out opinion for or against bypass surgery. So, I asked him, "Ed, what do you think of bypass surgery now? Is that good for people? Should we be doing that to people?" His reply: "It pays the bills!" And that was it. I could not persuade him to say anything more about the matter. He did offer that he was looking forward to an early retirement, but he had no more to say about bypass surgery.

One can only speculate about why the mass consciousness of doctors is not simply neutral to EDTA, but is, instead, openly hostile and disparaging. Otherwise open-minded docs will say absurd things like "I don't know anything about it except it is no good!" How can you know it is no good, if you know nothing about it? My guess is: it is a combination of unconsciousness, ignorance and pure capitalism on the part of both pharmaceutical companies and medical practitioners.

Many courageous physicians have faced censure from medical societies, loss of hospital privileges, and worse for administration of this incredibly effective and safe treatment. Those days are coming to an end, however, because of the massive evidence which has accumulated to validate the safety and effectiveness of EDTA and the power of ACAM, the medical society for chelating doctors.

Nevertheless, we cannot take this therapy for granted. The California Medical Board is striving, right now, 1996, to regulate the use of EDTA to the point that it will not be available for the conditions for which most people need it. The Board is evenly split on whether to do this or not with (predictably) the vascular surgeon on the Board rabidly for suppression of chelation, despite the evidence of its effectiveness. As one of these rigid, righteous, closed-minded doctors said at a recent board meeting, "As long as chelation therapy was limited to being used by only a few docs, it did not need to be regulated, but now that it is becoming well-known, this ripoff therapy must be suppressed." What he did not say, that is clearly true, is he wants to stamp out the competition to his enormous coronary bypass fees. This meeting was open to the public, and the room was full of hundreds of people whose lives had been saved by chelation, one of whom shouted out "Coronary bypass is the real ripoff!"

Let me quote this surgeon a little more. "If EDTA is so good, let them prove it. Proof is not so hard to get! Let them prove it with controlled, double-blind, placebo studies and then publish these results in the top peer-reviewed journals." He apparently had an attack of attention deficit disorder when these very studies had been presented to the Board only a few minutes before.

Only a few of the thousands of fine studies on EDTA have been published in what were once the distinguished journals of medical research. The reason for this: the pharmaceutical industry bought these journals out with "donations" and advertising dollars years ago. Studies on the uses of EDTA threaten the profits of the pharmaceutical industry with its panoply of patented, toxic, synthetic drugs and the surgical industry with its dangerous unnecessary interventions such as bypass surgery. These studies simply are not allowed to be published in what were once the best medical journals, but that now are disrespected by doctors who are knowledgeable about the political process behind these publications.

Indeed, the surgical, pharmaceutical and hospital industries would like to stamp out chelation therapy. I am sure some people at MacDonald's would like to outlaw other restaurants and make the Big Mac the required "food" for every person on the planet. Quality meals, like quality medical care, are not served at every standardized outlet.

A Vignette

Ten days ago one of my patients finished his course of chelation therapy. He went back for a visit to his cardiologist, who had recommended angioplasty and who strongly opposes chelation therapy. This man informed my patient that chelation therapy is dangerous, unproven, a financial ripoff and then insisted that my patient get back on his Mevacor (a toxic synthetic drug for lowering cholesterol). He then mailed to me a nasty little "progress note." A few days later my patient dropped by my office for a chat and pointed out that as a result of chelation therapy his blood pressure is down, his diabetes is under control, his arrythmia is no longer present, and he has a new-found experience of well-being.

When informed by his cardiologist that my fee was a ripoff, my patient reports that he leaned toward that doctor and asked "Just how much does angioplasty cost?" My patient received no answer, and then tried to explain the benefits he experienced from chelation, but the doctor did not want to hear it. Any chelation therapist can tell you several such stories.

My patient did not receive a straight reply that the cost is $20,000 for a two-hour angioplasty — which often is a failure, and if it failed a coronary bypass would have been recommended, costing $50,000. Furthermore, 2% and 5% of patients, respectively, do not surivive these procedures. Contrast that with the fact that people simply do not die, nor are they injured, from properly administered chelation therapy. Also, contrast my fee of less than $2,300 for 25 three-hour chelation treatments — which typically are successful. Remember, *chelation therapy* is supposed to be a financial ripoff and dangerous, according to this doctor.

I am proud to be a physician. I studied and worked hard for my degree. The only time I am embarassed to be a doctor is when I see performances like this one by a colleague. Ignorance and prejudice do not have to go together, yet they do when perceived financial competition is added to the brew. Nevertheless, I expect — and usually get — more from my colleagues. In this case, I am embarassed that this man has the same degree I have. I know better than to hope this doctor will change. The facts do not matter to righteous, closed minds. Things will change, but as a result of people like that growing rich, old, retired, and replaced — by a new generation of enlightened doctors.

Insurance Politics

As of this writing, insurance companies, including Medicare, will not cover the cost of chelation therapy with EDTA, even though the cost is only around $3,000 compared to $15,000 for angioplasty and $50,000 for a bypass. The excuse is, EDTA is not an "accepted" therapy. What that actually means is: not accepted by cardiovascular surgeons who compete with chelation therapy and not accepted by the drug industry, which depends on people remaining sick and taking loads of synthetic drugs, and not accepted by the leading medical journals, which have been bought out by the pharmaceutical and surgical industries.

What is most strange, on the surface, is the fact that insurance companies do not cover the costs of chelation, even though they will shell out for coronary bypass which costs fifteen times as much and treats only two, three or four of the hundreds of arteries in the body. However, if you consider how widespread is the incidence of atherosclerosis, the number of insured people who would need EDTA as a preventive measure is truly astounding, and the cost of covering those people is clearly outside what is possible for any insurance carrier.

Perhaps Medicare and the insurance companies have thought rather deeply into what it would cost to cover chelation therapy.

Nevertheless, if you are willing to have your treatment and then sue your insurance company for coverage, you probably will win, provided you present the facts about EDTA clearly. Historically this has been the case. I have a stack of several hundred scientific articles on EDTA, and I am prepared to prove my point in any forum.

How To Locate A Chelating Doctor

If you have a condition you think might benefit from EDTA, and you do not live close enough to visit my offices, you should call:

The American College for Advancement in Medicine (ACAM)
23121 Verdugo Dr.
Laguna Hills, CA 92653
(800) 532-3688

> **Throughout this book, I have attempted to give you sources from which to locate physicians who offer the kind of therapies about which I write. If you are unable to locate a doctor from this information, you may contact my office for a referral. See page 358 for instructions on making contact with my office.**

Sources

Clarke NE, Clark CN, Mosher RE The "in vivo" disolution of metastatic calcium: An approach to atherosclerosis. Am J Med Sci 1955;229:142-149.

Clarke NE, Clark CN, Mosher RE Treatment of angina pectoris with disodium ethylene diamine tetraacetic acid. Am J Med Sci 1956;232:654-666.

Lamar CP   Chelation therapy of occulsive artherosclerosis. J Am Geriatr Soc 1966;14:272-293.

Bjorksten J The cross-linkage theory of aging as a predictive indicator. Rejuvenation 1980:8:59-66.

Blumer W, Reich T Leaded gasoline - a cause of cancer. Environmental International, 1980;3:456-471.

Casdorph HR, Farr CH EDTA chelation therapy III: Treatment of peripheral arterial occlusion, an alternative to amputation. J Holistic Med 1983;5(1):3-15.

Selhub J, et al. Association between plasma homocysteine concentrations and extracranial carotid artery stenosis. N Eng J of Med 1995; 332:286-291.

INTRAVENOUS HYRDROGEN PEROXIDE THERAPY

In nonorganic chemistry (that chemistry not involving carbon-based molecules) there are only two basic types of chemical reactions: oxidation and reduction. An oxidation reaction removes negative charge by removing electrons. A reduction reaction adds negative charge by adding electrons. Whether a reaction is reductive or oxidative depends on one's point of view.

For example, when iron and oxygen react together, iron is the reducing agent and oxygen is the oxidizing agent. So, if you are studying iron, the reaction is an oxidation reaction (electrons have been removed by the oxygen). If you are studying oxygen the reaction is a reduction reaction (electrons have been added by the iron). In reality, this is a reduction/oxidation, or redox reaction.

Iron + Oxygen (with electrons to contribute) = Iron reacted with Oxygen (electrons contributed to Iron), or:

$$Iron + oxygen + water = rust$$

(Rust is mixed iron oxide and iron hydroxide.)

Iron reacted with oxygen is known as "rust." Iron is changed into something entirely different through this redox reaction with oxygen. Iron is an industrially useful substance. From iron, steel can be made. No one has found a decent use for rust.

This demonstrates the power of oxygen. Oxygen has the ability to accept electrons from atoms of other elements, thus combining with these other atoms, forming a new compound. Oxygen has this action with many different elements and molecules. (Molecules are made from more than one atom.) Anywhere oxygen comes into contact with an atom or molecule that has electrons to contribute (they are not tightly bound in the atom or molecule), oxygen will take those available electrons and transform that atom or molecule into a compound called an "oxide."

This fact is the foundation of bio-oxidative medicine. Bio-oxidative medicine is the addition of oxygen directly to the tissues of the body in the form of singlet oxygen (lone oxygen atoms) in a highly reactive state.

In living systems oxygen (as O_2) is transported by hemoglobin, a protein found in red blood cells. This is a highly efficient way of conducting oxygen from the lungs to the tissues of the body and insuring it does not react with anything along the way. Because it is bound by hemoglobin, it is unable to react to anything else until it is released by the hemoglobin (which then picks up carbon dioxide and transports it to the lungs).

In bio-oxidative medicine, oxygen is introduced directly into the body as hydrogen peroxide (H_2O_2) or as ozone (O_3). Although ozone is used safely and with great benefit throughout

Europe and in many other parts of the world, the medical establishment in the United States refuses to recognize it as a valid therapy and actively persecutes doctors who use it. Luckily, hydrogen peroxide is not treated in this way, even though it is an equally powerful oxidative approach.

The chemical reaction looks like this:

$$H_2O_2 \rightarrow H_2O + O^-$$

This is chemical shorthand to indicate that in the body, hydrogen peroxide is converted to water and singlet oxygen. This singlet oxygen located at the end of this reaction is a powerful oxidizing agent. It is the active agent in hydrogen peroxide therapy.

Hydrogen peroxide is infused into the circulatory system through a vein in the arm. It drips in over a ninety-minute period. Five cc of pharmaceutical-grade, three-percent hydrogen peroxide are put in 500 cc five percent glucose in water as a carrier solution. Two grams of magnesium chloride are added to prevent vein sclerosis.

In the blood, it encounters two enzymes: catalase and cytochrome-C. Catalase drives the above reaction to completion immediately. That part of the hydrogen peroxide that binds with cytochrome-C, however, is not allowed to become water and singlet oxygen for a period of forty minutes. After forty minutes of being bound to cytochrome-C this enzyme begins to act like catalase and breaks down the hydrogen peroxide to water and singlet oxygen. By this time, the hydrogen peroxide/cytochrome-C complex has been spread throughout the body. In this way the benefits of hydrogen peroxide are made available to all cells.

The effect of singlet oxygen in the human body is twofold. **It kills, or severely inhibits the growth of, anaerobic organisms** (bacteria and viruses that use carbon dioxide for fuel and leave oxygen as a by-product). This action is immediate, on contact with the anaerobic organism. Anaerobic bacteria are pathogens, the organisms which cause disease. All viruses are anaerobic.

Aerobic bacteria (those that burn oxygen for fuel and leave carbon dioxide as a by-product — as humans do) found in the human intestine are friendly bacteria, which aid in digestion. These organisms thrive in the presence of hydrogen peroxide.

The second effect of hydrogen peroxide is that it provides singlet oxygen, which, in turn, transforms biological waste products and industrial toxins into inert substances by oxidizing them. This makes them easy to handle for the kidneys and liver. It doubles the rate of enzymatic metabolism in the mitochondria within each cell, thus enabling the body to cleanse itself of toxins and still have plenty of energy to handle the business of living from moment to moment. This increase in metabolism probably accounts for some of the antibacterial, antifungal, and antiviral effects of hydrogen peroxide.

By the way, approximately 125,000 Americans die yearly from drugs approved for safety by the FDA. Some of these deaths are due to individual unique ("idiopathic") reactions. Bruce Lee, a martial artist without equal, and a promising actor with a brilliant career in front of him, died in 1973 in the prime of life at age 32 from taking an FDA-approved headache pill, Equagesic. Any time a drug is synthesized in the laboratory and not derived from nature, this kind of reaction is a possibility.

There are uncounted hundreds of thousands of lives lost each year from toxicity well-known to the FDA, toxicity which is printed right on the package insert which comes with the drug. Most of these drugs are "chemotherapeutic agents," like AZT and Tamoxifen, designed to treat (not really) terminal conditions. They do not work to cure these conditions, but they do treat the conditions, getting rid of the patient by destroying the immune system—no more disease, but no more patient either.

What happens after a new drug is developed, tested and approved is that an advertising blitz is aimed at doctors to persuade them to prescribe this new "miracle" drug. Doctors do listen to this sort of thing. They cannot avoid listening, because drug company sales representatives by the thousands fan out across the country delivering literature on the new "miracle" drug to doctors' offices. They leave free samples to get doctors in the habit of prescribing this drug. They make appointments with doctor to bend his/her ear with a high-pressured sales speech.

Doctors hate this, and they love it. They hate to give up their time to the drug reps, they hate the high pressured presentations, and they love the free samples. This transaction between drug reps and doctors is a major source of the continuing medical education which doctors receive. This is their main line to learning what is "new," and what is new is considered to be what is better! Such folly!

So how does hydrogen peroxide work? How can something so simple and so common as H_2O_2 be responsible for the outlandish claims made for it and the outrageous results reported by people suffering from such diverse disorders?

There has been much written about the possible benefits of shark cartilage in the treatment of cancer recently. The reasoning goes that because sharks do not get cancer they must have a secret, which may be contained in their cartilage. It is conveniently overlooked that whales don't get cancer, dolphins don't get cancer, starfish don't get cancer, octopi don't get cancer. In fact, none of the creatures of the sea (except those living in polluted water) get cancer. There may be something to shark cartilage. Sharks can live in polluted water and still are cancer resistant. The most common denominator is that all these creatures swim in sea water, which is rich in H_2O_2.

Were it not for industrial pollutants, herbicides, pesticides and food additives, we might be able to add "and human beings do not get cancer." However, even if we stopped polluting the environment and ourselves right now, we still would have environmental contaminants in our air and food chains for hundreds of years, so the diseases caused by these things likely are to be around for at least that long. The task now is to see if we can find some means of treatment and protection from this disaster until we can finally clean up our planet.

The most fundamental feature of a cancer cell is that it is relatively anaerobic. It needs sixty percent less oxygen than a normal healthy cell. It does very poorly in the presence of excess oxygen. All of this points toward the oxidative therapies as a decent treatment for cancer and a decent preventative measure as well. Apparently, cancer is the cell's attempt to survive under conditions of a low supply of oxygen. If your cells are well oxygenated, they have no reason to transform into cancer cells. It may be that the way toxins promote cancer is by interfering with the use of oxygen by cells.

Most diseases we assume inherent to being human are results of the polluted chemical soup we all live in during this modern industrial age. Anything which allows the body to cleanse itself of these toxins will deliver you to the pristine condition of health you were meant to enjoy. Fasting will help, a pure diet of plant origin will help, vitamin supplementation will help, EDTA will help, intestinal cleanse programs and colon therapy will help, and so will hydrogen peroxide. Any of these approaches will help cleanse your body of toxins such as pesticides and preservatives, which are laced into the food you buy off the grocery store shelf.

When toxins are released from the cells of the body, they must cross the space between those cells and the outside. Ultimately, they exit the body through the lungs, the liver, the kidneys, and the pores of the skin. Detoxification can feel temporarily worse than the disease. It may be accompanied by headache, fatigue, grouchiness, insomnia and body pains for days or even, in very diseased states, weeks. Hydrogen peroxide is no exception. Be prepared for these kinds of results on your trip to a clear state of health.

People have been traveling to the baths at Lourdes, in southwest France at the base of the Pyrenees Mountains, since 1858 when a girl is said to have seen there a vision of the Virgin Mary. The waters at the baths in Lourdes are believed by many people to have miracle healing powers. Perhaps it is no coincidence these waters are loaded with, you guessed it, hydrogen peroxide. People go there to bathe in and drink the water.

How does one take hydrogen peroxide? You can go to Lourdes, or you can go to a good organic grocery store and buy a bottle of food grade (35%) hydrogen peroxide, dilute it and drink it, or bath in it. If you go to Lourdes, be prepared to shell out thousands of dollars. If you go to the grocery store, be prepared to pay a few dollars. Be sure to dilute it, because the 35% solution will cause burning of the skin on application, or internal damage, if you try to drink it.

If you take it orally, you should dilute it approximately ten drops in an eight ounce glass of water, two or three times each day, on an empty stomach (three hours after your last meal). If you take it with food in your stomach, the hydrogen peroxide will react with the food, and you will not get the benefit from it. Even if you take it on an empty stomach it reacts to the cells of the stomach wall, as well as whatever food fragments still are present, and you receive not only hydrogen peroxide into your circulation, but also oxidation products of H_2O_2 plus sluffed off cells from the lining of your stomach and miscellaneous food.

Because of these considerations I cannot, and I do not, recommend you take H_2O_2 by mouth. I believe intravenous H_2O_2 to be far superior to the oral route of administration. However, because people do report good results with the oral route, I cannot recommend you absolutely do not take it by mouth. This is a gray area.

To benefit your body, the H_2O_2 must reach your circulation, where it can be broken down by catalase and bound by cytochrome-C for distribution throughout your body in the following forty minutes. You should not eat anything for at least twenty minutes after taking the H_2O_2.

You will notice hydrogen peroxide, even in this very dilute state, tastes terrible. It makes many people nauseated. You may be able to mask this effect by taking it with fresh lemon or berry juice or with aloe vera juice.

You also can bathe in hydrogen peroxide by putting a pint in your bath water. Be sure to stir it up well before getting in to avoid burning your skin. Many people with arthritis swear by this treatment.

If you are confronting a serious illness, or if oral and topical applications are not getting the job done, you can turn to intravenous infusion of hydrogen peroxide. Intravenous H_2O_2 is far more powerful than the oral ingestion or topical application. For this form of treatment, you must find a physician who is familiar with the proper preparation of pharmaceutical grade H_2O_2 in a bottle of sterile, isotonic intravenous fluid.

The infusion lasts ninety minutes. You will notice a warm feeling during treatment, not much more. The main effect of hydrogen peroxide infusions is that you regain your health. Treatments are one to three times per week, occasionally five times per week for an acute illness and, just as with chelation therapy with EDTA, the number of treatments needed depends on the nature of the illness with which you are dealing. From ten to fifty treatments will get the job done in most cases, and you should be able to maintain on oral hydrogen peroxide or the occasional intravenous infusion after that.

As I alluded to above, there is an exciting new development in the treatment of vascular disease, Chelox Therapy, which involves the combination of treatment with EDTA and H_2O_2, not in the same infusion, or even on the same day for that matter, but separated by at least one day. These two therapies work in different ways and cross react with each other, causing a thirty percent incidence of intravenous thrombosis. They can be given in combination to the same patient but not on the same day. The combination of these two therapies, given correctly, has been found to be more powerful than either one used alone.

Many fine doctors offer hydrogen peroxide therapy in the U.S. and Canada. However, most of the progressive approaches in medicine have a particular champion who assumes the responsibility to spread the information to other doctors. Dr. Charles Farr, M.D., of Oklahoma, is such a champion for hydrogen peroxide therapy. He has established the International Bio-oxidative Medicine Society. If you want to locate a doctor who offers hydrogen peroxide therapy, write for a referral to:

The International Bio-oxidative Medicine Society
P.O. Box 891954
Oklahoma City, OK 73189

Or, see page 358 for instructions on contacting my office for a referral.

Sources

Oliver TH, Cantab BC, Murphy DV, Influenzal pneumonia: the intravenous injection of hydrogen peroxide. Lancet 1920;1:432-433.

Root RK, Metcalf J, Oshino N, et al. H_2O_2 release from human granulocytes during phagocytosis. J Clin Invest 1975;55:945-955.

Finney JW, Jay BE, Race GJ, et al. Removal of cholesterol and other lipids from experimental animals and human atheromatous arteries by dilute hydrogen peroxide. Angiology 1966;17:223-228.

Urschel HC, Finney JW, Morale AR, et al. Cardiac resuscitation with hydrogen peroxide. Circ 1965;31 (suppl II);II-210.

Urschel HC, Finney JW, Balla GA, et al. Protection of the ischemic heart with DMSO alone or with hydrogen peroxide. Ann NY Adad. Sci. 1967; 151:231-241.

Gorren AC, Dekker H, Wever R Kinetic investigations of the reaction of cytochrome C oxidase by hydrogen peroxide. Biochem Biophys Acta 1986; 852(1):81-92.

Nathan CF, Cohn ZA Antitumor effects of hydrogen peroxide in vivo. J Exp Med 1981;154:1539-1553.

Manakata T, Semba U, Shibuya Y, et al. Induction of interferon-gamma production by human natural killer cells stimulated by hydrogen peroxide. J Immunol 1985;134(4):2449-2455.

Lebedev LV, Levin AO, Romankova MP, et al. Regional oxygenation in the treatment of severe destructive forms of obliterating diseases of the extremity arteries. Vestn Khir 1984;132:85-88.

PROLOTHERAPY

One out of three people, at some time in life, experiences spinal disease significant enough to lead to professional treatment. In America alone, $7.4 billion are spent on drugs every year to treat pain originating in the spine. This amounts to an average of $30 for each person, each year. Every day, one out of five people in Western countries (and probably worldwide) suffer from debilitating spinal pain.

Loss of work time in America amounts to $80 billion each year! Fifteen million Americans consult a physician for backache or neckache every year, paying these physicians a total of $20 billion. And what do we get for our money? Do we get a cure? Not exactly. The truth is, physicians in general have no effective treatment for spinal aches to offer you. Physicians typically offer the following palliative treatments, in this order:

1. anti-inflammatory medications (some of which are effective for no more than a few days, but also cost a fortune),
2. cortisone injections (causing dramatic but, alas, only temporary relief),
3. surgery and more anti-inflammatory medications, including more cortisone, resulting in damaged and iatrogenically (doctor induced) degenerated joints.

All of this leaves you in the poorhouse as soon as you are discharged from the hospital and, in more than half the cases, leaves you worse off than you were before surgery! Hundreds of thousands of careers have been destroyed by this misguided approach to joint disease of the back and neck.

Let us take a look at what spinal disease really is, so we can see why the standard medical/surgical approach is the only thing worse than spinal ache itself. The human spine is made of 24 individual, movable vertebrae, and nine fused vertebrae. Each articulates with the one above and below it. There are seven cervical vertebrae, twelve thoracic vertebrae and five lumbar vertebrae, the last of which articulates with the sacrum. The sacrum is formed in the embryo by the fusion of five vertebrae. At the end of the sacrum is the coccyx consisting of four vertebrae fused together, which represent what is left of the tail of our simian ancestors. The coccyx is made of four tiny, fused vertebrae and moves independently of the sacrum. It is the so-called "tail bone" which can easily be damaged when one falls backward to the sitting position. Each vertebrae of the spine, whether fused or not, has corresponding nerve roots in the spinal cord. The total number is therefore $7 + 12 + 5 + 5 + 4 = 33$.

While problems of the spinal column can occur at any level, the most common area to be affected is the low back with the neck running a close second. As the body ages, the ligaments which hold the vertebrae together become weaker, predisposing you to a greater risk of back and neck injuries with each passing year. Athletic people, and people who perform heavy labor for a living, are most likely to experience an injury due to ripping and tearing of these increasingly fragile ligaments.

Disk degeneration is a natural phenomenon, eventually present in everyone. It should be considered normal, and it is not, by itself, a cause of back or neck pain. The proof of this assertion is the fact many people have degenerated intervertebral discs, but no pain. Many doctors are not aware of this fact, and they will point to an x-ray revealing disc degeneration and tell you the cause of your back or neck pain has been found. Do not believe it!

The cause of back and neck pain is the instability of vertebrae, which results from weakened and/or damaged ligaments. The vertebrae are held in their proper position in relationship to each other by muscles and by ligaments. Muscles alone are not able to do the job. Nevertheless, they can help, and this is the rational basis of exercise as a treatment for an unstable back or neck.

Strong ligaments are necessary for a stable spine. However, instability is not, in itself, the cause of pain. The cause of pain is inflammation. Inflammation happens when vertebrae rub against each other in an abnormal way due to the presence of damaged ligaments. This is why anti-inflammatory agents, including cortisone, can result in temporary relief of pain. However, since the underlying condition is not treated with anti-inflammatory agents, this suppression of symptoms is like putting your finger in a dike. The flood will come sooner or later.

When it does, your doctor may recommend surgery, specifically: fusion of the vertebrae. This is an attempt to create stability in an artificial way, replacing two to five (rarely more) vertebrae with a single structure made by fusing together all these vertebrae, substituting the strength of these fused vertebrae for the lost strength of aging, damaged ligaments. Occasionally this maneuver is successful in the treatment of pain. However, there is a cost: decreased mobility. When vertebrae are fused together, the spine is less flexible than before. In more than one-half of the cases, pain is still present, and mobility also is compromised. Clearly the standard medical/surgical model of treatment of spinal problems is not the way to go, with the possible exception of the treatment of blunt trauma which requires surgical correction of fractured vertebrae to relieve acute pressure on the spinal cord. Even though medication/surgery is not the way to go in most cases involving back and neck pain, you will be recommended these treatments anyway because, in general, this is all doctors know to do. Even they will tell you chances of a real cure are slim with surgery and nonexistent with medication.

Nonsurgical reconstructive therapy — also referred to as "prolotherapy" or "proliferative therapy" — evolved out of a treatment pioneered by H. I. Biegeleisen called "sclerotherapy," which was originally used to treat varicose veins. Prolotherapy involves the injection of an "irritant" solution into the area where ligaments are weak and/or damaged. Over the next few days, cells called "macrophages," literally *big eaters*, are attracted into the area by the presence of this irritant solution. Once they arrive, these macrophages pick up the irritant solution and carry it away for disposal (they are the garbage men of the body). As the macrophages are finishing their job, the body sends in "fibroblasts," literally *connective tissue builders*, to lay down fibrous tissue wherever they detect damage to connective tissue such as ligaments.

The doctor's job is to introduce the irritant solution into the places where ligaments are weak or damaged. If properly placed, this causes the repair of ligaments, and the result can be a supporting structure for the spine up to forty percent stronger than the original! This new supporting structure pulls the vertebrae back into close relationship with each other correcting instability and therefore putting an end to inflammation. When inflammation disappears, so does pain! Stability is restored along with mobility.

That is the long and short of prolotherapy. Studies demonstrate it effects marked improvement in 92% of cases and, if properly administered, does not violate the first rule of medicine: do no harm. These claims cannot be matched by standard medical/surgical treatment methods.

Not only that, this treatment is relatively inexpensive. While a typical surgical procedure on your back or neck can cost $5,000 and more, a single treatment with prolotherapy will cost between $90 and $200. Usually not more than ten to fifteen treatments are necessary to bring a typical back or neck pain syndrome under control — permanently!

If you have a neck or back condition, which you think might benefit from prolotherapy, and you do not live close enough to visit my offices, contact:

The American Association of Orthopedic Medicine
435 No. Michigan Ave., Ste. 1717
Chicago, IL 60611
(800) 992-2063

Or, see page 358 for instructions on contacting my office for a referral.

Sources

Biegeleisen, H. I. *Varicose Veins, Related Diseases and Sclerotherapy, A Guide for Practitioners* ISBN 0-920792-18-9 Eden Press, Montreal Quebec, 1984

Shuman D Sclerotherapy Osteopathic Annals Dec 1978 6;12:10-14.

Gedney EH Disk syndrome Osteopathic Prof 18 1951 12:11-15.

Hackett GS Ligament and tendon relaxation treated by prolotherapy, third addition 1958.

Hackett GS Low back pain Indust Med and Surg Sept. 1959, pp. 416-419.

Ongley ML, Klein RG, Dorman TA, Eek BC, Hubert L A new approach to the treatment of low back pain: diagnosis and prognosis The Lancet 1987; 143-146.

Witt I, Vestergaard A, Rosenklint A A comparative analysis of x-ray findings of the lumbar spine in patients with and without lumbar pain Spine 9;1984: 298-300.

NUTRITIONAL MEDICINE

The Standardized Allopathic Approach

The practice of standardized allopathic medicine involves diagnosis and suppression of disease with specific "cures," when they are available. Standardized allopathic medicine does not attempt to actually cure disease, but rather to simply suppress the expression of disease symptoms.

For example, if you have a headache, and you take a pill for it — aspirin, ibuprofen, acetaminophen, etc. — the cause of the headache, perhaps a congested colon badly in need of a cleanse, an allergic condition, environmental toxin, or whatever, has not been dealt with. If you have a runny nose and take an antihistamine, you may suppress the runny nose, but whatever caused the problem in the first place has not been diagnosed or treated. If you are nervous, and the doctor prescribes a tranquilizer, you may not be nervous anymore but the cause of the nervousness remains unknown. If you have gallstones, the doctor cuts them out, but you never know what went wrong with your body to produce gallstones.

If you stop the drug in any one of these three situations (headache, runny nose, nervousness), the symptom will return. So you either remain on the drug or experience the symptom, take your choice. If you take the drug, you can be sure you are, at best, stressing your body to get rid of the drug which is, as far as the body is concerned, a foreign chemical. At worst you are putting a carcinogen or teratogen (causing cancer or birth defects) into your body, which has not yet been identified as a carcinogen or teratogen.

The classic, but by no means only, example of this is Thalidomide in the 1960s. Touted as a breakthrough anti-anxiety agent, originating in Europe, it was taken by millions, including pregnant women. Many of these women, about 5,000 in the U.S. alone, then gave birth to babies with phocomelia, a condition featuring short or absent arms. Thalidomide was approved by the FDA, the same government agency which bans substances natural to, and already found in nature and the human body — for example L-Tryptophan (on the thin excuse that a contaminated batch from Japan once caused some problems.) L-tryptophan is a wonderful antidepressant and sleep-inducing agent, but it would compete with the newer antidepressants, and cause the pharmaceutical industry serious loss of income. The FDA will not allow it, despite that, for many people, it is the only thing that works. This is a thorn in the side of holistic doctors who prefer to recommend safe substances, found in nature, which handle the basic cause of an illness.

In contrast, if an allopathic doctor does not understand the illness, but if the symptoms are, nevertheless, successfully suppressed with drugs, the doctor is likely to proclaim a "cure," even in the presence of unpleasant side effects and who-knows-what long-term damage.

This applies to many diseases for which patients come to doctors' offices; for example: acne, cataracts, bursitis, congestive heart failure, diabetes, emphysema, fatigue, glaucoma, osteoarthritis, rheumatoid arthritis, hypertension, PMS, scleroderma and a host of others.

These all are diseases which are not understood by standardized medicine, yet there are synthetic drugs available to suppress the associated symptoms.

The doctor rarely pays attention to the diet which may be contributing to the disease process, and if there is a comment made, it reflects the training the doctor received in grade school, because he or she did not receive any significant training in nutrition in medical school. Then comes the prescription for an expensive, laboratory-created, synthetic drug featuring a molecule often made to resemble a molecule which works better and is found in nature but cannot be patented (the progestins for natural progesterone, for example).

Many diseases, like gallstones, can be handled with nutritional medicine rather than surgery with less expense, less physical pain and less risk. No one should submit to surgery without first finding out if the disease can be handled in another way. The surgeon will not always tell you and may not always know. *Caveat emptor:* let the buyer beware.

The Nutritional Medicine Approach

Nutritional medicine, on the other hand, rejects the use of synthetic drugs on the basis that nature makes better pharmaceuticals than the lab of man can ever make. The first natural pharmaceuticals we concern ourselves with are the foods and liquids which are ingested. Averaged out over your life, food, air and water are the most powerful medicines you will take, and an adequate intake of healthy food is the beginning of nutritional health. For many people, especially those under the age of forty, this is all that is required for a healthy body.

While your nutritional doctor can advise you about a healthy diet, it is up to you to learn what is health promoting and to convert this knowledge into a pleasurable lifestyle. This subject is dealt with in depth on pages 145-158 of this book.

Most disease, in the view of the nutritional doctor, is an outcome of many years of unbalanced nutrition. It is possible many diseases represent starvation states of specific enzyme systems in the body. Aging may have a lot to do with a progressive loss of enzyme systems which leaves the body with a limited repertoire of pathways to produce the energy required of living processes. This loss of enzyme systems may be due to suboptimal levels of vitamins and minerals in the body, ingestion of chemical-laced, processed food, or the taking of synthetic drugs, all over a long period of time.

Much research needs to be done in this area. However, vested capitalist interests (pharmaceutical companies and government) have no interest in spending money to find out things which, if made known, will result in decreased profits for the pharmaceutical and processed food industries and, in the long run, the surgical industry and the government itself.

The FDA/pharmaceutical industry/surgical industry/food industry complex is an "Old Boys' Club." People frequently make career moves from one of these organizations to the next, and they do not leave their professional bias behind them. The FDA was commissioned to represent the interests of the people. It is very questionable that they do, or ever did.

The NIH (National Institutes of Health), where most of our tax dollars for medical research are spent, sits out on the periphery of this situation. A couple of years ago, under intense public pressure, they established a small corner (about one percent) of their mighty organization to study progressive medicine. Vitamins and minerals are being studied through the NIH, but very slowly.

Vitamins and minerals, by definition, cannot be manufactured in the body. Therefore, vitamin and mineral deficiencies become a real possibility. There are other substances, not strictly vitamins or minerals, which can be manufactured in the body (niacinamide and glucosamine for example), but as we age we are able to make less than is necessary for perfect functioning. These kinds of substances have important roles in nutritional medicine.

Most vitamins are less well absorbed as we age. Therefore, just when we need more of them, we are getting less (same situation as many hormones). Premature aging, a common condition, has a lot to do with poor absorption of nutrients.

Vitamins and minerals may be taken orally, given as an injection in the muscle or infused directly into the venous system. Oral vitamins and minerals are important, and I believe everyone, especially people over forty, should be taking a well-rounded preparation of vitamins and minerals daily, even twice daily. I do, my wife does, and we offer it to each of our children as well. This is a great way to offer your body the maximum opportunity to remain healthy. I believe a healthy diet, exercise, adequate rest, and vitamin/mineral supplementation to be the best method of disease prevention available. If you live this kind of lifestyle, you may never need to visit my office.

Rationale for Parenteral (Intravenous and Intramuscular) Vitamin and Mineral Therapy

By the time symptoms of disease have made their appearance, it is sometimes too late for oral vitamins and minerals to make much difference. Nevertheless, these same vitamins and minerals, given intramuscularly or intravenously, can benefit many diseases. At first glance, this looks like a contradiction. If nutrients can be used to handle disease, it should not matter by which route they enter the body. However, there is a good reason why it does matter.

It is a fact of biology that all life, except for viruses, is composed of cells and cell products. When we attempt to bring a disease under control, what we are really trying to do is provide cells with all the nutrients they need to get the job done. If the cells are not healthy, we are not healthy, since our bodies are composed entirely of cells and cell products.

So we approach the problem of curing disease as a problem of "the cell." We think of the health of a single cell to clarify our thinking, understanding "the cell" is actually billions of cells. We want to provide the cell what it needs to exist in a healthy condition. What the cell needs to be maximally healthy is always found in nature and is never found in a pharmaceutical lab test tube.

However, to work these nutrients must be passed by the cell, through the cell wall, to the inside of the cell. This is called "transport" and constitutes work done by the cell and thus requires energy. The best nutrient formula does no good when the nutrients remain in the extracellular space (outside the cell), circulating around the body, waiting to be filtered out by the kidneys.

There is another method by which nutrients enter cells: by absorption. Nutrients slip through the wall without requiring the participation of the cell or any work from the cell. The cell wall is thus said to be "semipermeable"; i.e., it will keep out all but a small percentage of nutrients unless they are actively transported from the outside of the cell to the inside. Absorption is a minor method of nutrient entry into cells, under ordinary conditions. It depends on a "concentration gradient," as the biochemists call it; i.e., it depends on nutrients being in a higher concentration on the outside of the cell compared to the inside of the cell. Now comes the point: if the cell is sick, it does not perform its functions well. One of these functions which it does not perform well is transport of nutrients across the cell wall. Therefore, we have a Catch-22: the cell is sick and does not transport well. What is needed to make the cell healthy is nutrients inside the cell; however, the cell is too sick to transport the nutrients in sufficient quantity to create health. What to do?

The answer is simple: give nutrients in a concentration high enough to force those nutrients into the cell by means of a high concentration gradient and the ability of the cell wall to absorb without expending its energy on active transport. When given in high concentration, IV or IM nutrients enter the cell by shear force of numbers. Highly concentrated on the outside, the "semipermeable" cell wall admits the nutrients due to the high concentration gradient which has been created.

Therefore, if the cell can only absorb ten percent of what it needs under conditions of usual concentration, and we increase the concentration of nutrient available by 1000% (ten times the usual), we automatically increase absorption to 100% [10% (0.10) x 1000 = 100%] of normal. Then, provided we introduced the proper nutrients, the cell becomes healthy and able to transport needed nutrients when those nutrients are in usual concentrations. The numbers used here are not meant to be accurate for any particular nutrient but simply to demonstrate the principle involved.

The only way to increase the concentration of a nutrient by this "1000%" is by intravenous or intramuscular administration. Why is this? Because the cells of the stomach and intestine can transport and absorb only so fast, and this is not fast enough to create a high concentration gradient throughout the body. IV and IM administration bypasses the stomach and produces an instant large increase in concentration, which is presented to every cell in the body. The intravenous route is especially useful for this purpose, because no time is required for absorption from an injection site in a muscle.

It is not always necessary to resort to the "parenteral" (intravenous or intramuscular) routes of administration, and we do not do this unless it is necessary. Many diseases can be handled by large oral doses of vitamins and minerals, but when this is not effective, parenteral administration provides a real benefit.

Because the effects on normal body function of synthetic drugs are unpredictable, especially when given parentally, there is a great fear of this route of administration. Most people have known or heard of someone who has died from an IM or IV synthetic drug. The situation is different with vitamins and minerals. These substances are natural to the body and, when given in proper doses by an experienced physician, are as safe as the day is long. "Idiosyncratic" reactions, which often happen with synthetic drugs, do not happen with substances which are natural to the body.

Formal research into the effects of large doses of vitamins on disease states is not progressing as fast as you might think. Vitamins and minerals are not patentable items, and therefore no great profits are be made in their preparation and sale. Pharmaceutical companies do not come loose from their billions of dollars earmarked for research if there is not a large profit to be made.

What research there is, is being done by clinicians, the people who render care directly to patients. This research is done on an empirical, clinical basis: try it, and see if it works. If it works, tell your colleagues, so their patients can benefit. Two such clinicians who are making a big contribution in this area are Dr. Jonathan Wright and Dr. Alan Gaby. They share their knowledge with other doctors through periodic seminars. Some of the following information I have learned from these two excellent doctors.

Some Examples

I want to give some examples of diseases treatable by vitamins and minerals to bring these principles to life for you. This is by no means a complete discussion. A complete discussion would be at least two more rather thick books. I give you these examples to demonstrate some principles.

These examples are not meant for you to take and try to treat yourself. I strongly recommend you consult a doctor experienced in nutritional medicine, if you have an illness you want treated nutritionally. Do not try to give yourself an intramuscular or intravenous injection. These are procedures which are safe in professional hands but which can damage your health if not done properly.

Treatment of Arrhythmia

With age and disease processes the electrical conduction system of the heart sometimes develops a problem conducting the electrical impulse. This condition is called "arrhythmia" and is classified among the "conduction defects" of the heart.

Nutritional doctors who have dealt with this problem have found they often are able to clear up arrhythmia without drugs through intravenous administration of trace minerals. It is thought by these doctors that the problem lies in the inability of the heart cells to retain and concentrate trace minerals, which are essential to proper electrical conduction in the heart.

These minerals are selenium, magnesium, manganese, copper, chromium, zinc and calcium. The last mineral, calcium, is not a trace mineral, however it is necessary to have sufficient calcium for correction of arrhythmia. Your nutritional doctor knows the proper dosage and frequency of each of these minerals to give you intravenously.

Treatment of Glaucoma

Glaucoma is a condition in which pressure builds up in the eye because certain structures in the eye have lost the ability to maintain the normal circulation of fluid through the eye. This fluid, which is called "aqueous humor," is filtered out of the blood, but the mechanism for putting it back into the blood is damaged. The increased pressure of glaucoma can lead to eventual blindness. The important mineral in treating glaucoma is chromium, and the important vitamin is thiamin. In addition, a substance known as "ACE," which stands for "adrenal cortical extract," has been found to be very useful.

E. M. Josephson, M.D., reported in 1935 on the use of ACE for the treatment of glaucoma. He achieved dramatic improvement in intraocular pressures in all of his cases from 30-40+ down to 10-20 which is the normal range! He also noted ACE administration caused a sharp rise in visual acuity in primary simple glaucoma which had not responded to ordinary treatment. He attributed this success in treatment to the normalization of capillary permeability, which eliminated edema of the ocular tissues. In other words, the ability of the eye to rid itself of used aqueous humor was restored. He was impressed with the promptness of the response. Within twenty minutes after administration of ACE, in one case, vision rose from 20/100 to 20/30 without correction.

Unfortunately, because of bad experience with excessive doses of steroids in the 1950s, the American medical establishment became phobic of the use of steroids, and included everything containing steroids into this phobic mix. (Factually speaking, anything which is naturally made by the body, given in doses similar to the doses the body normally makes for itself, including the adrenal steroids, is perfectly safe.)

Nevertheless, this phobia of steroids became institutionalized, and pharmaceutical companies which had made ACE for forty years, without any problems when given in proper dosages, have been forbidden by the FDA to make and sell ACE. After forty years of use, it was proclaimed a "new drug" by the FDA (figure that out), and it costs about $220 million to research a "new" drug to bring it to market. Since it is no longer patentable, no pharmaceutical company will put up the money for the research.

Some small labs around the U.S. offer ACE but the best ACE is European, particularly a product called "Maxi-cortex" from Italy. If you travel to Europe, you can buy Maxi-cortex across the counter and bring it back for administration by your nutritional doctor. However, your doctor is forbidden by FDA regulations to import ACE for you.

In addition, the person with glaucoma should do an elimination diet to discover allergens, which may be associated with glaucoma and also should take vitamin C to bowel tolerance, as well as oral thiamin and chromium.

Treatment of High Blood Pressure

The most important mineral in the correction of high blood pressure is magnesium, and the most important vitamin is pyridoxine. A mixture of the two is given over a thirty minute period. This should be done as often as necessary to obtain control of the blood pressure, then cut back to a maintenance frequency, perhaps once every week or ten days. This may be a bit inconvenient, but the safety and freedom from side effects such as nausea and dizziness, common with antihypertensive drugs, makes it well worth the trouble, not to mention freedom from the as yet undiscovered dangers of taking these synthetic drugs.

The diet with hypertension should be strict high fiber, no salt, sugar, caffeine, or alcohol. It should be heavy on garlic and onions and contain no meat or animal products, including no dairy. Take daily flaxseed oil, biotin, co-enzyme Q_{10}, vitamin E, calcium and magnesium. Several herb teas also are effective to lower blood pressure.

Treatment of Macular Degeneration

The important minerals in the treatment of macular degeneration are zinc and selenium. This should be combined with trace minerals and given IV twice weekly for eight weeks. At that point, the dosage can be doubled and the frequency halved to once each week. This should be supplemented with oral doses of taurine, an amino acid which nourishes the retina, as well as oral zinc, selenium and vitamin E.

Some people experience dramatically improved vision when this regime is first instituted, and over half have a marked improvement in vision overall. Even though not everyone experiences improvement, treatment is well worth doing, given that standard medicine has nothing to offer people with macular degeneration.

These are just a few examples in rough outline form to give you an idea of what is possible. The means to treat many of the most common diseases by natural methods is at hand. One has only to overcome the allopathic paradigm of disease as an attack from the outside, requiring a bodyguard in the form of a synthetic drug, and adopt the idea of disease as an imbalance frequently caused by a deficiency of nutrients.

When you find yourself making that appointment for an allopathic doc, or when you find yourself reaching for those over-the-counter synthetic, symptom-suppressing drugs, stop a minute, and ask yourself if you wouldn't rather heal by natural means.

Here is a list of imbalance states for which there is real hope for great benefit using nutrient therapy:

Acne	Acne Rosacea
Arrhythmia	Alopecia
Angina	Anxiety
Aphthous Ulcers	Asthma
Atherosclerosis	Benign Prostatic Hypertrophy
Bursitis	Cataracts
Cervical Dysplasia	Chronic Fatigue
Diabetes	Congestive Heart Disease
Eczema	Emphysema
Erythema	Fatigue
Gingivitis	Fibrocystic Breast Disease
Gallbladder (Stones and Infection)	Glaucoma
Hepatitis	Viral Infections
Heel Spurs	Hypercholesterolemia
Herpes	Hypoadrenalism
High Blood Pressure	Irritable Bowel
Infections (Bacterial and Viral)	Kidney Stones
Lupus	Macular Degeneration
Menorrhagia	Multiple Sclerosis
Nausea of Pregnancy	Osteoarthritis
Osteoporosis	Otitis Media
Peptic Ulcers	Peyronie's Disease
PMS	Psoriasis
Recurrent Infections	Reynaud's Disease
Rheumatoid Arthritis	Sciatica
Scleroderma	Tinnitus
Toothache	Ulcerative Colitis

DENTAL AMALGAM MERCURY POISONING

Although technically speaking, dental amalgams are not in the general ken of medicine — but rather dentistry — the problem is so widespread, I would be seriously remiss not to bring it to your attention. The problem of dental amalgams is the problem of mercury poisoning.

Mercury is a natural element, a toxic heavy metal, which is highly volatile, the vapor form having the ability to kill cells outright rather than merely do damage. Mercury is used in thermometers and also is known as "quicksilver." The breakage of a mercury thermometer is a potential, although usually unrecognized, medical emergency. Once exposed to air, mercury vaporizes rapidly. If inhaled it makes its way into the tissues of the body in minutes. A large dose can be lethal.

Like all heavy metals, mercury is found in two basic forms: inorganic and organic. Inorganic mercury is found in nature. Organic mercury has passed through a living system of some sort and has come out in the chelated form.

One particularly dangerous form of mercury is methylated mercury, which is produced by the chelating systems of certain bacteria. If inorganic mercury is found in your amalgams and these bacteria are found in your digestive tract, the inorganic mercury will eventually make its way to the bacteria where it will be converted to methylated mercury and from there make its way to your brain! Methylated mercury is hundreds of times more toxic than inorganic mercury and has a particular affinity for the brain where the symptom complex can include mild to severe intellectual impairment and/or emotional impairment. Only chelation therapy can fully and reliably remove this toxin from your body.

An ounce of prevention is surely worth a pound of cure. It is much better to never have amalgams put in. If you already have them I heartily recommend you have them removed as soon as possible.

Amalgam, or what dentist sometimes call "silver fillings," is made from fifty percent mercury, thirty-five percent silver and fifteen percent tin, or tin mixed with copper, and a trace of zinc. This blend is easy for a dentist to work with, and it is much less expensive than gold. It also lasts a long time. Until the mid-1980s dentists assumed no mercury vapor was released from amalgam fillings. Since then, studies have proven a significant level of mercury vapor is released by simply chewing your food.

The federal agency responsible for regulation of allowable levels of substances at the workplace has established 50 ug./cc as the maximum allowable level of mercury vapor in the workplace. The average level of mercury vapor in the mouths of people with amalgams varies between 50 and 150 ug./cc. When removed from your mouth, dental amalgam is considered a toxic waste by the Environmental Protection Agency and must be handled in a certain way to protect dental office personnel from mercury poisoning. This is the same stuff, unchanged, which just came out of your tooth!

There are over 125 known symptoms of mercury toxicity. Most of them are vague and nonspecific. It is not known what role mercury toxicity may play in MS (multiple sclerosis) and ALS (amyotrophic lateral sclerosis or Lou Gehrig's Disease), however Dr. Hal Huggins, a dentist in Colorado Springs, Colorado has developed a protocol for amalgam removal and replacement, and in treating large numbers of MS and ALS patients has noticed improvement of symptoms in 91%. People who were wheelchair bound often get up and walk, sometimes on the same day as amalgam removal!

This rather amazing result is thought to be due to removal of oral galvanic activity and its effect on the base of the brain. You probably have heard of people whose dental amalgams serve as radio antennas. Some of these people actually can hear the local radio stations in their mouths. This much induced electrical activity must have an effect on the brain, and judging from the results of amalgam removal in some cases, this electrical activity must somehow cause or potentiate paralysis.

Other people have nervous system symptoms such as anxiety, insomnia, depression, loss of appetite, and these people also demonstrate a high incidence of recovery from these troublesome symptoms after removal of dental amalgams. Many people with severe longstanding depression are benefited by amalgam removal and chelation.

When a physician hears these vague symptoms from a patient he/she may not even consider mercury toxicity, because these symptoms can be caused by many other conditions and illnesses. Also, the patient forgets to mention the new amalgams, and the doctor usually doesn't ask. The dentist, of course, doesn't even hear about these symptoms, because the patient thinks of the dentist as the tooth doctor, and the symptoms of mercury poisoning seem to have nothing to do with teeth.

It is necessary to be aware of a diagnosis before it is possible to make that diagnosis, and the doctor usually does not even suspect the diagnosis of mercury toxicity. Many people, who actually are poisoned with mercury, are thought of as chronic complainers by their doctors who try to lend a sympathetic ear but actually ignore the complaints, because they do not know what else to do. Many a patient with a mouth full of amalgams has heard these words: "It's all in your head." Of course, that is right, if you remember the mouthful of amalgams *is* in the head and jaw.

A few of the symptoms which are possible from mercury poisoning are vomiting, gastritis, colitis, excessive salivation, abdominal pain, depression, anger, sleep disturbance, headaches, heart attack, dizziness, speech disorders, leg cramps, clumsiness, bad breath, fatigue and irritability — just to name some of the 125 which have been documented so far. The official American Dental Association position on amalgam is that not enough mercury is released to pose a hazard — this despite hard evidence to the contrary. Dental schools have long taught the rationalization that the mercury is bound to the silver in the amalgam and does not escape to poison the patient. This is wrong.

In the U.S., dentistry, as a profession, does not question this party line. They respect authority as represented by their trade union, the ADA, too much to be objective about the matter.

Of course, there are exceptions. My dentist is a fellow named Allan Liles, and he is very aware of the truth of this matter. With his good information I have written some of this chapter. However, if you talk to the typical dentist in the U.S., that person will tell you not to worry about your amalgams.

In Europe, as usual in such things, there is much more awareness about this issue. Dentists in Europe recommend against using amalgams and suggest the use of composite (a plastic substance) or gold to fill teeth recently deprived of their rot.

Most dentists in the U.S. will drill out your amalgams and replace them, if you insist. However, I would not have anyone work on my amalgams who does not really understand the dangers involved. If a dentist does not take this issue seriously, he or she may not be diligent in getting the last bit of amalgam out of each filling before covering it over with gold or composite.

If you already have symptoms of mercury toxicity, these symptoms are coming from mercury already vaporized from your amalgams and now residing in the tissues of your body, particularly in your brain cells. The amalgams represent a source of future further intoxication and, for that reason, should be removed. However, to rid your body of the mercury which is causing the symptoms, only a course of chelation therapy will do the job. Chelation therapy with EDTA has myriad benefits for your health, aside from removing mercury. However, if removing mercury is the only thing you want to get done, the best chelating agent for mercury, by far, is 2,3 dimercapto-1-propane-sulfonic acid or DMPS for short. Two to four treatments with DMPS, lasting a few minutes each, will usually do the job, and the result can be confirmed with pre- and post-treatment measurement of urine mercury concentration.

Remember, mercury enters the body through inhalation. It is not necessary to touch the stuff. People who should be concerned about mercury intoxication, aside from those with dental amalgams in their mouths, are dentists, dental assistants, dental office personnel — anyone who has been around the use of amalgam; people living in the vicinity of mercury mines — even if those mines have been closed for years; people living around volcanoes — active or dormant. I recommend that people in all these categories be tested for mercury.

However, a serum or urine mercury level is an inadequate test, because mercury does not like to come out of the cells in which it is stored. A proper test is conducted with DMPS, which liberates a large amount of mercury. Urine mercury concentration, according to Godfrey and Campbell, shows a sixty-fold increase after DMPS administration in people with amalgam, a thirty-fold increase in dental personnel without amalgams, and only a ten-fold increase in people who have had their amalgams removed followed by a course of

DMSO: Dimethylsulfoxide

To exist, life must have a space in which to exist. Water is that space. All life, at least on this planet, is water based. The atoms and molecules which conduct the life process react with each other in water as the solvent. It is hard to imagine life without water. However, life might be possible in the presence of another solvent with qualities equal or superior to water. It may be that water is the solvent used by life on earth simply because it is here in much greater quantities than any other solvent.

A "solvent" is a carrier solution meaning that it has the capacity to accommodate other atoms and molecules in such a way that they are in "solution." What it means to be in solution is that the atoms and molecules are separated from each other by the solvent. When atoms and molecules are thus separated, they are said to be "carried" by the solvent, or "in solution." For example, water is an excellent solvent for salt. If you put a teaspoon of table salt in a glass of water and stir, soon you are unable to see the salt. It has gone into solution, i.e., the atoms of sodium and chloride are separated from each other and held apart by dihydrous oxygen (water).

Industrial chemists are always interested in finding new and more effective solvents. The perfect solvent, in an industrial sense, is that solvent which has the ability to put almost anything into solution in high concentration, is cheap, safe and smells good. Dimethyl sulfoxide (DMSO), except for the smell good apart, is just such a solvent.

Dimethyl sulfoxide (DMSO) was first synthesized in 1866 by the Russian scientist Alexander Saytzeff. Dr. Saytzeff reported his findings in a German chemistry journal in 1867. From there DMSO languished unnoticed in obscurity for 81 years! After World War II, chemists began to take note of the remarkable versatility of DMSO. They noticed it could dissolve almost anything and carry it in solution.

In the 1960s, medical research with DMSO showed it could not only dissolve substances, but it could also penetrate human skin and carry the dissolved substances along with it! This is remarkable, because human skin is inpenetrable to most substances.

It was also shown to relieve pain and swelling, relax muscles, relieve arthritis, improve blood supply and slow the growth of bacteria. It relieves the pain of sprains and even of broken bones. It enhances the effectiveness of other pharmacological agents. If you apply DMSO to a bruise, the bruise dissolves and disappears in a matter of minutes! If you apply it to the jaw after wisdom tooth removal, all pain and swelling is prevented! The pain of acute gout can be handled with the application of 5 cc of seventy percent DMSO in water four times each day. Application to a fever blister results in rapid resolution of this problem. DMSO also relieves the pain of minor burns and if applied soon after the burn happens, will decrease the tissue damage suffered. DMSO speeds all healing, approximately doubling or tripling all healing responses.

All applications should be done with a cotton swab allowing sufficient time after the solution is painted on to allow for absorption through the skin before covering with clothes. Remember, DMSO is a powerful solvent, and it will take the dye right out of your clothes and deposit it in your skin where you will have to wait for it to grow out.

The skin of the face, neck and intertriginous zones (where skin rubs against skin) are highly sensitive to DMSO and should be exposed only to dilute solutions of fifty percent (half and half with distilled water) or less. Any skin irritation associated with the application of DMSO can be treated topically with aloe vera gel.

In the states in which it is legal to do so, doctors experienced with DMSO treat the symptoms of cancer, atherosclerosis, Parkinson's disease, multiple sclerosis and arthritis with an intravenous push of up to 20 cc of a 25% solution of DMSO. An alternative method is to put 50-100 cc in 500 cc of saline or five percent dextrose, and drip it in over a two- to three-hour period with or without EDTA. Only doctors who are trained and experienced in this form of therapy should administer it.

DMSO, although it is not approved by the FDA for anything except an obscure bladder condition (interstitial cystitis), is widely used in sports medicine. Professional sports in particular are obligated to use DMSO to get their athletes recovered from injury and back on the playing field. Each team knows the competition will use it, and this would mean a tremendous advantage for the other team, if it were to be ignored. Combine that with the fact that DMSO is as safe as it is effective (unlike large-dose steroid injections, which were once commonly used in professional sports) and its use becomes mandatory in professional sports medicine.

When you consider the fact that DMSO is not a new and patentable drug, is cheap, safe and effective, and knowing what you should know about the medical establishment in the U.S., you could predict with your eyes closed that there is a propaganda campaign against DMSO. The FDA has done nothing except drag its feet in DMSO research since October 25, 1963 when the first research application to study DMSO was filed with that agency.

Despite the rejection of DMSO by the American medical establishment, this simple solvent is far from finished. Legally, it can only be sold as a solvent, but sufferers of osteoarthritis and rheumatoid arthritis are using it with regularity, usually having heard of it from a friend and fellow arthritis sufferer. Only medical grade — never industrial grade — should be used on the human body due to the acetone and acid contaminants present in the industrial grade product. Grocery stores which specialize in organically grown foods and health food stores are the most likely places to find medical grade DMSO. A bottle will cost you only a few dollars and will save hundreds, even thousands of dollars in doctor and pharmacy bills. No wonder the medical establishment is lined up against it!

The only medical grade DMSO is available from Terra Pharmaceuticals, in Buena Park, California. It is distributed through Research Industries, of Salt Lake City, Utah. Once obtained from Terra Pharmaceuticals distributors slap on their own brand name. Rimso and

Metabisulfite as an antioxidant. These additives take away its anesthetic power. This is useful, because GH3 is not designed to be used as an anesthetic. Once in the body, procaine breaks down into its component parts, para-aminobenzoic acid (PABA) and diethylaminoethanol (DEAE) which, as we know, occur as products of normal body metabolism.

Procaine has been proven to extend the life span of laboratory rats by 21%, as well as Nematodes, a kind of worm used for drug testing. Many people believe it extends the life of all cells, including those of human beings. This is backed up by Dr. Aslan's studies, which document an average of 29% increase in longevity with the use of GH3. GH3 also is useful in the treatment of depression in the elderly and in the treatment of arthritis, sexual impotence and elevated serum cholesterol.

People who take it, however, including Dr. Aslan, do so because of the strong possibility that Gerovital slows down the aging process and because of the strong quality it has to return a person to the experience of being young and vigorous. This latter quality is particularly strong in people over 45 years old. How, then, does Gerovital work?

There is an enzyme, present in cells throughout the body, called "monoamine oxidase" (abbreviated "MAO"). The major function of this enzyme is to destroy norepinephrine. Norepinephrine is an important transmitter of impulses between nerves. It is important that norepinephrine be held within a narrow range of concentration in the body, otherwise convulsions and death would be the result. Therefore, MAO is an important, even vital, part of body chemistry. It helps hold norepinephrin within that narrow range by destroying excess.

However, at age 45 MAO begins to be produced in greater amounts than before, and this results in a dramatic lowering of norepinephrine. The effect on the mind and body is remarkable — in many people youth and vitality begin to be ushered out the door at age 45 and old age begins to set in. Gerovital prevents this. Still, how does Gerovital work, and why does it have no undesirable side effects?

As it turns out, procaine is a weak, reversible, competitive MAO inhibitor. This means it competes with MAO without destroying it, so when norepinephrine becomes elevated and MAO is needed, it is still present and able to do its job. Until then, procaine holds it in check, allowing normal, healthy, youthful levels of norepinephrine. Procaine does this by occupying the spot on the cell membrane ordinarily occupied by MAO.

When norepinephrine becomes elevated, procaine (in some way not understood) stands down, allowing MAO to assume its position and do its job. This is how GH3 works. There are other MAO inhibitors available. However, they work by destroying MAO and this often tips the scales too far in the direction of a flood of norepinephrine, which can have severe, even fatal, results.

This leaves the question of why there are no side effects to the procaine in GH3. Aside from the fact it is a reversible MAO inhibitor, it also is made of molecules (PABA and DEAE) which are normal in the metabolism of the body. Therefore, procaine is easily metabolized into the body's normal chemistry when it is broken down into its component molecules.

In Europe (not in the U.S. because of an FDA ban — isn't that predictable!), GH3 is given by injection or as a tablet. The tablet is enteric coated to enable it to pass through the stomach without contact with stomach acid, which would destroy its usefulness to the body. The treatment regime recommended by Dr. Aslan is ten mg injected three times per week for four weeks (12 injections). Then there is a rest period of two to four weeks, and another round of three injections per week for four weeks is given. Sometimes oral GH3 is given at this point.

Other people have different ways of administering GH3. I prefer one injection every five days. I find the results wear off after about five days. To me, it makes no sense to say GH3 can, possibly, reverse aging and then take it only sometimes. That kind of rationale works well to support the idea of a clinic where people come and receive GH3, pay a load of money for it and then go home. The body, in my view, is not an automobile which is good for 40,000 miles after a change of tires, but rather requires frequent maintenance.

All of the above is the good news. The bad news, at least in the U.S., is that Gerovital is not available. The Food and Drug Administration has not approved Gerovital, and it is therefore illegal to sell the European preparation. The reasons for this failure to approve Gerovital are not clear, but you can be sure it has something to do with protecting drug company profits. I have reviewed the literature on Gerovital, and the consensus among investigators is that Gerovital is safe and effective. Suffice it to say, there are more factors influencing the FDA in the process of approving a drug than its proven safety and effectiveness.

In Europe and Mexico, however, every pharmacy sells Gerovital or Gero-H3-Aslan, another brand name. A prescription is not required in most countries, and you can simply walk in and buy it. It also is quite inexpensive, about $3 per vial. If you do not live in Europe or Mexico, in order to have the European preparation of Gerovital, you must travel there.

Despite the solid and extensive basis of scientific studies in support of the usefulness of Gerovital, the FDA has banned the sale of the European preparations in the U.S. There is an exception to this, if you live in Nevada, where the state legislature has over-ruled the FDA and passed a law making Gerovital and Gero-H3-Aslan legal. (It is a little known fact that state legislatures can over-ride the policies of the federal government in areas affecting the health and welfare of their citizens.)

However, it is possible for a doctor to write a prescription for "GH3" (Gerovital) which can be made by a compounding pharmacy directly from Ana Aslan's original formula. The price is reasonable, and it can be supplied in oral or injectable form. In the U.S., the trick is to find a doctor who is familiar with Gerovital, as it has been so long suppressed by the FDA, standardized medicine has not yet discovered it.

As far as dosage goes, I believe each person is different, and the proper dosage should be determined by the way your body responds. Intermittent series of treatments, which has been traditional with Gerovital, make no sense to me. If the preparation works (and it does) then you should take a maintenance dosage. One side effect you should watch for is mild thyroid suppression. If this occurs, it is easily corrected (see page 65).

If you are 45 or over, you can experience benefit from Gerovital or GH3. This benefit is nothing more or less than the prevention or correction of premature aging.

See page 358 for instructions on contacting my office for a referral to a doctor familiar with Gerovital.

Sources

Abrams A, Tobin SS, Gordon P, Pechtel C, Hilkevitch A The effect of a European procaine preparation in an aged population J Geront, 20:139, 1965.

Bailey, Herber *GH3, Will It Keep You Young Longer*? A Bantam Book paperback March 1977 ISBN 0-553-14460-X Out of print and hard to find — try a used book store. By far the best reference if you can find it.

Berryman JAW, Forbes HAW, Simpson-White R Trial of procaine in old age and chronic degenerative disorders Brit Med J, 2:1683, 1961.

Clinical Psychiatry News Gerovital H3 is called effective for treating adult depression Vol 3, No 3, March 1975.

Fee SR, Clark ANG Trial of procaine in aged Brit Med J, 2:1680, 1961.

Friedman OL An investigation of Gerovital H3 (procaine hydrochloride) in treatment of organic brain syndrome Gerontologist, Vol. 3, Sept. 1963.

Isaacs B Trials of procaine in aged patients Brit Med J, 1:188, 1962.

Kral VA, Cahn C, Deutsch M, Mueller H, Solyom L Procaine (Novocaine) treatment of patients with senile and arteriosclerotic brain disease Can Med Assoc J, 87:1109, 1962.

MacFarland MD, The nature of monoamine oxidase produced by Gerovital H3 Paper presented at the 26th annual scientific meeting of the gerontological society Nov. 1973.

May RH, Rutland MB, Bylenga ND, Peppel HH Prolonged procaine therapy in geriatric psychiatric patients Geriatrics 17:161, 1962.

Pfeiffer CC et. al Stimulant effects of DEAE Science, Vol. 126, No. 3274, 1957.

Zuckerman BM, Fagerson IS, Kisiel MJ Age pigment studies on the nematode *Caenorhabditis briggsae* Paper presented at the 4th annual meeting of the American Aging Association, Sept. 1974.

CONTROL OF AGING

THROUGH CORRECTION

OF HORMONE

IMBALANCE

SLOWING AND REVERSING THE EFFECTS OF AGING

We live in an age of expansion in all areas of human knowledge. The total amount of information which is available doubles every five years. Medicine is no exception. The average doctor completed training fifteen years ago. That means the amount of information a person needs to know to be a top-flight medical expert has doubled three times since then. Let us do some math: 1 x 2 x 2 x 2 = 8. The amount of medical information available to the practice of medicine is now eight times what it was in 1981!

Needless to say, most doctors are far out of date in their knowledge of medicine. Those of us who try to keep up, realize how far behind we really are. Those who do not try to keep up, do not realize how far behind they are, because they usually are too preoccupied with the business aspect of the practice of medicine.

With doctors this busy, and hopelessly far behind, many people are shifting responsibility for learning about the latest developments in matters of health to themselves. I am in philosophical agreement with this transformation, and I see progressive, holistic doctors in the role of facilitators of this change. My job is to provide you with the latest information in matters affecting your health.

Prevention of Abnormal (Premature) Aging

The advice for a person under 35 is fundamentally different than advice for an older person. Eat right, exercise, avoid toxic substances (nicotine, alcohol, caffeine, etc.), drink lots of filtered or distilled water and get plenty of sleep. Of course, this all applies to the over 35 group as well, but there is more to the task of staying young after you are no longer young. I divide aging up into minimal aging, normal aging and abnormal aging.

Minimal Aging

Minimal aging is what occurs when you take the best possible care of your body, including utilizing modern nutritional science. People who do this typically look ten to twenty years younger than their chronological age.

Normal Aging

Normal aging happens when you are taking the best care of your body, but you are not taking advantage of what is offered by modern nutritional and medical science to maintain your youth: vitamins, minerals, hormonal therapy, etc.

Abnormal Aging

Abnormal aging comes from abuse of the body: smoking, drinking, subjecting yourself to stress, etc. If slowing the aging process is what you want, and if you are going to choose a doctor to help you, I suggest that you ask that doctor's age, then step back and take a long look at that person. If this person is not looking a lot younger than the stated age, look elsewhere for someone who knows and practices the information of anti-aging.

Slowing the Effects of Normal Aging

Here is the sad fact of the matter: nature designed you to be healthy long enough to have children and care for them until they reach an age old enough to survive on their own. From a species survival standpoint, that is what your body is for. After age forty, nature doesn't give a rip about you, because you have lived long enough to have fulfilled your reproductive purposes.

This is true throughout the animal kingdom. Many species die immediately after having laid the egg, fertilized the eggs, given birth, etc. From an evolutionary standpoint, it is no surprise we grow old. Nature wants us out of the way, so there will be room for the next generations. So, after age forty, you are on your own: nature is not going to protect you, and you will have to do it for yourself, if you want to grow old and wise.

The body doesn't have the courtesy to break down all at once, it goes down the drain system by system. This gives us the opportunity to deal with it and repair each breakdown as it happens or, better yet, prevent it before it happens.

After accounting for the ill effects of a poor diet and lack of exercise, the manner in which the body deteriorates can be traced to the failure of the endocrine and exocrine glands. "Glands" are structures in the body which secrete something vital for life.

The Endocrine Glands

"Endocrine" glands secrete directly into the blood and circulate immediately throughout the body. "Endo" means inside, thus denoting that these glands place their secretions inside the body, namely into the blood stream. Such a secretion is a "hormone" (derived from a Greek word meaning "to stimulate"). Hormones are the language the body speaks between its various parts, letting the various organs know if they need to speed up or slow down, make more of this or less of that. It is an exquisite biochemical symphony.

Blood circulates throughout the body in sixty seconds. Therefore, it takes approximately sixty seconds for a hormone to reach any other part of the body.

The endocrine glands are the following:

PITUITARY

thyroid	adrenals
parathyroids	pancreas
thymus	ovaries/testes

The pituitary is listed on top and in capital letters, because it is the so-called "master" endocrine gland. It serves to regulate the other endocrine glands. It produces a variety of "trophic hormones" which tell the other endocrine glands to speed up, work harder.

As we age, and the endocrine glands decrease their function, the pituitary begins to whip them like tired horses. This contributes to the development of a state of exhaustion. It is plain and clear to me that normal aging (as distinguished from abnormal aging from poor diet and lack of exercise) is caused by the gradual decline of the endocrine glands with a resulting decrease in circulating hormones. What causes this gradual decline in the endocrine glands probably is the effect of free radical pathology. (See discussion on antioxidants, beginning on page 124.) This, in itself, is something which can be slowed down by proper diet and supplements.

Aging cells become more and more resistant to the effects of hormones, and therefore just at that time in life when the body needs a boost in hormone levels, it gets a decrease instead. The hormone secretions of the endocrine glands not only effect the health and well-being of the rest of the body, but they also are dependent on each other to maintain health. Thus, when the thyroid gland takes a nosedive, and the basal metabolic rate is slowed down, this, in turn, slows down the functioning of all the other endocrine glands. When the parathyroids age, they no longer hold calcium metabolism within the boundaries required for maximal health. When the thymus partially degenerates (which it does by age twenty) the immune system is no longer the lion it once was. When the pancreas puts out less insulin, all the other endocrine glands are denied easy access to glucose, because insulin helps drive glucose into cells. Glucose is an important energy source for the functioning of all the cells of the body.

The adrenal glands are responsible for regulating the body's response to stress through regulation of protein, carbohydrate and mineral metabolism, as well as powering up the immune system in conditions of stress. When the adrenals are exhausted, the other glands are unable to cooperate in reducing the effects of stress, and the body is more susceptible to infections. The adrenals become exhausted through constant exposure to stress from any source. This is an extremely common condition in our society.

The testes and adrenals in men and the adrenals alone in women make testosterone (or TNAS, the natural anabolic steroid as I like to call it), and this hormone is responsible for maintaining aerobic metabolism and preventing the body from resorting to the far less efficient anaerobic metabolism.

The ovaries and adrenals in women and the adrenals alone in men make estrogen, which lends softness and pliability to tissues without sacrificing strength. When estrogen production wanes, the connective tissue component of all organs (including the endocrine glands) suffer. The point is: all the endocrine glands work together and depend upon each other, and the failure of one of them affects the rest as well.

Endocrine gland failure is inevitable, and it is part of what I call "normal" aging. Warding off *abnormal* aging is done by proper diet, exercise and sleep. Slowing down *normal* aging is possible through timely recognition and correction of endocrine failure — and there is the rub.

Traditionally, doctors have relied on laboratory tests to diagnose deficiencies. That works well for the under 35 age group. However, after 35 or 40, the amount of hormone needed to maintain a youthful condition goes up progressively. Therefore, if you have a set of symptoms which could be attributed to hormone deficiency, you may go to the doctor, be sent for lab tests and then be told there is nothing wrong with you — you are just getting old.

Well, that is true, you are getting old, except it is not true that nothing is wrong with you. What is wrong with you is: you are getting old. Doctors say you are just getting old when they cannot correct a problem. Does it make sense to keep saying that when the means are at hand to correct the problem?

While it may be true that the endocrine glands are getting old and will not put out as much hormone as needed to keep the rest of the body young, that does not mean we should lie down and learn to live with it. If we can rejuvenate or supplement the endocrine glands, and if that rejuvenation or supplementation is safe and creates an enhanced experience of health and well being, as well as increased longevity, why shouldn't we do it? While it is true that our ancestors had to live with degeneration of the endocrine system, it does not necessarily follow that we should retrace their footsteps.

We can now go to the health food store and buy "glandulars," preparations made from animal endocrine organs containing the precursor molecules necessary to power up the various endocrine organs. (See page 139 for a discussion of glandulars.) This works, up to a point, and is especially effective to prevent aging of the endocrine organs and, to some degree, reverse it. When it no longer works, it is now possible to supplement with the actual hormones themselves. See the chapters on the individual endocrine organs for details, pages 67-113.

Where the Doctor Fits In

The contribution the doctor can make is the correct diagnosis, based on clinical symptoms and physical examination, of which endocrine organs are weak. Your doc should also know the correct replacement dose(s) of hormone(s) which are required and have the courage to prescribe them whether or not the lab tests reveal a hormone level consistent with low endocrine function for a 35-year-old (or younger) person.

If you want to roll back the clock and completely rejuvenate your body, it is necessary to become familiar with, consider closely the health of, and then fully support the function of each and every endocrine (and exocrine — see below) gland. This is known as a "glandular workup" — in which we test and examine each gland in your body and then bring each gland up to youthful function.

The Exocrine Glands

The "exocrine" glands secrete outside the body. The inside of the gut (stomach, small and large intestines) is considered to be outside the body. If you drink a glass of water that water is not on the "inside" of you until it is absorbed through the walls of your stomach and intestines into the blood stream. The same goes for food.

Here is a list of the digestive exocrine glands.

salivary glands	liver	specialized cells in the wall of
stomach	pancreas	the small intestine

The function of most of the exocrine glands has to do with digestion of food. Sweat glands help regulate the balance of salts within the body and keep the body cool, as well, during times of heat stress.

Immediately upon ingestion of food, your exocrine glands go to work to digest that food. The salivary glands of the mouth secrete amylase to begin the breakdown of starches (complex carbohydrates). When the food reaches the stomach the parietal cells pour forth hydrochloric acid at a pH of 2! This is stronger than battery acid, and it is combined with pepsin, which begins to break down protein.

After about two hours, the food is moved on to the duodenum where the acid nature of this chyme (as it is called) stimulates the secretion of an enzyme from the duodenum called "secretin." Secretin is then absorbed and carried by the blood stream throughout the body. When it reaches the pancreas, it stimulates the secretion of lipase, proteinase and more amylase to digest fat, protein and complex carbohydrates respectively.

The presence of fat in the chyme stimulates liver production of bile containing emulsifying agents. These act like a kind of soap to separate the molecules of fat, so that they can be worked on and digested by lipase.

When chyme is broken down to individual molecules, it is absorbed directly into the blood stream through the wall of the gut. From there it is taken directly through the liver by the portal venous system, so that anything requiring immediate detoxification and/or excretion can be dealt with. The chyme progresses through the small intestine and, as the pH returns to neutral, bacteria take over to help in further digestion. If conditions are normal most of these bacteria are aerobic and friendly.

When the food reaches the colon it begins the conversion to fecal matter through dehydration. The colon absorbs water from the chyme, and bacteria finish the digestive process and produce vitamin E in the process. If all goes optimally, defecation occurs within 24 hours of ingestion and this defines the "transit time." This is the normal situation. Unfortunately, few people are normal. Here are some of the things which can go wrong.

Hypochlorhydria

The most common thing which goes wrong is hypochlorhydria. It is impossible to overemphasize the subtle yet devastating results of hypochlorhydria, or underproduction of stomach acid. The entire digestive process depends on a healthy load of acid being dumped on the food when it arrives in the stomach. If this does not happen, protein digestion is incomplete. Remember that acid is necessary to trigger secretin release from the duodenum, which, in turn, provokes the pancreas to produce lipase, proteinase and amylase. If acid is deficient, this response is muted, and digestion of not only protein, but also fat and carbohydrate is compromised.

The presence of undigested food causes an overgrowth of unfriendly bacteria in the lower small intestine and in the colon. The toxins produced by these bacteria are absorbed, and the liver works overtime trying to straighten the situation out. The final result is poor digestion and inadequate absorption of nutrients (even in the face of a healthy diet) and also a toxic condition caused by overgrowth of unfriendly bacteria (a condition called "dysbiosis"). Many symptoms result from this toxicity: headaches, fatigue, hypertension, gas, muscle aches and pain, insomnia, personality changes, irritation and more.

The frequency of hypochlorhydria in the population is fifteen percent. Among people who feel ill enough to show up at a doctor's office, fully fifty percent are affected. By age forty, forty percent of all people are affected, and by age sixty, fifty percent have hypochlorhydria. A person over age forty who comes to a doctor's office has about a ninety percent probability of having hypochlorhydria. It is easily the most underdiagnosed and misdiagnosed condition in medicine. (See page 202 for more details.)

Pancreatic Incompetence

The pancreas is, as the acid producing parietal cells of the stomach also are, especially sensitive to toxins. One of the toxins to which the pancreas is especially sensitive is alcohol. Many people are unable to fully digest their food, because the pancreas is not producing sufficient amylase, lipase and proteinase. This is diagnosed by measuring circulating levels of these enzymes and also by stool analysis for completeness of digestion.

Liver Incompetence

When the liver is damaged, it ceases to put out a healthy complement of bile salts, and this causes a failure of emulsification of fats leading to poor digestion of fats.

Colonic Incompetence

The frequently overlooked colon is equally important to health as any of the other organs of digestion. With age, a low fiber diet and low intake of water, it may slow down and stasis of food occurs, thereby allowing unfriendly bacteria to multiply, producing toxic material which leads to fatigue, headache, anxiety, insomnia, etc.

Butyric acid is a substance which serves as the energy source for the cells of the colon, so ingestion of this substance tends to regenerate a tired colon. Also, colon therapy is valuable to help the colon; but unless more fiber and water is presented to the colon, colon therapy will be of only temporary benefit. There is a variety of plant derived colon stimulants, such as aloe vera leaves, which serve to power up the colon. Psyllium husks (not powder) are an excellent source of supplementary fiber.

Discussion

There is a variety of other, much more uncommon conditions, which can affect digestion, but I will omit them here and stick to those conditions which are so common as to be accepted by the medical establishment as normal, or at least not worthy of attention.

I believe that poor digestion is behind most of the diseases of aging — including cancer and vascular disease. Genetics may play a role, but something like a five percent role compared to a 95% role played by food selection and life style emphasizing exercise, rest, nutritional supplementation, and perfect digestion. I also believe that much of the degeneration of the endocrine glands is related to poor digestion. Nothing could be more important to the prevention of abnormal and normal aging than attention to the efficiency of digestion.

Inevitable Aging

If the endocrine and exocrine organs are managed appropriately this leaves us with the last type of aging: inevitable aging. This is a kind of change in the genes apparently regulated by a genetic "clock" of some kind, which ticks inexorably to a final conclusion. If it is true that what I am calling inevitable aging is a function of some kind of genetic clock, we will have to wait until our knowledge of genetics is sufficient to devise a prevention of inevitable aging.

Of course, when that time comes, we will have to rename this kind of aging, since it will no longer be inevitable. Presumably at that time, we also will have the ability to reverse the genetic clock, so that a person has the choice to grow younger instead of older.

In that utopian world, one would be able to choose his favorite age and progress or regress to that age and then remain there. Once this can be done, it will bring up an enormous philosophical debate. Should it be done? Who will have access to this technology and on what criteria? We may find that people do not want to live forever, and then we will be confronted with the Kevorkian Enigma with a new twist: should healthy people who could live forever be allowed to choose to die? And should doctors assist them?

THYROID REPLACEMENT THERAPY

The thyroid gland is an endocrine gland, meaning that it secretes its hormones directly into the blood stream. It is shaped like a butterfly and located under the skin just below the larynx (Adam's apple). In the normal state it is not visible but can be palpated, felt, by the experienced examiner.

The thyroid gland puts out two hormones known as "T3," or "tri-iodo-thyronine" and "T4," also known as "thyroxin." These two hormones together regulate the rate at which the cells of the body use oxygen; that is to say they regulate the metabolic rate. Metabolism produces heat, and so T3 and T4 also regulate body temperature. A third hormone is produced, di-iodo-tyrosine, which may potentiate T3 and/or T4.

Two abnormal conditions are possible with thyroid function, namely *hyper*thyroidism, when too much T3 and/or T4 are produced, and *hypo*thyroidism when too little T3 and/or T4 are produced.

Hyperthyroidism

*Hyper*thyroidism is treated with radioactive iodine, which is taken up by the thyroid gland. It destroys, in a dose-dependent fashion, a portion of the cells of the gland. The other treatment of hyperthyroidism is surgical removal of part or all of the gland. In either case, there is subsequent administration of thyroid replacement to fix the hypothyroid condition caused by the radioactive or surgical destruction of the gland. Hyperthyroidism gained national prominence when not only Barbara Bush, but then her husband, the president and the first dog all came down with this condition in the space of thirteen months.

Hypothyroidism

*Hypo*thyroidism was first described in 1873 in England, and the English have continued to break new ground in the discovery of further aspects and treatments of thyroid dysfunction since that time. From the turn of the century until 1940, doctors treated hypothyroidism based on symptomatology and clinical acumen, sometimes aided with a basal metabolic rate test, which most doctors recognized as flawed.

In 1940, the PBI or protein bound iodine test was developed. What you need to know about allopathic doctors is that they attend the Church of the Holy Lab Test on a regular basis. Beginning in 1940, patients who did not have an abnormal PBI were not given thyroid replacement therapy, even if they had symptoms of hypothyroidism and had already been benefiting from thyroid replacement before the appearance of the new messiah, the PBI. These people were cut off from the therapy they needed because of blind faith in the PBI lab test. The PBI, or protein bound iodine test, after 27 years as the Holy Grail of thyroid disease diagnosis, was shown to be relatively useless in 1967.

Because hypothyroidism is the more common condition, we will focus on it here. Because both T3 and T4 contain iodine, iodine deficiency can account for hypothyroidism. In such a case, iodine replacement may completely handle the problem. More commonly there is either a failure to produce enough thyroid hormone or there is some defect in the body's use of thyroid hormone. The final effect of thyroid hormone occurs inside each cell, and this is a place we have no way to measure T3 and T4 levels. Therefore, blood tests for T3 and T4 often are not useful in evaluating the presence or absence of thyroid dysfunction.

If there is a deficiency of thyroid hormone, it can be caused by either a failure of the pituitary gland to produce sufficient TSH (thyroid stimulating hormone), or a primary failure of the thyroid gland itself. TSH is the hormone which affects only the thyroid gland and commands it to produce T3 and T4. Regardless of whether the failure is in the thyroid gland or the pituitary gland, the result is the same (hypothyroidism), and the treatment is the same: replacement of thyroid hormone.

Deficiency of thyroid hormone is called "goiter" when the cause is insufficient dietary iodine, and it is called "myxedema" when there is a primary failure of either the pituitary or the thyroid itself. In goiter, the thyroid gland is typically hypertrophied, or overgrown and is easily palpated and seen on examination. By contrast, in myxedema the thyroid gland appears normal. Myxedema means literally "mucus swelling," so-called because the swelling of tissues is produced by the presence inside the cells of excess quantities of mucus, also called "mucopolysaccharide" in polite scientific circles, or "snot" by my kids. Whereas ordinary edema is caused by the presence of excess water between the cells and can be "pitted" by applying pressure with, for example, your finger, myxedematous edema is caused by mucus inside the cells which cannot be squeezed out and therefore cannot be pitted. Myxedematous edema therefore also is called "non-pitting edema."

The big problem in thyroid disease is making the diagnosis. For many years the basal metabolic rate was used as the index to make or refute a diagnosis. However, it soon became apparent that finding the true *basal* metabolic rate was near impossible, because almost any disturbance, physical or mental, would raise the metabolic rate. The only accurate BMR is that taken immediately upon awakening before the patient has aroused from bed. That requires the person doing the testing to be present when the person wakes up in the morning, a rather impractical requirement.

For many years, the PBI, or protein bound iodine, was the test most commonly used — but it proved to be quite inaccurate. Then T4 and later T3, tests became available, but these tests only measure circulating levels of the thyroid hormones and say nothing about the amounts of T3 and T4 available inside the cells. Therefore, these tests are not completely reliable in making a diagnosis.

The T3 and T4 tests pick up eighty percent of cases of hypothyroidism, which leaves twenty percent of the patients out of luck. That is, out of luck until Dr. Broda O. Barnes, who spent his entire adult life doing thyroid gland research and working with people with thyroid dysfunction, developed a simple but highly accurate test called the "basal temperature test."

Take a mercury thermometer to bed with you when you retire for the night, shake it down and leave it at your bedside. When you wake up in the morning, place it in your armpit, and hold it snugly for ten minutes. Then read it. A temperature above 98.2 Fahrenheit indicates hyperthyroidism and a temperature below 97.8 indicates hypothyroidism. This test is more accurate than any of the expensive tests mentioned above, much to the displeasure of the lab test industry.

A man can take this test on any given morning as can any woman before menarche or after menopause. However, a woman in her childbearing years, unless pregnant, should take the test on the second and third day of her cycle. Otherwise, there are other affects on body temperature which influence the outcome. Three readings are necessary to determine if you can benefit from thyroid replacement therapy.

Other conditions can lower body temperature. Starvation will do it. Cachexia, the wasting away associated with some chronic illnesses, also will lower body temperature. So will hypoadrenalism. However, with these exceptions, the basal temperature is a reliable indicator of thyroid dysfunction. Because it is free and easy to administer, I suggest you test yourself periodically — whether or not you have noticed symptoms.

Ah symptoms! There is the rub. Few doctors would miss a case of classic hypothyroidism. The pictures of cretinism in children and myxedema in adults seem to wear a large name tag reading "hypothyroidism." Nevertheless, most cases of hypothyroidism are not so severe that these unmistakable pictures are produced. Let us look at the symptoms commonly seen.

Fatigue

Fatigue leads the list. A person feeling just plain dog-tired despite adequate rest should be considered hypothyroid until proven otherwise by the basal temperature test. Fatigue affects a person in diverse ways. It makes some people tense, irritable: grouchy for no apparent reason. It causes others to withdraw, and still others become depressed. Some individuals expend what energy they have on their favorite activity and, after that, are just too knocked out to participate in anything, including normal conversation.

Anemia

People with hypothyroidism become anemic because of hypothermia. Most red blood cells are made in the bone marrow located in the proximal portion of the long bones of the body, because that is where temperature is highest. However, when body temperature drops, even these areas have difficulty producing red blood cells, even in the presence of sufficient iron and vitamins. On examination, the red blood cells are found to be normal in size, shape and hemoglobin concentration. There simply are not enough of them. Anemia contributes to fatigue.

Slowing of the Heart

In addition, the heart slows down and delivers up to forty percent less blood. This results in less oxygen being delivered to the tissues and contributes further to fatigue. Normal activities feel like going to war.

Toxic Buildup

When metabolism slows down, the rate at which waste products are broken down and eliminated also slows down resulting in a buildup of toxic products. This accounts for most of the symptoms of hypothyroidism discussed here.

Delayed Healing

The body is in a constant state of repair. The act of living and moving about carries with it the inevitable small cuts, scratches, bumps, bruises, etc. The body is designed to heal these minor wounds so quickly and efficiently that you hardly notice their presence. When metabolism slows down in hypothyroidism (or for any other cause), wound healing also slows down. You become aware of these minor wounds, because they sit there for several days longer than they should. Delayed wound healing, regardless of the age of the person should make you think of hypothyroidism and a basal temperature test should be done.

Headache

It may be that brain swelling is part of this edema, and this may explain why hypothyroidism is so commonly present in people complaining of migraine and tension headaches. Many conditions can cause headache, but hypothyroidism should be at the top of the list when evaluating chronic headaches — especially those which happen when fatigue is pronounced.

Emotional Disorders

Every emotional disorder can be brought on or simulated by thyroid dysfunction. Hypothyroidism slows the thought process, produces depression and sometimes hallucinations, delusions and even paranoia. Slowness of thought and activity is a hallmark of this disease. When present and untreated from early childhood, the final outcome of severe hypothyroidism is idiocy, growth failure and early death in the late teens or early twenties. In adulthood, a change in personality or depression, fatigue, uncharacteristic irritability, or a change in sleep pattern should raise a suspicion of thyroid dysfunction.

Hyperactivity of Childhood

During childhood, hyperactivity and a short attention span are typical of hypothyroidism. These children often are treated with Ritalin, an amphetamine-like drug, or amphetamines themselves. Apparently, this solves the problem of fatigue for the child and allows for better concentration and less hyperactivity. The more appropriate treatment, of course, would be thyroid replacement.

Milder hypothyroidism can allow growth to be normal and even produce extreme height due to a delayed closing of the epiphyses where bone elongation takes place during growth. Tall hypothyroid patients are not rare.

Susceptibility to Infections

It only makes sense that if the metabolic rate is slowed, the response to bacterial or viral invasion also will be slowed. So it is no surprise to find out that the person with hypothyroidism is unusually susceptible to infection.

In the age of antibiotics, we do not think of infections with the same fear which gripped the heart of a person in the middle ages, or even earlier in this century. Dr. Broda O. Barnes, a doctor and researcher with a lifetime of experience, reports that the hypothyroid patient, often so susceptible to repeated infections, when given thyroid replacement therapy suddenly stops coming down with infections. He reports that this is effective against both bacteria and viruses. There is an association with the now popular, in-the-public-eye, "yeast syndrome." Hypothyroidism should be looked for in any patient who has the yeast syndrome for he/she may have the more fundamental disorder of hypothyroidism, which lowers resistance to yeast as to all infectious agents.

The advent of antibiotics saved the lives of many hypothyroid people beginning in the 1920s. Many of these people would have died from infections except for antibiotics. It can be hypothesized that many of these people lived to reproduce and have children who also are hypothyroid. This may be why we are seeing so much clinical hypothyroidism, up to forty percent of the population by Dr. Barnes' estimation. Whatever the reason, Dr. Barnes figures that the incidence of hypothyroidism has increased from twenty to forty percent since the dawn of the age of antibiotics. My guess is that it has a lot more to do with the inhibition of iodine by chlorine, flourine, and bromine levels present in our water supply.

Skin Diseases

The most common skin finding in hypothyroidism is dry, flaky skin. However, skin disease of almost any kind should raise suspicion of hypothyroidism. Circulation to the skin is decreased, as it is to the rest of the body, and also the production of mucopolysaccharides is increased dramatically in the skin. These two factors together predispose the patient to acne, impetigo, erysipelas, cellulitis, eczema, psoriasis and ichthyosis (fish scale skin). Often these conditions are relieved with thyroid extract. The same is true for the syndrome of "winter itch," in which the skin below the elbows and knees itches severely during the winter. Even some cases of lupus involving the skin clear up with thyroid extract, and when they clear up, the disease does not progress to systemic involvement of the internal organs.

Anyone with a skin disease should at least have a basal temperature test and, if found to be below 97.8, thyroid should be prescribed. This may help the skin disease, and even if it doesn't the patient will have been done a service. Regarding the skin disease, it may take up to six months to get results, so do not become prematurely discouraged if the problem doesn't respond immediately.

Disturbed Menstrual Flow

Another common symptom of hypothyroidism is dysfunction of the female cycle. In children, the onset of menses may be delayed or, paradoxically, it may come years early with hypothyroidism. At the other end, menopause may happen much too early or much too late. During childbearing years the menstrual cycle may be upset in just about any pattern imaginable. The most common condition is that of irregular bleeding. The lining of the uterus, the endometrium, just like other tissues in the body, requires thyroid hormone for proper growth and function.

Infertility

Hypothyroidism is a common cause of infertility in women and incompetent sperm in men. Many childless couples have the misfortune to be hypothyroid (one or both partners) and yet not have an abnormal lab value (T3 or T4 test) to convince the doctor to prescribe thyroid replacement therapy.

High Blood Pressure

Hypertension is another disorder associated with hypothyroidism (as well as with *hyper*thyroidism). If hypertension is present, along with a lower than normal basal temperature, the hypertension will almost always come down with thyroid replacement therapy alone. When this type of hypertension is treated with anti-hypertensive medications alone — without thyroid replacement — the blood pressure does not come down, and the doctor brands this patient as having "refractive hypertension." That term only means that the hypertension is refractive (resistant) to the treatment which the doctor knows to prescribe.

Premature Presbyopia

Some people, between the ages of 35 and 55, when they receive thyroid replacement therapy, will experience the return of the ability to focus for reading without the necessity of wearing reading glasses. Based on this observation, I assert that one of the symptoms of thyroid deficiency is the premature loss of the ability to focus for reading. The technical term for this condition is "presbyopia," literally "old seeing."

Dr. Barnes' Epidemiological Studies

Dr. Barnes did an extensive analysis of the autopsy records of people who died in Graz, Austria in the years 1930 and 1970, plus selected years in between — around 70,000 cases in all. Graz is a city with a stable population of around 230,000 people. There is only one hospital, the National Hospital (Landskrankenhaus), and by a two-hundred-year-old royal decree, everyone who dies in the National Hospital must have an autopsy. About seventy percent of deaths in Graz occur in the National Hospital.

Dr. Barnes noticed that after World War II, the incidence of death from coronary artery disease went almost to zero. After the war, the incidence went back to prewar levels. He believes that people who would have died from heart attacks later in life died prematurely during the war — primarily from infectious diseases, because antibiotics were generally unavailable during that time. After the return of availability of antibiotics, the same people who would have died of infectious disease again began to die of coronary artery disease.

In the cases from the year 1930, the great majority of deaths in Graz were caused by tuberculosis. Tuberculosis kills its victims at the average age of forty (recall Wolfgang Amadeus Mozart — dead at age forty from tuberculosis).

Dr. Barnes is one of those people who thinks for himself. He looked at the evidence, as follows: prior to the era of antibiotics, coronary artery disease was almost unknown. A certain segment of the population was susceptible to tuberculosis and infections in general, and they died young from infectious disease, primarily tuberculosis. Then came antibiotics and an entirely new population of people appeared: people who were susceptible to both infection and to coronary artery disease; except now they were enabled to live long enough to die from the slower of the two diseases: coronary artery disease.

Coronary artery disease kills its victims at the average age of 66, 26 years later than the previous big killer, tuberculosis. Dr. Barnes noticed that the death rate from coronary artery disease in 1970 was ten times that of 1930. Statistically, the death rate would be expected to be double, not ten times the 1930 rate. The only way he could explain this to himself was that the people who were saved from tuberculosis were almost all dying of coronary artery disease, and the people who did not need saving from tuberculosis were not susceptible to coronary artery disease either. They would die at an older age of something else.

Dr. Barnes combined this insight with his vast clinical experience of thousands of people treated with thyroid replacement therapy and realized that the incidence of both infection and coronary artery disease is dramatically reduced by thyroid replacement. This led to the realization that thyroid deficiency is the common denominator in both susceptibility to infection and coronary artery disease. In other words, there is a segment of the population (about forty percent according to Dr. Barnes) which accounted for almost all deaths from infectious disease before the invention of antibiotics and is now destined to account for almost all of the mortality statistics related to heart attacks, and these same people are hypothyroid.

Dr. Barnes' advice to you is to take your morning basal temperature, and determine if you are one of those people and, if you are, find a doctor who will prescribe thyroid replacement therapy for you.

Ah, but there is the rub, for while the incidence of hypothyroidism was well appreciated before the invention of blood lab tests for the disease, now most doctors think it is rare. Remember, almost all doctors attend The Church of the Holy Lab Test on a regular basis. If the clinical picture presented by the patient conflicts with the Holy Lab Test, the clinical picture is ignored. According to this point of view, you cannot be hypothyroid unless you have a low T3 and/or T4 blood level.

So, if you have hypothyroidism, unless you have the proper lab result, you will have to become a discriminating consumer and conduct a search for a qualified physician. If I were you, I would call up armed with knowledge, and boldly ask to speak to the doctor *before* making an appointment. Ask the right questions. How common is hypothyroidism? Do you know about the taking of basal temperature? How reliable are lab tests in diagnosing hypothyroidism? Do you know of the work of Dr. Broda O. Barnes? Get the right answers or do not waste your time and money with that doctor.

If you think about it, Dr. Barnes' ideas dovetail nicely with what we now know about the mechanism of coronary, nay any, artery disease. We now believe this to be a free radical disease. Excess hydroxyl radicals left over from lipid peroxidation cause tiny areas of inflammation, then necrosis (tissue death), in the walls of arteries. When the body tries to repair this necrosis it forms a scar tissue and incorporates into the scar tissue calcium and cholesterol. The body's natural defense to this process is to produce antioxidants, which neutralize hydroxyl free radicals before they can do damage. Thyroid hormones regulate the rate of metabolism and, when in inadequate supply, the rate at which antioxidants are produced would, of course, be slower. Therefore, there would be less antioxidants around to do the job and atherosclerosis would proceed more rapidly.

The sequence is clear. Low thyroid function → decreased antioxidant production → vascular lesions → scar (plaque) formation → eventual artery blockage → heart attack or → stroke ("brain attack," as it is now called), or → gangrene, or → any set of symptoms caused, or contributed to, by decreased blood flow to organs.

It also makes sense that low thyroid function would make one susceptible to infection. The entire chemical factory we know as the immune system, is running only as fast as the amount of thyroid hormone which penetrates the immune system cells. Therefore, low thyroid → depressed and slowed immunity → increased likelihood of infection. It all fits together so well!

Arthritis

Hypothyroidism predisposes a person to arthritis, and thyroid replacement therapy often brings arthritic symptoms under control. In severe cases of arthritis it may be necessary to add a small dose of prednisone — from five mg. every other day up to five mg. twice daily. (I prefer natural hormones for hormone therapy, but this may be the one place prednisone, a synthetic hormone, should be used — only in low doses and only because the effect of cortisone treatment in arthritis wears off after a few days.) Some of the ill side effects of prednisone are due to its thyroid-suppressing effect and can be avoided, at least at low doses of prednisone, by supplementing thyroid hormone to the level required to maintain the basal temperature between 97.8 and 98.2.

Where gouty arthritis is concerned, thyroid replacement also helps here. Gout is caused by an inability to metabolize uric acid and the accumulation of uric acid, notably in the drainage system of the kidneys (as stones) and in the joints, especially the big toe. If the basal temperature (and thus the basal metabolic rate) is low, naturally the body is even less able to metabolize uric acid. Although thyroid replacement is not specific to gout, it is a valuable adjunct to the treatment of this painful disease.

Again the problem is that doctors rely on unreliable laboratory tests to determine the presence or absence of need for thyroid replacement therapy, when the only reliable test is the basal temperature.

Diabetes and Hypothyroidism

The symptoms of diabetes are related to the poor control of blood sugar present in this disease due to either inadequate insulin production from the pancreas or a resistance in the cells of the body to the effect of insulin. It is as if, in some people, the body becomes immune to the effects of insulin. Before the discovery of insulin, the diagnosis of diabetes was a death sentence. The average person lived less than five years after diagnosis, and the usual cause of death was tuberculosis. One could say that part of being a diabetic was a weakness toward contracting and dying from tuberculosis.

Insulin was isolated by Canadian doctors Banting and Best in 1922, and for a few years the medical world was optimistic that diabetes would be cured. What happened instead was that controlling blood sugar with insulin allowed diabetics to live longer lives. This revealed aspects of diabetes, which previously had been no problem, because the diabetic died before they could appear. Diabetics were observed to develop atherosclerosis far earlier than non-diabetics, and this became the major killer of diabetics later in life, by heart attack or stroke. However, they die at a much younger average age than do other sufferers of atherosclerosis. It has been discovered that even before the onset of diabetes, the diabetic-to-be is developing atherosclerosis at an accelerated rate.

A weakness to tuberculosis and early atherosclerosis: just like hypothyroidism! And, indeed, if you check the diabetic for a low basal temperature, it often turns out that hypothyroidism is present. It has long been known that the classical test for diabetes, the GTT or glucose tolerance test, cannot distinguish between diabetes and hypothyroidism. However, sometimes doctors forget this and fail to collect the basal temperature (or worse yet rely on the T3/T4 tests) and thus treat hypothyroid patients for diabetes, which they do not have!

Also, many true diabetics also have hypothyroidism, which is overlooked and not treated for the same reasons.

The complications of diabetes, such as cataracts, heart disease (and atherosclerosis in general) and kidney disease are not present in the diabetic, if that diabetic is producing plenty of thyroid hormone. These complications also can be prevented in the diabetic patient who also is hypothyroid, simply by adding thyroid replacement therapy. The point is that whenever diabetes is suspected, it should always be distinguished from hypothyroidism. This can be done by testing not only glucose tolerance but also insulin tolerance. A GTT should never be ordered alone. Second, even if a person is correctly diagnosed with diabetes, hypothyroidism should always be suspected anyway, and a basal temperature should be done with thyroid replacement, if indicated by a low reading. Many "prediabetics" are actually undiagnosed hypothyroid cases and, if not recognized as such, the opportunity to treat with thyroid and thus prevent atherosclerosis will be lost.

Lung Cancer and Emphysema

It appears from the extensive epidemiologic studies conducted by Broda Barnes on deaths occurring in Graz, Austria, that there are two other diseases to which there is a shared susceptibility, along with the susceptibility to tuberculosis, and those are lung cancer and emphysema. His data indicate that people who have tuberculosis are twenty times more likely also to have lung cancer than the average person.

As regards emphysema, part of the cause of this disease is chronic bronchitis, i.e., repeated infections of the bronchi. People who finally end up with emphysema are people who smoke and/or have had multiple infections of their breathing tubes. Infections produce coughing in the presence of obstruction of the airways by mucus. Coughing into obstructed lung tubes causes the pressure in those tubes to back up into the alveoli, the tiny sacs in the lungs where oxygen and carbon dioxide are exchanged. When the walls of these sacs rupture under pressure from coughing and scar tissue forms this is called "emphysema."

As we already have seen, people who are especially susceptible to infections are more likely to be hypothyroid, and the addition of thyroid replacement therapy raises resistance to infection to normal levels. This protects against bronchitis and therefore against the eventual development of emphysema.

Dosage and Administration

Thyroid hormone comes as an extract of whole thyroid tissue in pill form. In children under six, we begin with 1/4 grain thyroid extract daily. From age six to thirteen, the beginning dose is 1/2 grain daily. Above thirteen, the proper beginning dose is one grain daily. In each case, the beginning dose is maintained for two months. Results are not immediate and require two months for full expression. If the basal temperature is not in the normal range at the end of two months, we increase the dosages by the same amount as the initial dose: small children, 1/2 grain; larger children, one grain; teenagers and adults, two grains.

We then follow the same procedure using the basal temperature as our guide. Rarely are higher doses necessary but when they are, we use the same procedure. It is important to use the lowest dose which gets the job done, because this preserves what thyroid production is naturally present, as well as the pituitary gland's role in fine tuning the production of this endogenous thyroid hormone. Treatment should not be rushed. Loading up on large doses of thyroid extract in the beginning of therapy accomplishes nothing except to make the patient ill. Time is required for the body to adjust to this therapy.

While it is possible to buy T3 (Synthyroid) and T4 (thyroxin) separately I believe it is best to use the whole extract, which contains T3, T4 and di-iodo-tyrosine. This is the way nature designed thyroid, and I am not one to second-guess nature.

Final Recommendation

Everyone should take a periodic check of his or her basal temperature. It is easy and free, and the information gained, if acted on, may make a world of difference. To repeat, simply get a mercury thermometer, shake it down, and lay it by your bedside. When you awake in the morning, before you get up, place it in your armpit and keep it snugly there for ten minutes. Then take the reading and record it.

See page 358 for instructions on contacting my office for a referral to a doctor familiar with this approach to the treatment of thyroid dysfunction.

Sources

Barnes BO, Barnes CW Heart attack rareness in thyroid treated patients. Charles C. Thomas; Springfield, IL 1972.

Barnes BO, Galton L Hypothyroidism: the unsuspected illness. Harper & Row Publishers; New York, NY 1976.

Barnes BO Headache - etiology and treatment. Federation proceeding 1947; 6:73.

Barnes BO Etiology and treatment of lowered resistance to upper respiratory infections. Federation Proceedings 1942;69:808.

Barnes BO The treatment of menstrual disorders in general practice. Arizona Medicine 1949;6:33.

Barnes BO, Ratzenhofer M One factor in increase in bronchial carcinoma. JAMA 1960;174:2229.

THE NATURAL ANABOLIC STEROID (TNAS)

To understand the value of the use of testosterone in modern medicine, it is necessary to expand our thinking. Testosterone is not simply "the male sex hormone." It is perhaps even unfortunate that it was first discovered in animal testes and thus named "testosterone," implying that it comes only from the testes and thus associating it exclusively with sexual function. Testosterone is best termed The Natural Anabolic Steroid, or TNAS.

The biochemical name of TNAS is a jaw-breaker, and I will write it only once: cyclo-pentano-perhydro-phenanthrene. The hyphens are my addition to this mouthful and help us pronounce this long string of letters. No wonder they named it something else!

The interaction between TNAS and the cell is to increase protein production. TNAS commands the DNA structure of each cell to increase production of RNA. RNA, in turn, migrates from the nucleus into the main body (cytoplasm) of the cell where it increases protein synthesis. Thus, TNAS increases lean body weight at the expense of fatty tissue. Food that would be stored as fat is stored as muscle.

The Natural Anabolic Steroid, or TNAS, should not be confused with synthetic anabolic steroids, which have given such a black eye to steroid therapy. While it is true that synthetic anabolic steroids do increase muscle mass, especially when combined with exercise, they also have a host of potential harmful side effects, especially to the heart. The use of synthetic anabolic steroids by athletes, with associated deaths, has put a large barrier in the public consciousness to the legitimate use of TNAS in medicine. TNAS does not have the life threatening side effects of the synthetic anabolic steroids, because it is a natural hormone made in nature's lab. Therein is the problem for capitalistic pharmaceuticals: no big profits are realizable from a substance from a natural, therefore nonpatentable, source. From the patient's standpoint, however, TNAS is a God-send: a powerful natural element with a large safety factor.

TNAS is made in women as well as in men. The major site of production is the adrenal gland. Castration does not end a man's TNAS production, and women produce sufficient quantities of TNAS. In women, TNAS and estrogens work together to maintain health and positive nitrogen balance (the production of at least as much muscle tissue as is lost each day). Therefore, TNAS is necessary for the maintenance of health in women, as well as men.

Anaerobic Metabolism

To understand the value of TNAS, we must understand the principles of aerobic and anaerobic metabolism. When life first began on the earth, it used what was available for energy. That substance, which was most available in the early atmosphere, was carbon dioxide, or CO_2. This CO_2 was in plentiful supply, and every time another volcano erupted it spewed millions of tons more of CO_2 into the atmosphere.

Heart disease can be expected in these four; however, that leaves the other four people with no identifiable risk factors (not age and not family history) who will die of heart disease before age 65. These people simply develop anaerobic metabolism at an early age of sufficient degree to cause damage to the heart muscle.

The common medical explanation for a heart attack is that a coronary artery is partially blocked by atherosclerotic lesions. Turbulence in blood flow, produced by this partial blockage, leads to thrombosis (clotting) and complete blockage of the coronary artery, resulting in loss of blood supply to the heart muscle supplied by that artery. Thus, the muscle is said to die due to loss of blood supply.

That explanation held up until someone demonstrated that approximately half of heart attacks happen *before* coronary thrombosis and not after. In some cases heart attack has happened, and there is no blood clot present. This brings up the possibility that the thrombosis which happens inside the coronary vessels and death of heart muscle have a *common* cause and are not causally related to each other.

It is well-known that TNAS has a powerful "fibrinolytic" effect. That means that it tends to prevent blood clots, and when they happen it breaks them up. A lowered level of TNAS, therefore, predisposes to blood clots. Therefore, the blood clot which forms in the coronary artery and the death of surrounding heart muscle may both be caused by lowered levels of TNAS.

If thrombosis often has a common cause with "heart attack" (death of heart muscle fibers), rather than being the cause of heart attack, what is the true cause? When that question came up, someone postulated that coronary spasm (the coronary artery squeezing itself shut) may cause heart attack in the absence of thrombosis, even in the absence of any vessel disease. In other words, the blood vessel chokes the heart muscle to death and then relaxes leaving no evidence of what happened.

Radiographic films have been made of this process happening while the heart circulation is being examined with dyes and x-ray. So we know that it can happen while the heart circulation is being examined with dyes and x-ray. We do not know, however, that it can happen when the heart circulation is not being examined with dyes and x-ray. Because of this, I suggest you decline to have your heart circulation examined with dyes and x-ray ("angiograms" they are called).

The other possibility is that the heart attack originates in the heart muscle itself due to a shift to anaerobic metabolism. This makes some theoretical sense in that the heart is the only muscle in the body which is not allowed to take a break and rest. It must contract fifty to eighty times per minute to sustain life. If it goes on a break, you die. This kind of demand is not made on any other muscle. If there is a shift to anaerobic metabolism in the heart muscle, it may just work itself to death in short order, even with a sufficient blood supply. Remember aerobic metabolism depends not only on oxygen supply but oxygen utilization as well.

All muscles store energy in the form of adenosine triphosphate (ATP). ATP is made from adenosine monophosphate (AMP) by the addition of two phosphate groups, a process called "phosphorylation." In anaerobic metabolism, phosphorylation proceeds at a slower pace, resulting in a bottleneck effect at the level of two phosphate groups (adenosine diphosphate or ADP). Lowering the ATP level to less than fifty percent of normal results in irreversible tissue death. In some heart attacks, this is what happens. The muscle simply dies in a region of the heart, and this causes clotting in the coronary arteries. What was once considered the cause of a heart attack is sometimes the effect. The cart goes before the horse.

The major function of TNAS is to maintain aerobic metabolism. As we age, we not only receive a decreasing supply of TNAS, but also cells become resistant to the effects of all hormones. Thus, for TNAS to produce the same result in a sixty year old person as it does in a twenty year old person, there must be a higher level of TNAS in the older person.

The cause of heart disease is complex but it is clear that a shift from aerobic to anaerobic metabolism plays an important part.

Treatment of Heart Disease with TNAS

Thus, the theoretical basis for treatment of heart disease with TNAS is solid and, although in the United States, this treatment is not in vogue, probably due to blind prejudice against the word "testosterone," the use of TNAS for heart disease in Denmark is decades old. Dr. Jens Moeller has used TNAS in the treatment of angina in Copenhagen with great success for over forty years.

Dr. Moeller has discovered that tissue resistance to TNAS in the older person sometimes requires the administration of several times the usual dose of TNAS for symptom relief of the pain of angina. Dr. Moeller is the president of the European Organization for the Control of Circulatory Disease. He is an original thinker and a courageous physician who points out some very interesting things in his ironically misnamed 1987 compendium "Cholesterol." This should be required reading for any physician who treats vascular disease.

Cortisol and the Catecholamines

In normal metabolism there is a balance between protein synthesis and breakdown. TNAS encourages protein synthesis, and an adrenal hormone named "cortisol" (hydrocortisone) acts antagonistically and encourages the breakdown of protein. The breakdown of protein also is encouraged through chronic tension and anxiety (as many underweight worriers can tell you) through the production of the catecholamines — adrenalin and noradrenalin (also called "epinephrine" and "norepinephrine"). Stress raises both cortisol and catecholamine levels and, if stress becomes constant, the hormonal balance between TNAS, cortisol and the catecholamine is upset. Indeed, this balance is upset by the aging process itself, by the decreased production of TNAS and the increased production of the catecholamines, which occurs with age.

This is the root cause of stress-induced heart attacks: the shift toward anaerobic metabolism caused by the domination of the effects of cortisol and the catecholamines over TNAS. When this condition becomes chronic, angina may begin, because the heart muscle is unable to utilize the oxygen in the usual efficient manner. In experimental animals, administration of excess cortisol alone has been shown to produce death of heart muscle. Excess catecholamines can cause the heart to go into ventricular fibrillation, which results in death rather quickly. This can happen when there is a very upsetting event—a person is literally scared to death.

While most people are not subjected to catastrophic levels of cortisol or the catecholamines, the aging heart is subject to a hormone imbalance which is harmful, even in the absence of vascular disease. One solution is to shift metabolism back toward the aerobic condition through the administration of TNAS, thus restoring the balance which has been lost.

The Great Cholesterol Hoax

Cholesterol, despite the vilification of this substance by the medical establishment, is simply an innocent bystander in the biochemical drama of vascular disease. Cholesterol is made constantly in the liver and is essential for life itself. It is the precursor for the male and female sex hormones and the adrenal cortical hormones as well. The body uses cholesterol to make these hormones.

When metabolism becomes relatively anaerobic, the enzyme systems which alter cholesterol to make these hormones are unable to function normally. This results in the accumulation of cholesterol. Thus, an increased cholesterol level is a signal that metabolism has shifted toward the anaerobic and alerts us that we should do what is necessary to deliver more oxygen to the tissues and also to condition the tissues to use that oxygen more efficiently.

Cholesterol is made in the liver from acetyl-CoA, which also is used by aerobic metabolism in the Krebs Cycle. When the Krebs Cycle is not functioning well, acetyl-CoA builds up, and the production of cholesterol is accelerated, because the raw building block material, acetyl-CoA, is in abnormal excess due to the fact that it is not being used at the normal rate by the Krebs Cycle.

Therefore, cholesterol level is only a marker and not the cause of the problem itself. Giving the person a drug to inhibit the production of cholesterol, while yielding great profits for the pharmaceutical manufacturers of these substances, does nothing to lower overall death rate. The studies which show evidence that lowering cholesterol in this manner lowers the incidence of heart disease or death from heart attack were sponsored by the drug companies which make the drugs. This introduces investigator bias. Also, other studies demonstrate increased death rate due to automobile accident and suicide in people taking cholesterol lowering drugs. Draw your own conclusions.

The mesmerization of the public with the idea that cholesterol is somehow the cause of vascular disease has been called "The Great Cholesterol Hoax" by some writers. It is a marketing creation, which makes enormous wealth for the food and pharmaceutical industries. It also gives doctors something to do to feel useful: help you drive your cholesterol level down by artificial means.

If one takes those actions which promote aerobic metabolism it is true that the cholesterol level will drop naturally, with no medications to force it down and no dietary changes. These actions include regular aerobic exercise and a revitalization of the hormone system. An important part of this revitalization is the administration of the appropriate amount of TNAS. I am not saying that a low-fat diet, vitamins, etc., are of no value. I do say, however, that compared to aerobic exercise and hormone balance, they are running only a close third and fourth in importance. Ideally, one would make all these changes sooner rather than later and at the very latest when the first signs of vascular/metabolic dysfunction appear.

The Great Fat Hoax

While it is true that the reduced dietary consumption of fat is proper for maximum health, it is not the fat itself which is the problem. Toxic materials, such as herbicides, pesticides and preservatives are stored in concentrated form in animal fat. If then you eat this animal fat, you eat these toxins in concentrated form, and most of it ends up stored in the fat of your body. From there the name of the game is "Slow Poison." If you can obtain organically produced meat, you could consider it good food, if eaten in a balanced way with the other food groups. Otherwise, adopt a low- or no-animal-fat diet.

To summarize, TNAS favorably influences the enzymes which power up the Krebs Cycle, and it thus powers up aerobic metabolism, making anaerobic metabolism less necessary and less present. The administration of TNAS lowers cholesterol in the absence of any other medical or lifestyle changes, demonstrating that a shift back to aerobic metabolism has occurred. The dominating influence of cortisol and the catecholamines from aging and stress is reversed, and the probability of a catastrophic cardiovascular accident is greatly decreased. This is the obviously sensible route to take when dealing with "vascular" disease, be it of the heart, the brain, the kidneys or the extremities. Replacement of vessels with plastic tubes should be absolutely abhorrent to anyone with a medical degree or, indeed, to anyone with knowledge of the behavior of living tissues. Blood vessels are made of living cells. They are not made of plastic and not made of a plastic-like substance. They derive from the same tissues in the embryo which give rise to the red blood cells. Therefore, they are friendly to red blood cells and can allow the passage of these cells without harm. The same cannot be said of plastic substitutes for blood vessels.

The surgical replacement of an artery with a vein is a little less insult to common sense, however not much less. Arteries are designed to withstand many times the pressure for which a vein is designed. Veins in the natural ungrafted state are supplied with blood through tiny arterioles, which feed capillary systems within the vein walls themselves. When a vein is cut from the leg to be grafted into the heart, it is ripped away from its blood supply. This blood supply cannot be replaced, and the vein must therefore derive what little oxygen it can from the blood which passes through it. Although this seems like it should work, it does not. Therefore, a vein will eventually (usually sooner rather than later) develop anaerobic changes and clog when grafted into the arterial system.

In short, surgical intervention in the cardiovascular system is almost never justified when the alternatives are given proper consideration. Chelation therapy, hydrogen peroxide therapy, and hormone therapy along with lifestyle changes yield better and longer-lasting results for a fraction of the cost of surgery and at almost no risk compared to the extreme risk involved in surgery. Even the diagnostic procedures leading up to surgery carry an unacceptable risk when compared to the alternatives.

Adult Onset Diabetes

The aches and pains of growing old are due to anaerobic metabolism. If anaerobic metabolism predominates in the upper back and shoulders there will be intermittent or constant aching in that area. This usually is conceived of as tension, but when anaerobic metabolism is converted back to aerobic metabolism by TNAS, this pain promptly disappears.

The pancreas is made up of two populations of cells. The cells of the Isles of Langerhans are of two types: beta cells (which produce insulin) and the alpha cells (which produce glucagon, a hormone which balances insulin). The Isles of Langerhans (named after the guy who first described them) makes up an endocrine gland which is embedded in a second population of cells. This second population of cells constitutes an exocrine gland, secreting its products not into the blood stream but into the gut. This secretion contains enzymes to digest food.

When anaerobic metabolism strikes the pancreas, the result is poor digestion and/or adult ("maturity") onset diabetes. It is typical for a person to both have diabetes and cardiovascular disease, because the root cause is the same: anaerobic metabolism. This is not the case with juvenile onset diabetes, and in this disease TNAS is not a good treatment. It is a mistake to attack adult-onset diabetes, or any of the diseases of anaerobic metabolism as if they were isolated diseases. The control of blood sugar is a nice goal but if the patient dies of a heart attack in the interim, it is not much comfort to the family that he died with a correct blood sugar. Administration of TNAS, along with correct balancing of protein and carbohydrate intake at 7:10 on a caloric basis, normalizes the glucose tolerance test in adult-onset diabetes after only a few weeks of treatment.

The administration of oral hypoglycemic agents may have the same effects but ignores the root cause of adult-onset diabetes, allowing cardiovascular disease to progress unimpeded. Diabetes should always alert the physician to the presence of CVD, even if there are not symptoms yet present. Adult-onset diabetes should be considered a signal of cardiovascular disease and treated as such. To do less is to ignore the onrushing train while dodging the bicycle crossing the tracks.

Fibrinolytic Activity of TNAS

A major consideration in managing heart disease is the prevention of thrombosis, which can cause the occlusion of coronary arteries already compromised by atherosclerosis. When the possibility of thrombosis is a threat to life, doctors often prescribe "blood thinners" to prevent thrombosis. Again, the root cause of the problem is ignored. When cardiovascular disease is properly treated with TNAS, the patient also is protected from thrombosis by the powerful "fibrinolytic" (clot-breaking) activity of TNAS. This makes the administration of synthetic drugs, such as coumadin, unjustifiable. Many patients have died from the treatment where coumadin is concerned. An overdose of coumadin can occur quite accidentally and, if it does, the patient cannot form clots when needed. Therefore, spontaneous internal bleeding becomes a threat to life.

Once again, when the patient dies of spontaneous internal bleeding or from the inability to form a clot and heal a severe cut, it is little comfort to the family to know that he was well-protected from heart attack when he died.

Postsurgical Use of TNAS

When surgery is necessary, it is important for the surgeon to know that the stress of surgery drives up cortisol and catecholamine levels and drives the level of TNAS down. Thus, the patient is a sitting duck for a leg vein thrombosis followed by the breaking loose of this thrombosis in the large veins of the legs and abdomen, with the subsequent migration of this thrombosis to the heart — where death can quickly ensue. When a thrombosis breaks loose it is called an "embolus" and may quickly lead to death. The postoperative administration of TNAS not only speeds healing, but also protects the patient from the hazard of thrombosis and subsequent embolism.

Dosage

The correct dose of TNAS for a man with refractory angina is 250 mg testosterone enanthate three times in the first few weeks until pain is controlled. After that the patient should be titrated to the smallest effective dose, which might be between 200-1000 mg. per week. Women are more easily managed and require only 100 mg. per week in the first few weeks. This lower dose usually avoids the masculinizing effects of TNAS (hirsutism, lowered voice), but not always. Some men experience an increase in aggressive feelings and should be warned in advance of this possibility. The patient is informed of the possible side effects before treatment and asked to sign a release acknowledging having received this information. Once TNAS therapy is begun, the aerobic pathways, through which hormones are created from cholesterol, are empowered, and the result is an increase in endogenous hormones, including TNAS itself.

To find the compounding pharmacist closest to you, contact:

Professionals and Patients for Customized Care
10925 Kinghurst #508
Houston, TX 77099
(800)435-1412

> **Or, see page 358 for instructions on contacting my office for a referral.**

Sources

Kumada T, Abiko Y Enhancement of fibrinolytic, and thrombolytic potential in the rat by treatment with an anabolic steroid, furazabol. Thrombos. Haemostas. (Stuttg.). 36,1976

Moeller J Cholesterol Springer-Verlag Berlin Heidelberg New York London Paris Tokyo ISBN 0-387-17097-9 (U.S.) 1987

Allison SP, Prowse K, Chamberlain MJ Failure of insulin response to glucose load during operation and after myocardial infarct. Lancet I.292:478-481;1967

Allison SP, Tomlin PJ, Chamberlain MJ Some effects of anaesthesia and surgery on carbohydrate and fat metabolism. Br J Anaesth 41:588-593;1969

Breier C, Muelberger V, Drexel H, Herold M, Lisch H-J, Knapp E, Braunsteiner H Essential role of post-heparin lipoprotein lipase activity and of plasma testosterone in coronary artery disease. Lancet June 1:1242-1244;1985

Carruthers M Danish experiences in the treatment of advanced circulatory disease with anabolic steroids. Bullitin EOCCD 6;1980

Ehrlich JC, Shinohara Y Low incidence of coronary thrombosis in myocardial infarction. Archives of Pathology 78:432-444;1964

Fuller JH, Shiply MJ, Rose G, Jarrett RJ, Keen H Coronary heart disease risk and impaired glucose tolerance. Lancet I:1973-1976;1980

Gaardner A, Jonsen J, Laland S, Hellem A, Owren PA Adenosine diphosphate in red cells as a factor in the adhesiveness in human blood platlets. Nature (London) 192:531-532;1961

Moeller J The concentration of cholesterol and testosterone in the blood of male patients with circulatory diseases. Bullitin EOCCD 1:1-4;1977

Tweedle D, Walton C, Johnston IDA The effect of an anabolic steroid on post-operative nitrogen balance. Br J Clin Pract 27/4:130-132;1973

D H E A: Dihydroepiandosterone

I believe the body is made to function perfectly when it is provided with the right nutrients and a clean environment, free of environmental toxins. Unfortunately, the invention of processed food, combined with the rush of modern life have converged to a state of malnutrition in a large percentage of people.

Add to this the inescapable presence of industrial toxins, heavy metals, chlorine and fluoride in our public water supply, pesticide residue and liberal amounts of preservatives in processed food, not to mention increasing levels of CO_2 and decreasing levels of O_2 in the atmosphere, along with airborne industrial pollutants, and it is no surprise to learn that the incidence of all degenerative diseases, including cancer, have tripled since the year 1900.

Despite the fact that life expectancy has increased by about 25 years since 1900, the life expectancy of a person fifty years old is only one year more than it was in 1900. The increase in overall life expectancy is due primarily to the conquest of transmittable diseases in children.

Modern medicine has met with abject failure regarding the diseases which occur in adulthood. As for prevention of illness, modern medicine has abandoned that field to others — except for the perpetuation of the simple-minded idea that cholesterol is somehow responsible for vascular disease.

So the consideration that the body should function perfectly is merely a theoretical construct, because the conditions of perfect nutrition and a clean environment do not exist in the modern world. One of the ways the body expresses its discomfort in these difficult times is hormonal imbalance.

The adrenal glands take a beating not only from chronic stress but also from various toxins, including tannic acid, found in coffee — even in decaffeinated coffee. A patient recently told me that her coffee intake was no problem, that she had been drinking only one cup of decaf each day for twenty years. A quick examination of those numbers reveals that 20 x 365 = 7300. Adding five cups of coffee for leap years, which have 366 days, and that comes out to 7,305 tannic acid assaults on her adrenal glands over the last twenty years! Because she also is slightly overweight and feeling run down despite seemingly healthy habits, I sent her for a DHEA level. The result came back low, as expected.

The adrenal glands are paired, and they are set just above the kidneys on each side as their name indicates (ad = above, renal = kidney). Some glands have greater ability to resist aging than others. The adrenal glands are not among the stronger of the endocrine glands. Normal aging results in a decrease of adrenal function until, in the octogenarian years, we find the adrenals essentially dead in most people.

As it turns out, proper adrenal function is essential to the correct functioning of all the other endocrine glands. Many hormones (six of them in all) are derived from a parent molecule

Therefore, progesterone levels are low from day 26 until ovulation, usually around day twelve. Then levels are high until day 26, unless pregnancy occurs in which case, levels are even higher throughout pregnancy.

Another function of progesterone is known only by what happens when it is no longer present in youthful levels. Because most progesterone is produced by the corpus luteum, and because there is no further corpus luteum formation after menopause, progesterone levels fall precipitously at menopause and remain low for the rest of a woman's life.

Not by coincidence, another thing happens concurrently around menopause and especially the next five to six years: demineralization of bones, which is called "osteoporosis." Osteoporosis can be *prevented* with the use of natural progesterone. It also can be *reversed* with the use of natural progesterone.

Much attention has been paid to the largely unsuccessful, or partially successful, attempt to prevent osteoporosis with estrogens. Because there is no large profit in natural progesterone, the drug companies have not alerted physicians to the value of this good medicine. Consequently, docs are out there following the party line: horse estrogen (Premarin), vitamin D and calcium for osteoporosis prevention.

Many women, who now are disabled with hip fractures and other debilitating complications of osteoporosis, followed that advice. That regime can slow down osteoporosis in some cases but has nothing like progesterone's power to prevent demineralization of bones and remineralize osteoporotic bones.

The fact that osteoporosis can be prevented and reversed with natural progesterone is not something which drug companies want you to know about, because there is not much money in natural progesterone. However, they would love to have you know about all the possible uses of their synthetic (patented) estrogens.

The major use of synthetic estrogens is, of course, for birth control, and they are combined with synthetic progesterone-like substances (called "progestins"). It is important to realize that progestins are synthetic — made in labs other than nature's lab — and are profoundly incompatible with the human body, as any woman who has taken BCPs can tell you. Here is a partial list of warnings to be found for your friendly BCP, found on the package insert and caused by the progestin content.

Possible side effects:

Birth defects
Loss of vision
Thrombophlebitis, embolism, cerebral thrombosis
Liver dysfunction, cholestatic jaundice
Breast or genital malignancy
Fluid retention, migraine, asthma, epilepsy

Heart and kidney dysfunction
Menstrual irregularities
Depression, nervousness, fatigue
Decreased glucose tolerance, may exacerbate diabetes
Breast tenderness, galactorrhea (flow of milk)
Skin eruptions
Acne, alopecia, hirsutism
Edema, weight changes
Cervical erosions
Pyrexia, nausea, insomnia, somnolence
Anaphylactic reaction (sever, life-threatening allergic reaction)
Hypertension

If you bother to read the fine print, you will see that almost every synthetic drug is sporting such a warning. Man's lab is just unable to compete with nature's lab. In the case of natural progesterone, given in proper doses, here is a list of possible adverse side effects:

None.

It is a short list; a list of nothing. There are no side effects — hard to believe, but true. The first tenet of medicine, part of the Hippocratic Oath, an oath taken by all doctors when they graduate from medical school, is, "First, do no harm," or *Premum non nocere* in the original Latin. Many doctors have forgotten this basic tenet of medicine under the hypnotic influence of a blizzard of propaganda from pharmaceutical companies touting their latest patented, money-making, synthetic nightmare.

Estrogen and progesterone exist and do their respective jobs in relation to each other and must be in a certain proportion to each other to work best. Estrogen acting in the absence of progesterone goes out of control in certain ways. Estrogen and progesterone mutually antagonize the effects of each other, thus making the cyclic nature of ovulation, fertilization, implantation and gestation possible in human reproduction. If fertilization and/or implantation do not occur, estrogen and progesterone are involved in resetting the system to try again one month later.

At around age 45 to 50, the woman's supply of oocytes (eggs cells) diminishes from millions at birth to around 1000. Because the major source of estrogen is the oocytes, this depletion of oocytes induces a condition of hypoestrogenemia — and thus menopause. So, age itself does not account for menopause, but rather the falling estrogen levels from the depletion of oocytes. Proper nutrition and avoidance of toxins delay menopause by preserving greater numbers of viable oocytes.

Even though estrogen levels fall at menopause, progesterone falls even more, because there is no longer the monthly creation of a corpus luteum to make progesterone. Because estrogen and progesterone balance each other, there comes to be a condition of estrogen dominance after menopause. The regulating hormones of the pituitary gland sense this imbalance and give the neurochemical command for more estrogen and progesterone. This creates an even larger imbalance, because the ability to make progesterone is so extremely compromised while there still are around 1000 eggs left to make estrogen. This imbalance accounts for the myriad symptoms and complaints seen in the doctor's office at this time of a woman's life.

The solution for this situation is natural progesterone along with a good diet and avoidance of toxins. Progesterone supplementation should be considered when there are signs of estrogen dominance: edema, swelling of breasts or fibrocystic disease, loss of sex drive, mood swings with depression, uterine fibroids, irregular or heavy menses, weight gain around hips and thighs and craving for sweets.

For the premenopausal woman who may be experiencing anovulatory (no eggs traveling down the Fallopian tubes) cycles, progesterone provides relief from estrogen dominance/progesterone deficiency between days twelve and 26. For the premenopausal woman, the symptoms of hot flashes, mood swings, etc., are eliminated. For the postmenopausal woman, the advantage of progesterone is a continuing good sex drive.

It is unlikely that estrogen supplementation will be needed since a good diet includes a number of phytoestrogens (estrogens of plant origin) and everyone is exposed to xenoestrogens of petrochemical origin from the environment. Also, progesterone sensitizes all estrogen receptors, so that there is a heightened response to estrogen which is present. If, after three months, there are neither hot flashes nor vaginal dryness, there is no need for estrogen.

The sources of progesterone are the wild yam and placentas harvested at birth. The synthetic substitutes for progesterone (the progestins) are made from the wild yam. The progesterone molecule is altered so that it can be patented.

Few doctors are even aware that natural progesterone is available and far safer than the pharmaceutical attempt at substitution for the real thing. At present, you cannot obtain USP progesterone from standard pharmacies. For this, you must find a compounding pharmacist. Most docs don't know how to find a compounding pharmacist, or even what they are!

Many pelvic diseases improve with progesterone therapy given before menopause. These include pelvic inflammatory disease (PID), vaginitis, Mittelschmerz (pain on ovulation), ovarian cysts and endometriosis.

PMS

Premenstrual syndrome (PMS) is a problem for many woman (and therefore many men) and involves physical and mental changes. PMS begins around seven to ten days before menses and brings a tidal wave of negative emotions for which husbands and boyfriends are sometimes blamed. The mental effects of PMS are so severe that they even have been used as a defense in court against the charge of murder! Some of the physical effects are a loss of interest in sex, headache, weight gain, back ache, breast tenderness and fatigue.

The treatment of PMS is notoriously unsuccessful. The need for an effective treatment is made clear by the many vitamin/mineral/supplement entries on the market for treatment of PMS. The symptoms of PMS read like a catalog description of estrogen dominance. If estrogen levels are higher than normal, or if progesterone levels are lower than normal, the stage is set for estrogen dominance. If there is an anovulatory cycle, the woman is exposed to an abnormal full month of estrogen effects, relatively unopposed by progesterone.

That PMS should occur at all, even in the absence of anovulatory cycles, is a comment on the effects of the industrial age on our immune systems and on our hormone systems as well. Nature did not design women to become physically and emotionally unstable every month. You can be sure that this syndrome has its origins in the toxic chemical soup in which we live in the modern world. (A similar situation holds for men in that progressively decreasing sperm counts and infertility among men is related to pollution.)

The treatment of PMS with progesterone is 100 to 200 mg. transdermally or 25-50 mg. by mouth from day fourteen to day 25 of the cycle.

Osteoporosis

Osteoporosis, the progressive demineralization of bone, causes 1.3 million fractures per year in the U.S., at an estimated cost of $10 billion. Thin white women fare worst and risk factors include smoking, vitamin D deficiency, calcium and/or magnesium deficiency, a meat-based diet, alcohol consumption and lack of exercise. Until now, the most effective therapy was "estrogen" (not the real human variety) with vitamin D replacement, and the best one could hope for was to slow the disease down and maybe even prevent it.

No hope has been offered to reverse osteoporosis with "estrogen" therapy. Also, the risk of cancer, as well as a panoply of other symptoms of estrogen dominance, mars the use of horse estrogen (Premarin) as well as synthetic estrogens. Despite the clear warnings attached to estrogen therapy, even outlined in the best textbooks of medicine, mainstream establishment medicine has stayed with "estrogen" therapy. This is a tribute to the power of pharmaceutical company propaganda. To handle a part of the risk of osteoporosis — which could be handled safely with natural human progesterone — the drug companies recommend that you take their products and increased your chances of dying of cancer.

Although there have been many therapies for osteoporosis over the years, the fact that none of them could reverse the condition gave testament to the fact that the cause of osteoporosis was simply not understood. Now, it appears that, in women at least, the cause is the loss of adequate progesterone supplies at menopause. This conclusion is arrived at by reverse logic, because replacement of progesterone has the power to reverse osteoporosis, and strengthen and remineralize fragile bone in the older woman.

Of course, the progression of osteoporosis is much more of a problem for women than it is for men. Men also experience osteoporosis, but typically about twenty years later than women and even then not to the extreme degree seen in women. We can hardly say that loss

may be insufficient for the stress to which that person is subjected. Resting (nonstress) levels bear little relationship to the adrenal glands' ability to increase production to counter the effects of stress. The diagnosis can be made with an ACTH challenge test. ACTH (adrenal corticotrophic hormone) is the pituitary hormone which commands the adrenal cortex to produce hormones. By giving a dose of ACTH, we expect to see a doubling of adrenal hormone output, at least. If this does not happen, adrenal fatigue is probable. In extreme adrenal fatigue, the levels actually fall, demonstrating the "whipped horse" phenomenon.

A person who becomes exhausted after stress, and remains exhausted, should be considered adrenal fatigued, until proven otherwise. The diagnosis can be suspected when the patient reports that he is exhausted for days after vigorous exercise. A person who used to run three miles, four times each week, who can no longer tolerate running one mile without being out of commission for days to weeks, is highly suspect of having fatigued adrenal glands. The methods listed below regenerate adrenal function, if the adrenals are not totally and permanently damaged.

Conditions Benefited

While tiredness is the most common presenting symptom of adrenal fatigue, it is by no means the only presenting condition. The failure to adjust to stress shows up in almost all body systems as disease states.

Let us discuss some of the conditions which are benefited by regenerating (or replacing) adrenal function. Like the discussion on thyroid hormone therapy, it is truly amazing to discover that all these conditions are related to adrenal fatigue, but it becomes less amazing when we consider the almost global responsibility the adrenal glands have in regulation of the body under conditions of stress.

Diseases of the Respiratory System

The common cold	Pleurisy (exudative)
Bronchial asthma	Tuberculosis
Allergic bronchitis of children	

Digestive Diseases

Gastritis	Hepatitis
Enteritis	Cholecystitis
Cyclic vomiting	Pancreatitis

Kidneys, Bladder and Urethra Disorders

Acute nephritis	Essential renal hematuria
Chronic nephritis	Acute hemorrhagic cystitis
Nephrotic syndrome	Allergic urethritis
Hemospermia	

Blood Disorders

Leucocytopenia

Thrombocytopenia

Purpura angiopathica

Hypoplastic anemia

Joint Diseases

Osteoarthritis

Arthralgia

Rheumatoid arthritis

Lumbago

Neuralgia

Scapulohumeral arthritis

Skin Diseases

Chronic eczema

Contact dermatitis

Acute urticaria

Urticaria perstans

Neurodermatitis

Pruritis

Prurigo

Exudative erythema
multiforme

Erythema nodosum

Psoriasis vulgaris

Herpes zoster

Herpes simplex

Chickenpox

Acne simplex

Strophulus infantum

Juvenile verruca plana

Pregnancy

Late toxemia

Vomiting

Lumbago

Bleeding

Eye Diseases

Kerato-conjunctivitis

Episcleritis

Post ocular neuritis

Glaucoma

Blepharoconjunctivitis

Chorioretinitis centralis

Blepharitis

Ears, Nose and Throat Disorders

Otitis media

Tinnitus

External eczema

Sinusitis

Meniere's syndrome

Catarrhal syringitis

Otitis externa

Allergic rhinitis

Pharyngitis

Stomatitis

Most of these diseases will abate with the use of glycyrrhiza (licorice tea two to four times each day). Abatement occurs between three days and four weeks with cessation of the chronic stress condition. In more severe cases of adrenal exhaustion, it may be necessary to employ ACE and/or hydrocortisone as described below.

These illnesses (and probably many more) should be considered to be manifestations of adrenal fatigue and the inability to mount the general adaptation response as described originally by Selye in 1936.

Treatment of Addison's Disease

In the case of true Addison's Disease, the only proper solution is a prescription for one of the hormones made exclusively by the adrenal cortices: hydrocortisone. President John F. Kennedy had Addison's Disease and was restored to full function when hydrocortisone became available in 1949. Except for hydrocortisone, he most certainly would not have had the energy required to run for political office leading to the presidency.

Treatment of Adrenal Fatigue

Addison's Disease is so rare, and adrenal fatigue so common, that I prefer to spend most of our space here on the latter. The use of adrenal glandular concentrates is easy, simple and economical and is the first thing I recommend. You can buy these at your health food or vitamin store without prescription.

Another easy, simple, effective, economical treatment is freshly made licorice tea two to four times each day. Licorice tea contains glycyrrhiza, mentioned above. By itself, or together with adrenal glandular concentrate, the effect is potent.

Glycyrrhiza works by blocking the breakdown of hydrocortisone in the liver. Therefore, the hydrocortisone level becomes higher, and this slows down the production of ACTH from the pituitary gland, so the adrenals are given a much-needed rest. Thus, glycyrrhiza can be discontinued later when the adrenal gland function is restored.

Glycyrrhiza also can be purchased in capsule form but it is probably more fun to drink the tea and, who knows, there may be something else in licorice tea which we don't know about that helps do the job.

Nevertheless, if your condition is too progressed to respond to these measures, you may need to visit your nutritional physician. To understand the treatment you may encounter there, we need to discuss a bit more about adrenal physiology.

Adrenal activity is regulated by the pituitary gland. When the adrenals become fatigued, the pituitary senses this fatigue in the form of lowered levels of hydrocortisone and releases ACTH (adrenal corticotrophic hormone).

ACTH commands the adrenals to perk up and produce more hormones. That works for a while, but the adrenals may become overworked and unable to respond — in which case, ACTH stimulation simply stresses them more and leads more quickly to fatigue.

However, the pituitary is unmerciful and continues to pour forth ACTH like a man whipping a tired horse to do work it is incapable of doing. If the adrenal gland can get just a bit of rest from the ACTH whip, it is allowed to regenerate. To this end, your doctor may give you intramuscular or intravenous ACE (adrenal cortical extract). This makes the pituitary think the adrenals are back on line, and it shuts down ACTH production. During this respite, the adrenals can recover some lost function.

Your ACE dose may be administered once, or daily for several days, or even several times in one day, depending on how fatigued your adrenals are. Of course, this should only be done in conjunction with adrenal glandular concentrate and glycyrrhiza by mouth.

Usually, a course of adrenal glandular concentrate, glycyrrhiza, and ACE is enough to jump-start a tired adrenal gland. In case your adrenals are too far gone for this to be effective, you may need to take a low dose of hydrocortisone by mouth.

Hydrocortisone has a checkered history in medicine. As mentioned earlier, when it became available in 1949 doctors had no idea what dose was "physiologic," i.e., natural. They guessed and, by and large, guessed wrong. While a physiologic dose is between twenty and forty mg. per day, divided into four doses, the usual dose given in the early days of adrenal steroid therapy was 100 to 200 mg. and in some cases much more. Anything, even a hormone natural to the body, is toxic in high doses. Even water, in excess, can kill you.

Predictably (in retrospect), many side effects were noted, and the medical establishment became phobic of hydrocortisone. This trend was heartily supported by the pharmaceutical houses, which were busy developing synthetic, patentable substitutes for hydrocortisone, the most famous of which is prednisone.

Since then, two generations of doctors have been trained to fear hydrocortisone while prescribing prednisone and its cousins with their many harsh side effects. The truth is that physiologic doses of hydrocortisone, in distinction to "pharmacologic" (i.e., arbitrarily large) doses, are highly effective and extraordinarily safe for a variety of conditions. Because they are natural adrenal hormones they are without adverse side effects when given in physiologic doses. The same cannot be said of prednisone and its unnatural cousins. For disease states brought on by stress, adrenal support or supplementation is clearly the safest and most natural approach.

See page 358 for instructions on contacting my office for a referral to a doctor experienced in the treatment of adrenal fatigue.

Sources

Jeffries W McK The present status of ACTH, cortisone, and related steroids in clinical medicine N Engl J Med 253:441-446;1955.

Thorn GW, Forsham PHM Metabolic changes in man following adrenal and pituitary hormone administration Recent Progress in Hormone Research, Vol. IV New York Acad. Pr. 1949:229-288.

Levitt MF, Bader ME Effect of corisone and ACTH on fluid and electrolyte distribution in man Am J Med 11:715-723;1951.

day. Creatine is excellent for treating the "dwindles" of old age — that condition in which old people literally shake with weakness. After a few weeks, the shaking stops as strength returns. It is a dramatic effect.

L-arginine has many beneficial effects, increased stamina being one of them. It also helps expand constricted blood vessels and protects from infectious agents entering through the mouth. Both of these actions are accounted for by the fact that the body produces nitric oxide from arginine. This also has a powerful effect on the prevention of cardiovascular disease and should be a mainstay of your preventive program, along with vitamin C.

Growth Hormone Production

However, for the best effect, there must be a youthful level of HGH ready for release, and for this you need a plentiful supply of circulating amino acids. You can achieve this by taking free-form amino acids, which are expensive, or you can achieve the same results by taking a thrice daily protein drink along with an enzyme preparation of proteinase, or at least containing proteinase. This splits protein into its amino acids immediately. I recommend organic soy protein powder.

Don't overdo it. Remember your recommended daily protein intake, expressed in grams, is eighty percent of your body weight expressed in kilograms. One pound = 0.454 kilograms. For example, if you weigh 150 pound, in kilos your weight is 150 x 0.454 = 68.1 kilograms. Your rcommended daily protein intake is 0.8 x 68.1 = 54.45 or about 50-60 grams.

If you are doing vigorous athletics and building/repairing muscle, it may be temporarily more, up to twice as much, but never more than that.

If I were you, given the extreme cost of laboratory-produced HGH, unless you are rich like Ross Perot, I would forget about external supplementation and use the above methods, expecially exercise, to make my own. Besides, what could be better for you than you own Human Growth Hormone?

See page 358 for instructions on contacting my office for a referral to a doctor familiar with HGH therapy.

Sources

Rudman D, et. al Effects of human growth hormone in men over sixty years old The New Engl J of Med July 5, 1990; vol 323:1-5.

Hall K, Sara VR Somatomedin levels in childhood, adolescence, and adult life J Clin Endocrinol Metab 1984; 13:91-112.

Cynober L Can arginine and ornithine support gut function? Gut 1994; suppl. 1:S12-S15.

Welbourne TC Increased plasma bicarbonate and growth hormone after oral glutamine load. Am J Clin Nutr 1995; 61:1058-1061.

EICOSANOID BALANCE

The evolution of life on earth is, to say the least, a fascinating subject of study. It seems to plod along, being the same for eon after eon, punctuated by transformational events. These transformational events create entirely new spaces — platforms for life to begin again, on which evolution can redefine itself. Each platform occurs at that point when, apparently, no further progress is possible.

The greatest transformation was, of course, from inanimate to living: the creation of life. Without this transformation, nothing further was possible. The invention of living is a miracle which dwarfs all other wonders in the universe. Somehow, living material arose out of random chemical reactions, perhaps by chance, more likely by the hand of God.

This living material then coated itself, separating itself from that out of which it came. This coat is called a "cell membrane." With this cell membrane, virus-like particles gave birth to intelligent, mobile, one cell animals. These animals evolved to the ceiling of the space provided by the cell membrane and there life remained for billions of years; apparently life was stymied at this level and could go no further. Then came the next great transformation: multicellular life.

They must have tried incessantly before they finally got it right. A language was required: a compatible chemical language, with which two cells could speak to and understand each other. This chemical language would allow them to stick together and cooperate as one.

It may have been a matter of nothing more than chance, that day when two cells met at the local coffee house and discovered that — *voila!* — they spoke compatible languages. Sticking together allowed them to live and reproduce as one and to divide the tasks of living between themselves — a happy marriage. Cooperation replaced domination at the cellular level, a transformation which is only now trying to happen between humans. It was so successful that soon other cells were applying for membership in the Multicellular Club.

This little communication system, this compatible biochemical language, was a good idea, and when nature has a good idea she always keeps it. Therefore we, as multicellular animals, still have this complex, elegant method by which our cells speak to each other.

This language cells speak to each other, we call the "crines." A common example is the language of the "endo-crines," the injection of chemical messengers into the blood by cells, to request action be taken at a distant location in the body. A "crine" is a chemical messenger, preceded by some letters which denote the nature and purpose of the crine. A crine is one type of "hormone," a word coined in 1905 by Ernest Starling, from the Greek *hormao*, meaning to put into quick motion, to excite, or to arouse.

In the case of one cell speaking to its neighbor, the hormone messenger is call a "paracrine" literally a beside messenger. There are also "intracrines" and "autocrines," hormones which

In the area of nutrition, never have so many said so much, knowing so little. Most people have tried several types of fad diets, ultimately becoming disappointed. People who are willing to be responsible for their health, who have thought about and read about the issue, know intuitively that food selection is the most important aspect of health. People are, therefore, paying attention, and when the "experts" speak about nutrition, these people are listening. If the experts advise a diet of rice, potatoes and cardboard, these good-intentioned people line up to buy it.

Paleo-pathology

Let us look at the facts. Skeletal remains demonstrate the remarkable change in stature which occurred when Cro-magnon man invented agriculture. Prior to agriculture, human beings were tall, about as tall, on average, as we are now. Then came agriculture and with it the production of abundant supplies of grains and cereals, items which were rare prior to agriculture.

Man shifted from a mixed diet of meat and vegetable food sources, which were hunted and gathered, to a diet composed almost entirely of cereal and grain. Height plummeted by about one foot and did not begin to recover until 200 years ago, when animal husbandry made it possible for people to have a bit of protein in their diet on a regular basis.

Egyptian Mummy Evidence

There are literally thousands of mummies left over from the age of the Pharoes, not just a few as you probably thought. Extensive studies have been performed on the bodies of these people who lived out their lives in agricultural society. When compared to bones from people from hunter gatherer societies, they demonstrate no clear difference in degenerative joint disease, but a clearly increased incidence of infection.

Hunter gatherers lived longer, and more of their children survived childhood, evidenced by the fact of fewer children found in their burial grounds. Another difference noted is in the rate of tooth decay, far more prevalent in agriculturalists. The diet in ancient Egypt was a modern nutritionist's heaven: fruits, vegetables, stone ground whole wheat bread, honey as well as olive, safflower, flaxseed and sesame oils, and only occasionally meat.

Heart disease was well-known in ancient Egypt and was commonly mentioned in their literature. Atherosclerosis is a common finding in mummies. Obesity, particularly abdominal obesity, was well-known as was extensive dental disease and parasitic infestation. It may have been good for society as a whole to develop agriculture. It allowed people to live in large cities, to devote their lives to learning and the arts rather than chasing food around. However, what is good for society as a whole may not be good for members as individuals, then or now. The Egyptian diet, the same sort of diet now considered perfect by conventional wisdom — a high-complex carbohydrate diet — caused a devastating decline in health in agricultural societies. Because we have the same biochemistry and physiology as our ancestors of a few thousand years ago, it stands to reason that we will not fare any better on this diet.

Only the individual who thinks for him/herself is going to survive the experts' advice and live a long and healthy life. The experts have been telling us for forty years to cut back on fat intake. Many people have done this to lose weight. Here are the results: in forty years the average percent of calories consumed as fat has fallen from 41% to 35%; in the same time period the number of people overweight has increased from 25% to 33%. How can this be? Weight gain is a straight proposition of number of calories consumed minus number of calories burned off in activity. People are eating more calories, but using carbohydrate sources for these calories. Ironically, many people are eating this way in an effort to lose weight, be more healthy and live longer. Meanwhile, the studies continue to pour in reporting that health and longevity decrease as the number of calories consumed and body weight increase.

The correlation between increasing levels of serum insulin, which goes up in response to the "healthy" high-complex carb diet, and the rate of coronary artery disease (CAD), is clear. As insulin goes up, so does the rate of CAD. Furthermore, if the disease is studied in terms of one-, two- or three-vessel disease, the number of arteries involved climbs steadily, in step with increasing serum insulin.

These studies force us to look again at what we believe about proper nutrition. What must happen for maximum health is the development of nutritional habits which lead to balancing of insulin and glucagon so that the most powerful hormones in the body, the eicosanoid prostaglandins, PGE-1 and PGE-2, are balanced. This requires attention to the amount of protein consumed in relationship to the amount of carbohydrate.

I believe that we must rely on the experience of hunger to tell us when to eat. However, we cannot rely on the experience of hunger to tell us what to eat until after the addiction to carbohydrate is overcome. To overcome the addiction to carbs requires the intentional balancing of protein and carbohydrate. Your appetite must be satisfied, or you will continue to suck down the carbs.

I also believe that we can afford to let the chips fall where they may in regard to fat. Fat comes associated with carbs and protein, so if we eat those items we are going to get essential fatty acids, and that is all we need. Despite all the hysteria about the importance of a low-fat diet, fat has nothing to do with the balancing of insulin and glucagon and the avoidance of hyperinsulinemia. Fat does not make you fat. Calories make you fat. Fat is the storage form of excess calories and the body will convert excess carbs to fat. As Dr. Barry Sears says, it is simple-minded and against common experience to believe the adage: "If no fat passes my lips, there will be no fat on my hips."

So, how much protein do you need? That is highly variable. For the average seventy-kilogram man at the average activity level, seventy grams per day, or even half that, is enough to sustain life, but insulin/glucagon, PGE-1/PGE-2 balance will not be optimal unless that protein is balanced correctly to carbohydrate intake at a 7:10 ratio.

A sedentary individual needs less protein, a body-builder needs more on those days he or she pumps iron. There is no hard and fast rule. If you consume so much protein you get a headache, that is definitely too much. If you consume so little you feel weak, that is definitely too little.

The U.S. government, which has an opinion about everything, has lowered its estimate from the old one gram per kilogram to around 50-60 grams per day for the seventy-kilogram man. When we say so and so many grams per day, that does not mean you should wait until bedtime and then eat exactly that much. The pancreas does not do a calculation at the end of the day and plan its insulin/glucagon output for the next day. Insulin and glucagon are made on a moment by moment basis based on circulating glucose and amino acid levels. Therefore each meal should be properly balanced 7:10, protein to carbs, even more protein with exercise, and less when you are being a couch potato.

If you balance your food intake consistently, at every meal, with ten grams of carbs to every seven grams of protein, your weight should, in time, take care of itself, provided you are not stuffing yourself for psychological reasons. If you eat because you are hungry and you stop eating when you are no longer hungry, that should, eventually, do the job. You will feel more satisfied on less calories, if you have the proper proportion of protein and if you let go of fat phobia. However, if eating is your substitute for sex, or what you do to avoid boredom, that is another story.

People who are very obese did not get that way overnight, and they should not try to drop weight overnight. The safest and most long-lasting weight loss comes with correct eating, not fanatical starvation, appetite suppressants, or fad diets. No one should have to suffer to lose weight. Those who do suffer to lose weight will gain it back, e.g., Oprah Winfrey.

Dyslipidemia

For those people with an apparent imbalance in their fat metabolism, with high cholesterol and triglyceride levels, this approach works also. Balancing food intake will bring these lab studies into the normal range much better than interfering with fat metabolism by the use of dangerous synthetic drugs like Mevacor, which are statistically associated with markedly increased accident, suicide and homicide rates! What the body does with excess carbs is convert them to fat stores in the body, using the circulation as a storage site.

Advice For Vegetarians

People who are vegetarians, particularly strict vegetarians, are especially susceptible to protein deficiency. However, a diet balanced in carbs and protein can easily be had by paying attention to sources of protein. The body does not know where the protein comes from, it only knows if there is too little or too much. Vegetable sources are just as good as, and often better than, animal sources.

My favorite source of protein is soy powder. It is ninety percent protein, rich in the isoflavones which are proven anticarcinogenic substances. The ten percent is made up of bromelain and lecithin. This food of the gods comes from a company named "Falcon" at (408) 462-1280. If your organic grocer does not carry it, ask them to call that number and order it.

I mix, with one-half rice milk and one-half filtered water, the amount of protein powder which equals about seventy percent of the weight of the carbs I eat with any particular meal. Put it all in a bottle and shake vigorously. If you are obese, and you want to lose weight, have your shake for breakfast and lunch and then allow yourself solid food at night. Drink whatever it takes to satisfy your appetite, but not more. At night, eat only what it takes to satisfy your appetite, but not more. Engage in this program only after consulting your physician.

Of course, you can be more conventional and simply eat tofu, which is also a soy bean product. Unless you are eating at home, you will do well to carry your protein powder or tofu with you, as most restaurants are not supplying these items.

See page 358 for instructions on contacting my office for a referral to a doctor familiar with the eicosanoid diet.

Sources

Reaven GM Role of insulin resistance in human diabetes. Diabetes 37:1595-1607, 1988.

Kaplan NM   The deadly quartet: upper body obesity, glucose intolerance, hypertriglyceridemia, and hypertension Arch Int Med 149:1514-20, 1989.

Karhapaa P, et. al Isolated low HDL cholesterol, an insulin resistant state Diabetes 43:411-17, 1994.

Bjorntorp P, et. al   The effect of physical training on insulin production in obesity Metabolism 19:631, 1970.

Rizza RA, et. al Production of insulin resistance by hyperinsulinemia in man Diabetologia 28:70-75, 1985.

O'Dea K Marked improvement in carbohydrate and lipid metabolism in diabetic Australian Aborigines after temporary reversion to traditional lifestyle Diabetes 33:596-603, 1984.

Baird I Safety of liquid-protein diets Lancet 1;1979:618

HEALTH

AND

NUTRITION

THE MICRONUTRIENTS: Oxidation, Free Radicals, Aging and Antioxidants

In recent years there has been intensive research into the phenomenon of aging. Until the 1950s, the predominate thinking in science was that aging is exclusively a phenomenon programmed into the genes, a kind of genetic clock with just so many ticks and, at the last tick, your time would be up, and there would be nothing to be done about it.

That paradigm has been replaced with the idea that aging is a complex phenomenon affected by many variables. Most of these variables are covered in this book. You could think of this book as an anti-aging course, although it is much more than that. Such areas as nutrition, emotions, aerobics, colon health, addictions, fasting, sugar, salt, internal organ health, relationships and sexuality now are well-known to be associated with vitality and longevity. Probably there is an internal clock ticking away, but there are many ways to wind that clock so that it ticks longer and with more vitality.

Curiously, one of the most powerful ways of rewinding the life clock is almost unknown to the general public. Does this term ring a bell: "Free radicals?" Probably not, unless you have made a point to educate yourself broadly in health matters. Dr. Denhan Harman first proposed the Free Radical Theory of aging and disease in 1959. For many years his theory was rejected, ignored, or disparaged by the medical establishment. Since then, Dr. Harman's ideas have been validated and expanded, particularly in the late eighties and early nineties.

Your body burns food for fuel just as a fireplace burns wood for fuel. In both cases it is literally a burning process. In the case of a fireplace the fire is more obvious. In your body, this burning occurs molecule by molecule, so that a fire does not erupt. Both processes — that in a fireplace and that in the cells of your body — burn oxygen, a process called "oxidation." In a fireplace, there are ashes left over after the fire. In your body, free radicals are left over. These are molecules which have an extra unpaired electron. This extra electron makes the free radical molecule highly reactive. These molecules act like flaming torches in relationship to the tissues of your body. Free radicals, at a molecular level, burn everything they touch. The type of free radical makes a world of difference. Oxygen free radicals, known as "oxides" and represented by the chemical symbol O^-, are cleansing and assist in breaking down toxins and killing pathogenic organisms. Hydroxyl free radicals, represented by the chemical shorthand OH^-, are damaging to cellular structures, particularly the cell membrane which holds the cell together.

The breakdown of fats in the body produces even more free radicals than does the breakdown of carbohydrates and proteins. When fat is left out at room temperature, free radicals are formed. We say the fat has gone "rancid" and is no longer edible. If you bite into a nut which has gone rancid, you spit it out immediately, because it tastes terrible. This is how a mouthful of hydroxyl free radicals tastes.

There are several categories of free radicals, which result from the oxidation of different kinds of foods. Cholesterol, fats and particularly unsaturated fats, are routinely oxidized to free radicals called "peroxides." Lipid peroxide attacks and destroys cell membranes.

Because hydroxyl free radicals are so damaging to the body, nature has designed a system to neutralize them. The body produces substances called "antioxidants," which convert hydroxyl free radicals into harmless molecules. Antioxidants are produced within the cells. The cells' ability to produce adequate amounts of antioxidants is determined by age, inheritance, nutrition and stress. People who produce higher than usual levels of natural antioxidants enjoy greater health and longevity. This connection has been researched and proven.

Free radicals affect the body as CDCs affect ozone in the upper atmosphere—a little goes a long way. When a free radical does its damage, it is not neutralized but able to continue doing further damage, creating more hydroxyl free radicals. If unchecked by antioxidants, hydroxyl free radicals act like a fire out of control.

In a young, healthy, well-nourished, nonstressed individual, sufficient amounts of antioxidants are produced in the cells to handle the challenge of hydroxyl free radicals. As a person grows older, the cells are less able to produce sufficient amounts of antioxidants. This circumstance is made worse when the person is on a high-fat, high-carbohydrate diet, or when the person is ill.

Any combination of these conditions can result in an imbalance, so that there are excess hydroxyl free radicals in the body. These hydroxyl free radicals attack the tissues and cause cell breakdown and inflammation. The most obvious result is arthritis and myositis (joint and muscle inflammation), but most investigators believe that excess hydroxyl free radicals play an important part in cancer, heart disease, cataracts and aging itself. It may be that hydroxyl free radicals attack the very systems which produce antioxidants and thus, over a period of years, weaken the body's ability to deal with hydroxyl free radicals. Most investigators believe that a constant barrage of hydroxyl free radicals damages the chromosomes themselves and may, in this way, speed up the aging process.

Whatever the cause, the production of antioxidants begins to decline at age twenty and, interestingly, this also is the time when visible aging begins. Until very recently, aging and the degenerative changes which go along with aging were thought to be inevitable. This may turn out not to be the case.

The word "antioxidant" refers to a broad range of substances, each designed to handle one type of an equally broad range of hydroxyl free radicals. Here is a list of vitamin antioxidants: vitamin A, vitamin C, vitamin E and beta-carotene. Beta-carotene is the precursor of the vitamin A molecule. It is made of two vitamin A molecules attached to each other.

Certain minerals empower these vitamin antioxidants, and these are selenium, copper, zinc and manganese. One amino acid is an especially powerful antioxidant: L-cysteine. Vitamin C often is added to processed food as a preservative. It works by preventing oxidation.

Biotec Foods, in Hawaii, is doing seminal research into extracting antioxidants identical to the body's own naturally occurring antioxidants from whole grain. These substances are known as superoxide dismutase (SOD), catalase (CAT), glutathione peroxidase (GT) and methionine reductase (MET).

Here are recommended steps to take to handle hydroxyl free radicals and stop aging almost in its tracks. If you are a real warrior for absolute health and vitality, here is what to do. Also, if you want to reverse a degenerative disease such as arthritis, here are the actions to take.

1. The first order of business is to stop swallowing hydroxyl free radicals. Free radicals are produced by frying foods in oil or fat. Do not eat fried foods.

2. The most powerful source of free radical formation is saturated fat. Eat a minimum of saturated fat in your diet.

3. Avoid consumption of rancid fat. Learn to identify rancid fat with your nose. You can do this by allowing cooking oil to set out for a few days. Sniff any fatty substance before you put it in your mouth. If it is rancid throw it away. This applies to nuts and not-so-fresh fried food of any kind.

4. Every day, eat a large salad and one or two carrots. This supplies beta-carotene, plus other carotenes as well, vitamin C and probably a variety of useful substances not yet discovered.

5. Take the following doses of antioxidants daily: vitamin A 10,000 IUs, vitamin C 5000 mg., vitamin E 800 IUs, beta-carotene 50,000 IUs, selenium 400 mcg., L-cysteine 1 gm. in morning and 1 gm. in afternoon, thiamine 150 mg. and 4-6 tabs of one of the grain-derived antioxidants made by Biotec Foods (see the previous paragraph).

6. Take a daily vitamin B complex supplement with two to three times the daily recommended level of vitamin Bs.

The issue of cost may come up for you as this will not be inexpensive. You have to ask yourself about the value increased vitality and longevity have for you, as well as consider the money you save by virtue of the diseases which you will not have.

If you are not a warrior, don't care to live to 140 with great vitality, and if you do not have a degenerative disease to deal with, follow steps one and two above and take two of the suggested antioxidants.

A Short History of Vitamins

The first vitamins were discovered in the 1930s. The general category of "vitamins" was defined as (1) substances found to be absolutely necessary for life (i.e., vital) and which (2) the body cannot synthesize on its own. The first few such substances discovered were amines (i.e., containing a nitrogen bound to three hydrogen atoms -NH_3). The first name given these substances was "vital amines" and this was later shortened to "vitamins." Subsequently, other substances were discovered which were not amines and yet were vital and which the body could not synthesize on its own. When these were discovered, the "e" was dropped, and the word became "vitamins."

Vitamins were given letters to go with their chemical names to simplify discussion about them. Not many people know what to say about "d-alpha tocopheryl succinate" but most people have some idea of what "vitamin E" is all about. When the "B" names were being handed out, several substances were give "B" names, which turned out not to be vitamins after all. Therefore, you have heard of vitamins B_1, B_2, B_3, B_5, B_6 and B_{12} but not 4, 7, 8, 9, 10 and 11. Those latter substances lie in the scrap heap of nutritional history.

So a vitamin is a substance which the body cannot synthesize on its own, yet which is necessary for life. Therefore, by definition, it is necessary to obtain all vitamins from outside the body. If a molecule can be synthesized in the body, it is not a vitamin. The single exception to this rule is vitamin D which can be synthesized in the skin, but only when exposed to sunlight and Niacin (B_3) which itself can be synthesized in the liver in small amounts.

There are thirteen vitamins in all, divided into the four fat soluble (A, D, E and K) and the nine water soluble (eight B vitamins and vitamin C). The fat soluble vitamins can be stored in the body and do not need to be ingested every day. Because they can be stored, it is possible to store too much and thus become toxic on these vitamins. The water soluble vitamins cannot be stored, with the exceptions of B_{12} and Folic Acid and must be consumed frequently for optimal health. However, these vitamins can be taken in large amounts without toxicity, because they are not stored and are easily eliminated.

"Nutritional supplements," which includes vitamins, is a term applied to substances extracted from foods or manufactured in the laboratory, to be presented to the body in concentrations which are not to be found in foods. The difference between those vitamins extracted from food sources and those manufactured by chemical processes in the laboratory is an important distinction, because vitamins manufactured in the laboratory, using artificial synthetic techniques, come without trace substances which make them work at their highest potential. They also come in the dextro- and levo- forms (so-called "right" and "left handed" molecules, which are the mirror images of each other), and the body can only use the levo-forms.

Some people think that if you consume a healthy diet, you have nothing to gain from vitamin supplements. If you are a young adult (under 24), and you eat a diet of fresh, raw, organically grown complex carbohydrates in great variety (with a balance of protein), and never stray from that diet, in my view, you have little to gain from supplements. However, if you are an older adult (24 or over), or if you sometimes stray from that kind of diet, you have a lot to gain from supplements. It is true that you can survive without supplements, even if you are on a diet of average nutritional value. However, I expect that you want more from life than mere survival. You want absolute health and vitality.

Even at that, it is still necessary to be very well educated about each supplement you take or you will be wasting your money on supplements you do not need. Also, if you are not very well educated about the purpose of each supplement, you will forget to take them — and supplements sitting in a bottle on your shelf give no benefit to your body.

Each vitamin should become a personal friend of yours. Since there are only thirteen of them this is not an impossible task.

Here is what you need to know. (By the way, I will not be listing animal sources of vitamins, as that might encourage you to eat and drink animal products, a practice definitely injurious to your health when considered over a long period of time.)

The Fat Soluble Vitamins

Vitamin A or Retinol / Provitamin A or Carotene (the first class of vitamin discovered)

Vitamin A is actually not, in the strictest sense, a vitamin, because it can be synthesized in the body. The real vitamin is carotene, which the body uses to make vitamin A. Beta-carotene is made of two vitamin A molecules covalently bonded. Carotene is present in carrots, broccoli, squash, spinach, kale and sweet potatoes.

The beta form of carotene is a powerful antioxidant. It is possible to obtain "vitamin" A, already synthesized in the bodies of animals, by consuming animal meat and animal products. However, I suggest you not put these kinds of toxins into your body and be happy with the carotene present in the aforementioned vegetables.

An abundant supply of carotene has the following effects on the body: moist, supple, youthful skin and mucous membranes, moist, well-lubricated eyes and good night vision. However, if you are treating a specific condition, which responds to vitamin A, as we sometimes do in nutritional medicine, only vitamin A will work. You will not get the same effect with beta-carotene.

Vitamin D (Calciferol)

Vitamin D, also called the "sunshine vitamin," is synthesized in the skin when sterols (present in many foods) migrate to the skin and are irradiated by sunlight. From there it travels to the liver where it is converted to 1-hydroxy-vitamin D and then to the kidney where it becomes 1-dihydroxy-vitamin D, the active form. Excessive sunlight is not necessary (unless you like to age your skin prematurely), and normal exposure to indirect sunlight will result in the synthesis of plenty of vitamin D. Therefore, strictly speaking, vitamin D is not a vitamin either in that it is not necessary to consume it. The only way to fall into insufficiency is to be generally malnourished and/or not exposed to an average amount of sunlight. It is possible to obtain vitamin D from animal sources; however, I recommend strongly against this. Sufficiency of vitamin D results in smooth calcium and phosphorus absorption and metabolism and thus healthy bones and teeth. It also has an anti-mitotic effect (prevents the excessive multiplication of cells) and 1-dihydroxy-vitamin D in a cream base is a very effective treatment of psoriasis.

Vitamin E (Tocopherol)

The major role of vitamin E is as an antioxidant preventing the oxidation of fats and vitamin A. Vitamin E neutralizes LDL or Low Density Lipo-proteins, also known colloquially as "bad cholesterol," and prevents it from oxidizing and damaging the walls of arteries. Vitamin E is found in vegetable oils, whole grains, cereal, bread, wheat germ and leafy green vegetables. An abundance of vitamin E is important for maximal sexual function, particularly in men. It has been found that a high blood level of vitamin E correlates better with cardiovascular health than does a low level of cholesterol.

To get the full effects of vitamin E, it is necessary to use the natural, non-synthetic form. Real "vitamin E" is actually eight related molecules: four tocopherols and four tocotrienols. What is commercially available in your vitamin store is synthetic alpha-tocopherol, perhaps mixed with a tiny portion of natural source, so the manufacturor can use the word "natural." There is only one source of all natural vitamin Es which I know of: a product called "Unique E" made by A. C. Grace Co. in Big Sandy, Texas. It is rarely found in stores and usually only available (unfortunately) through doctors' offices.

Vitamin Ks (K_1 and K_2): Menaquinone and Phytonadione

This vitamin aids in blood clotting, as it is essential to the formation of prothrombin, an enzyme which is, in turn, necessary for the formation of fibrin, the major constituent of a blood clot. Vitamin K is derived from leafy green vegetables and soybean oil. It also is synthesized in the colon by bacteria. A normal diet combined with unimpaired bacterial synthesis usually is sufficient to supply enough vitamin K.

The Water Soluble Vitamins

Vitamin C (Ascorbic Acid)

This well-known vitamin is important in the maintenance of collagen, the protein which holds most of the soft tissues of the body together. Along with B_6, it is also vital to the utilization of amino acids. It enhances the absorption of iron from vegetable sources. It inhibits the synthesis of nitrosamines, compounds implicated in cancer. Fruit sources are citrus fruits, fresh strawberries, cantaloupe, pineapples and guava. Vegetable sources are broccoli, Brussel sprouts, tomatoes, spinach, kale, green peppers, cabbage and turnips. Regular intake of vitamin C insures health of the soft tissues of the body and perhaps an ounce of cancer protection. There is ample research evidence that substantial doses of vitamin C, taken regularly over the course of years, prolong a person's life expectancy by lowering the probability of vascular disease. (The same is true of vitamin E.)

For all except four mammalian species, ascorbic acid is not a vitamin, because they make their own abundant supply. Man is one of the four exceptions. Of the four enzymes necessary to make vitamin C, man has the first three. Somewhere in our evolution, we lost that fourth enzyme, and ascorbic acid became a vitamin for us — we have to obtain it from our diet. Animals make that amount of vitamin C which would be the equivalent of four grams (4,000 mg.) daily for an average size human.

While the U. S. government RDA (recommended daily allowance, some say "recommended deficiency allowance") is 60 mg., this is merely the amount which will prevent death from scurvy. Optimal health requires the higher dose levels. This enzymatic defect in humans undoubedtly accounts for a shorter life span than we were designed to have.

One of the many functions of ascorbic acid in human biochemistry is to regenerate oxidized vitamin E which, in turn, serves to protect cell walls from oxidative damage.

The ascorbate form of ascorbic acid is the form which is effective in the treatment of colds and flu. Do not bother trying to treat a cold or flu with ascorbic acid. It will not work. The L- form is the bioactive form of vitamin C. The D-form is just so much stuff the body must get rid of. Synthetic ascorbic acid contains equal amounts of L- and and D- forms. Natural sources of vitamin C contain only the L- form. Read the label to know what you are getting. If it is not specified otherwise, assume it to be synthetic. If it doesn't say "ascorbate," assume it to be ascorbic acid.

Vitamin B_1 (Thiamine)

B_1 is a coenzyme, which serves as a catalyst in carbohydrate metabolism in the Kreb's cycle, enabling simple sugars to release their energy. B_1 also aids in the synthesis of neurotransmitters. Healthy sources of B_1 include leafy green vegetables, whole cereals, wheat germ, berries, nuts and legumes. Rice, for example, in its natural state, is rich in B_1; however, milling removes most of this vitamin. White flower and polished white rice are lacking in B_1. A plentiful supply of B_1 has a calming and focusing effect on the nervous system.

Vitamin B_2 (Riboflavin)

B_2 also is a coenzyme which serves as a catalyst in fats and proteins, as well as carbohydrates. It helps maintain healthy skin and mucous membranes. Sources include dark green vegetables, whole grain and mushrooms. A plentiful supply of B_2 results in soft, youthful skin, particularly around the nose and mouth.

Vitamin B$_3$ (Niacin)

B$_3$ also is a coenzyme serving as a catalyst for the release of energy from nutrients. It helps prevent sun damage to the skin, promotes healthy colon function and helps maintain balanced neurochemistry. Healthy sources of B$_3$ are whole grain, dried beans, peas and nuts. It has been found that B$_3$ can be synthesized in the liver from the amino acid tryptophan; therefore, it does not meet the strict criteria for being a vitamin. Nevertheless, a plentiful supply of B$_3$ reduces blood cholesterol and provides protection from the development of atherosclerosis.

Vitamin B$_5$ (Pantothenic Acid, Calcium Pantothenate, Panthenol)

This vitamin is necessary for the conversion of fat and sugar into energy, although its mechanism of action is not known. It is present in whole grains, wheat germ, bran, green vegetables and brewer's yeast. It also is synthesized by intestinal bacteria. This vitamin promotes wound healing and antibody formation.

Vitamin B$_6$ (Pyridoxine, Pyridoxal-5-phosphate)

Along with vitamin C, B$_6$ is necessary for the absorption and metabolism of amino acids and is necessary in proportion to the amount of protein and/or amino acids consumed. Healthy sources include whole grains, cereals, avocados, green beans, spinach and bananas. Plenty of pyridoxine allows you to enjoy the benefits of all the amino acids, as well as aiding in the formation of red blood cells, which are vital to the transport of oxygen to the tissues of the body. If you are treating an illness which responds to pyridoxine, e.g. the carpal tunnel syndrome, use the activated form of pyridoxine: pyridoxal-5-phosphate. It costs more, but it gets the job done.

Vitamin B$_{12}$ (Cobalamine, Cyanocobalamine, Hydroxycobalamine)

B$_{12}$ is necessary in small amounts for the formation of proteins, red blood cells, the function of the central nervous system (production of myelin — the stuff which serves as insulation for the "wires" of the brain, spinal cord and peripheral nerves) and maintenance of the inner lining of the intestinal tract. B$_{12}$ is not available from vegetable sources and is produced only by microbes (bacteria and algae). Microbes found in the mouth and intestine produce sufficient B$_{12}$ for most people. The body generally has stored a three to eight year supply of B$_{12}$. Since the introduction of techniques to kill micro-organisms associated with food, it has become possible, although extremely unlikely, that a strict vegetarian can develop B$_{12}$ deficiency. To guard against this, within three years of commencing a strict vegetarian diet, you should add tempe, miso, soy sauce, or tamari sauce to your diet on an occasional basis. These foods all contain B$_{12}$. It is true that B$_{12}$ is present in animal products, but when you look at what else also is present, you will want to choose to learn a little about these not-so-well-known oriental foods which contain B$_{12}$. An abundance of B$_{12}$ helps in the production of red blood cells, helps keep the nervous system running smoothly and helps maintain the integrity of the intestinal mucosa.

Folic Acid (Folacin, Folate, Vitamin B_c, or Vitamin M)

Folic Acid is a coenzyme needed for forming protein and hemoglobin. It is available from leafy green vegetables, legumes, nuts, whole grains and brewer's yeast. It is lost in cooking and when stored at room temperature. Your best source is a fresh green garden salad. Unlike the other water soluble vitamins, Folic Acid can be stored in the liver, so you do not need to eat it every day. An abundance of Folic Acid can improve lactation, act as an analgesic for pain, promote healthy, youthful skin and increase appetite in cases of debilitation.

Biotin (Coenzyme R or Vitamin H)

Biotin is another coenzyme, essential for the normal metabolism of fats and protein. It maintains healthy skin and is especially good for the health of hair follicles. The best natural sources are nuts, fruits, brewer's yeast and unpolished rice. This vitamin will rejuvenate hair follicles when taken by mouth or rubbed directly on the skin in a cream base. It may even regrow a few hairs, which have gone into early retirement. Hair will stand up straighter and recover a healthy sheen.

That concludes the discussion of the substances commonly accepted as vitamins. There are proponents claiming that several other substances are vitamins. Some of them may yet one day be classified as true vitamins; however, as yet, these claims are not proven. There is a strong capitalistic motivation for drug and nutrition companies to discover new vitamins, as there is a lot of money to be made in this endeavor. This motivation may lead to exaggerated claims. I will merely mention these substances for completeness; however, I do not believe it to be worth your time to focus a lot of attention on these items just yet. They are: orotic acid ("vitamin" B13), pangamic acid ("vitamin" B15), laetril ("vitamin" B17), choline, "vitamin" F, inositol, "vitamin" P, para-amino-benzoic acid (PABA), "vitamin" T and "vitamin" U.

Amino Acids

Amino acids are the building blocks of proteins. Your body needs amino acids, not proteins. The value in eating protein is that it is broken down into polypeptides by hydrochloric acid in the stomach and then into amino acids by digestive enzymes in the small intestine. These amino acids are then absorbed into the body through the small intestines. The wall of the small intestine, when in a healthy condition, will not allow anything larger than an individual molecule to pass through to the body. Once in the body, amino acids are used to build new proteins to do various jobs around the body. The body also has the ability to synthesize amino acids, to make them from scratch, except for eight amino acids, which must be supplied from the outside. These are called "essential amino acids," because they are essential for you to continue living. Their names are isoleucine, leucine, lysine, methionine, phenylalanine, threonine, tryptophan and valine. We place an "L-" in front of each to denote the natural form which is the only form used by the body for most purposes. For infants and children there is a ninth essential amino acid called "histidine." However, adults can synthesize histidine. It is important that these essential aminos be present in the proper proportion. A diet of vegetables and fruits supplies all the needed aminos and in the proper proportion. If you are eating this kind of diet you need not worry about amino acids.

However, you should consider another aspect of the aminos: their medicinal value as supplements. Taken in concentrated form, these substances can produce remarkably beneficial effects countering many of the effects of aging. Let us talk about them one by one.

L-tryptophan is used by the brain along with niacin (B_6) and magnesium to produce serotonin, a neurotransmitter. L-tryptophan can help induce natural sleep, reduce pain sensitivity, act as an antidepressant, reduce anxiety and aid in the control of alcoholism. Unfortunately, as of this writing, the FDA has taken the excuse of a contaminated batch of L-tryptophan from Japan to ban this valuable nutrient from the U.S. market. This is a moral crime aginst your right to health.

L-phenylalanine is an amino acid which is used by the body to produce the neurotransmitters norepinephrine and dopamine which promote alertness. L-phenylalanine can reduce hunger, increase sexual interest, improve memory and mental alertness and alleviate depression.

DL-phenylalanine (DLPA), not to be confused with plain phenylalanine, is a mixture of equal parts of the "D-" (synthetic) and "L-" (natural) phenylalanine. DL-phenylalanine inhibits the enzymes systems which destroy endorphins, and the resulting increased level of endorphins accounts for the effects of DLPA: pain relief and strong antidepressant action. DLPA is very useful in conditions of chronic pain such as arthritis, low back pain, neuralgia, etc. Some people, who do not respond to ordinary pain relievers, such as Empirin, do respond to DLPA. The analgesic effect of DLPA may require from four days to two weeks to manifest but once it does appear it is long lasting.

L-lysine is used to treat herpes simplex infections (cold sores), enhance concentration, aid in fat metabolism and alleviate some infertility problems. L-lysine inhibits the replicaton of the herpes virus and, while it does not kill the virus and wipe it out, it will suppress the symptoms in some people.

L-arginine and **L-ornithine** are best discussed together as they usually are prepared and sold in combination. L-ornithine is converted to arginine in the body and therefore serves as a back up supply of L-arginine. L-arginine is converted to nitric oxide by an enzyme called nitric oxide synthase. Nitric oxide serves to keep pathogens out of the digestive tract; it serves to dilate blood vessels, and it is a potent source of energy and a sexual stimulant as well.

Upper back tension responds particularly well to L-arginine/L-ornithine. Other effects of this dynamic duo are muscle building and fat burning (especially when combined with exercise) with overall weight loss, accelerated wound healing, tissue repair and strengthened tendons and ligaments. L-arginine/L-ornithine should be taken with vitamin C, vitamin B_6 and a good mineral supplement for maximum effect.

L-glutamine is the precursor of glutamic acid, which serves the brain by neutralizing excess ammonia (a byproduct of brain metabolism), thus creating a clearer space for brain activity. L-glutamine has been shown to improve IQ, alleviate fatigue, depression and impotence, as well as speed healing. It also is well-known to decrease the craving for alcohol and is a valuable adjunct in the treatment of alcoholism. These effects may be due to the HGH-releasing (human growth hormone-releasing) properties of the L- form of glutamine, which is, of course, popular with body-builders.

L-aspartic acid helps expel ammonia from the body. Ammonia is the major waste product of cell metabolism and is eliminated through the kidneys. The faster it is eliminated from the body the better you feel. Aspartic acid results in increased stamina (studies have proven this in athletes) and decreases fatigue. It is sold as L-aspartic Acid (the natural, non-synthetic form).

L-cysteine is a sulfur-containing amino acid and aids in detoxification by boosting the biosynthesis of the endogenous antioxidant, glutathione. Cysteine can chelate, and protect the body from, excess copper and other harmful metals. It also binds free radicals and serves as an antioxidant. It is best supplied as N-acytel-L-cysteine (or NAC), because a portion of straight cysteine is converted to cystine, which is not bioavailable.

L-methionine is another sulfur-containing amino and protects against certain tumors. It also helps in the treatment of some schizophrenics.

L-glycine aids in treatment of low pituitary gland function and is useful in the treatment of muscular dystrophy. It also is used in the treatment of hyperglycemia and hyperacidity of the stomach, as well as a biochemical disorder in which there is a Leucine imbalance, causing an offensive body and breath odor. L-glycine also has HGH-releasing properties similar to L-arginine.

L-trosine is effective as a mood elevator. It too has HGH-releasing properties similar to L-arginine.

L-taurine is useful in the treatment and prevention of macular degeneration. Macular degeneration is the slow wearing out of the retina of the eye, including the focal point on the retina, which is called the "macula," eventually leading to blindness. There are two types of macular degeneration: the accelerated type and the age-related type. We all have age-related macular degeneration (AMD) and if you live long enough you will go blind! That is the bad news. The good news is that you can slow down macular degeneration with taurine, perhaps to the point that something else gets you *before* you go blind.

I have not given you the recommended dosages of amino acids. For this information, consult the label. In general, four grams per day is a top dose of any individual amino acid, although there are exceptions. Consult your doctor of nutritional medicine for further advice.

Enzyme Co-factors (Minerals)

The body is powered by enzymes present in every living cell. Enzymes work by catalyzing (accelerating) chemical reactions. The body is a complex chemical soup with a fantastic number of chemical reactions possible. Most of the possible chemical reactions are incompatible with life. If they were to happen on a large scale, the chemical soup of life would simply self-destruct.

This is where enzymes come in. Enzymes can be thought of as matchmakers. Each enzyme is designed to bring together two particular molecules, so that those two molecules interact to produce a third (needed) molecule quickly and efficiently. In this way, the presence of enzymes favors the occurrence of certain reactions over others. The undesirable reactions do occur occasionally, but so rarely as to present no problem to the overall chemistry of the body. The presence of an enzyme makes the reaction it is designed to catalyze several thousand times more likely than it would be in the absence of the enzyme.

Enzymes cannot work, however, without co-factors, and each enzyme is designed to work with a particular co-factor. You have heard of these co-factors, they are called "minerals." Unless an enzyme is accompanied by its co-factor/mineral, or a substitute co-factor/mineral, it will simply sit around doing nothing. There are eighteen co-factor/minerals in human nutrition. They are, in alphabetical order: calcium, chlorine, chromium, cobalt, copper, fluorine, iodide, iron, magnesium, manganese, molybdenum, phosphorus, potassium, selenium, sodium, sulfur, vanadium and zinc. Some of these can substitute for each other, and in this way the body maintains a survival advantage in time of dietary imbalance.

Calcium

Calcium is the most plentiful co-factor/mineral in the body. All but a small percent is found in the bones and teeth. It functions, in relationship to phosphorus, to maintain the strength of the teeth and skeleton. It is in dynamic flux with twenty percent of bone calcium removed and replaced each year by cells known as "osteoclasts" and "osteoblasts" — literally bone breakers and bone builders. The optimum ratio of calcium to phosphorus is 2:1. Vitamin D is required for the absorption of calcium. Calcium also functions with magnesium to keep the heart healthy and the electrical rhythm of the heart pulsing regularly. Calcium also is important in the transmission of impulses between nerves throughout the body. Non-animal, healthy sources of calcium are soybeans, peanuts, walnuts, sunflower seeds, dried beans and green vegetables.

Chlorine

This co-factor/mineral regulates the acid-base balance of the body. It circulates in the blood in relationship to sodium and potassium. It aids enzyme systems in the liver to metabolize and dispose of toxic materials absorbed through the colon. It also functions with hydrogen to form hydrochloric acid, which digests food in the stomach.

Chromium

Chromium is the co-factor/mineral for the enzyme insulin. Insulin is derived from the Isles of Langerhans cells of the pancreas and is responsible for facilitating the entry of glucose into the cells. Without a sufficient supply of chromium, insulin cannot do its job. Chromium also functions in the transport of proteins from one location in the body to another. This is an important growth function and may be important in the prevention of atherosclerosis. Chromium also is important for the heart and blood vessels and is required to maintain a normal blood pressure. The best natural sources are corn oil and brewer's yeast.

Cobalt

Cobalt is the co-factor/mineral for vitamin B_{12} (cobalamine). It enables B_{12} to do its job in the construction of red blood cells. It is necessary in very small amounts and must be obtained from foods, as it is not built into supplements. Sea vegetables are rich in cobalt even though some writers claim that you have to eat animal products to get it. This is just not true. Cobalt is known to replace zinc in some enzyme systems.

Copper

Copper is a co-factor/mineral for a broad range of enzymes throughout the body. It is essential for hemoglobin synthesis and for the conversion of tyrosine into melanin (which protects the skin from sunburn). It also is essential for the utilization of vitamin C and therefore has a profound effect on the health of the elastic tissues of the body, such as ligaments and tendons. Copper is so abundant in nature that it is difficult for you to become deficient in this mineral. It is found in beans, whole wheat, prunes, leafy vegetables and in high concentration from use of copper cookware.

Iodine

Iodine is the co-factor/mineral involved in the enzyme systems which produce thyroxin, the thyroid hormone. Thus, two-thirds of the iodine in your body is concentrated in your thyroid gland. Iodine is necessary for thyroxin, and thyroxin is responsible for maintaining a normal metabolic rate in all the cells of the body. You can think of thyroxin as the accelerator pedal and the rest of your body as the car. As long as there is sufficient iodine, in the absence of thyroid disease, your body will run at a comfortable rate, not too fast, not too slow. Thyroxin also is responsible for the healthy growth of hair, nails, skin and teeth. Salt was fortified with iodine by law, until a few years ago when that law was repealed. That law was originally passed around the turn of the twentieth century (about 1910, if I remember correctly) to lower the incidence of goiter (a condition caused by iodine deficiency), particularly in the Midwest region of the U.S., around the Great Lakes and the inland mountains, where soil is iodine poor. Iodine is available in vegetables grown in iodine rich soil. It is especially present in kelp and onions. Sufficient iodine promotes a normal metabolic rate, proper growth, normal energy, normal mental acuity and healthy hair, nails, skin and teeth through its effect on thyroid homone output.

Iron

Iron is necessary for the construction of, and is actually part of, the hemoglobin molecule. Hemoglobin is necessary for the transport of oxygen around the body. Iron is a necessary part of myoglobin, the red protein in muscle cells. It also is used as a co-factor/mineral to enzymes involved in growth. This is obviously of importance in children who are growing. It is equally important in adult bodies, which are constantly replacing skin and intestinal tract cells. Iron is important in the enzymes of the immune system and is essential for maintaining normal resistance to infectious disease. Premenopausal women lose twice as much iron as men each month, due to menstruation, and therefore women are much more likely to have iron deficiency anemia. When you select an iron supplement you should avoid inorganic iron (ferrous sulfate), because it is not easily absorbed and destroys vitamin E as well. Choose the organic forms: ferrous gluconate, ferrous fumarate, ferrous citrate, or ferrous peptonate. Your best natural sources of iron are peaches, nuts, beans, asparagus and oatmeal. Sufficient iron results in healthy growth and replacement of cells, as well as a healthy amount of red blood cells, for the all-important job of transporting oxygen.

Magnesium

In the plant world, magnesium is the co-factor for chlorophyll, the molecule which has the unique ability to convert and store sunlight in chemical form for later use. Chlorophyll is green — therefore, the greener the vegetable, the more chlorophyll and thus the more magnesium present as well. In the human body, magnesium is the co-factor/mineral to enzymes involved in carbohydrate and protein metabolism. It also acts as an antagonist to calcium and tends to prevent calcium stones in the kidneys and gallbladder, as well as the calcium deposits of atherosclerosis. It is nature's original "calcium channel blocker." Magnesium also is involved in enzyme systems of the central nervous system and is required for proper function of the CNS. Alcohol depletes magnesium and this is a problem in alcoholism, which can lead to seizures. The best sources of magnesium are fresh green vegetables, the greener the better. Magnesium also is found in corn and apples. An abundant supply of magnesium promotes a healthy cardiovascular system and helps prevent calcium deposits and depression.

Manganese

Manganese is a co-factor/mineral involved in a great diversity of enzyme systems. It is important to the proper use of biotin, thiamine and vitamin C. It is important in the production of thyroxin, normal CNS function, proper digestion and sexual function. Proper sources include green veggies, whole grain cereals and tea. A plentiful supply promotes health in many areas of the body through good thyroid, CNS, digestive and sexual health.

Molybdenum

Molybdenum is the co-factor/mineral for the enzyme xanthine oxidase and is vital for iron utilization. It also is important in fat and carbohydrate metabolism. Supplements ordinarly contain no molybdenum — therefore, your dietary sources are very important. They are dark leafy green veggies, whole grains and legumes. A sufficient supply allows iron to be properly used and tends to prevent iron deficiency anemia.

Phosphorus

Phosphorus is widely distributed as a co-factor/mineral in the enzyme systems of the body. It is a component of bone and is in dynamic relationship to calcium. Its ratio to calcium should be 1:2. Phosphorus is present as phosphate in many food preservatives. Avoid food preservatives by consuming only fresh foods. Phosphorus is present in colas, consumed by so many people in the U.S. After age forty, the kidneys have more difficulty than before with phosphorus excretion, so that this advice, about fresh food and avoiding colas, is especially important. When excess phosphorus is present, the bones decalcify to release calcium in order to maintain the 2:1 ratio with phosphorus. If this continues over a few years, the result is osteoporosis. Women, particularly, should take note of these principles, as they are especially prone to osteoporosis after menopause. The problem with phosphorus is that, given food preservatives and colas, people are exposed to too much phosphorus. When vitamin D and calcium are in sufficient supply, and when foods heavy in phosphorus preservatives are avoided, there should be no problem.

Potassium

This co-factor/mineral is in dynamic relationship with sodium. Potassium is found primarily inside the cells and sodium primarily outside the cells. It is particularly important as a co-factor/mineral in glucose metabolism, also water and fluid balance, muscle (including heart muscle) action, transmission of impulses along nerves and in kidney function. Veggies and fruits are high in potassium. Sufficient potassium is necessary for the continuation of life. It also must be kept at just the right concentration, and the body is equipped with mechanisms to achieve this balance. Any significant deviation from this level can result in cardiac arrhythmias, fibrillation, seizures and death. You are well advised to maintain your potassium level.

Selenium

Selenium is synergistic with vitamin E. Together they are more powerful than the sum of both combined. Selenium is an antioxidant, as is vitamin E. Both serve to slow down hardening of tissues caused by oxidation of fats. Selenium concentrates in the male organs — seminal vesicles and testes — and is lost in the semen. Therefore, men have a higher requirement than women for selenium. Natural sources include veggies and grains. Sufficiency is associated with youthful elasticity of tissues, alleviation of hot flashes and menopausal stress and treatment of dandruff! It also is suspected that selenium provides some cancer protection.

Sodium

Sodium, as sodium chloride, was thoroughly discussed in an earlier part of this book. It is the most common of all minerals, and there is almost no possibility of ever becoming sodium deficient. There is every possibility of becoming overloaded with sodium. There is no instance in which it is advisable to supplement your sodium intake, except for adrenal fatigue or collapse (called Addison's disease). It is much more commonly needed to restrict sodium intake.

Sulfur

Sulfur is contained in the amino acids cysteine, cystine and methionine. These amino acids are, in turn, abundant in proteins. If you are ingesting sufficient protein, you have no worries about sulfur deficiency. A variety of fresh veggies will more than do the job. Sulfur is important in the construction of healthy skin and the two outgrowths of skin: hair and nails.

Zinc

Zinc is documented to participate as a co-factor/mineral in over eighty enzymes, thus it has many affects on the body. Zinc is necessary for protein synthesis, it governs the contractibility of muscles, is important in prostate health, helps in the formation of insulin, is important in brain function and is required for the synthesis of DNA. Good sources are whole grain products, brewer's yeast and pumpkin seeds. An abundant supply of zinc can accelerate the healing of wounds, help avoid prostate problems, stop the formation of white spots in the fingernails (the old ones will not disappear until they grow out), promote mental alertness, heighten the ability of bored taste buds to taste the goodness of food and aid in the treatment of infertility.

Glandulars and Live Cell Therapy

Glandulars are extracts of animal organs containing not only the hormones associated with those organs, but also other substances contained in those organs — some of which have yet to be isolated and identified. Glandular therapy is the oldest of supplement therapies, dating back thousands of years, having been used by the ancient Hindus, Egyptians and Greeks.

The theory behind glandulars is a deceptively simple: "like heals like." Therefore, to successfully employ a glandular, theoretically at least, one must only identify the function which one wants strengthened, know the gland associated with that function and administer the glandular extract associated with that gland.

Glandulars have a dramatic history with strong polarization on the question of their efficacy. There have been outrageous, and certainly unsupportable, claims for the miracle healing power of glandulars. The reaction of the mainstream medical community to this kind of activity has been a total repudiation of glandulars. The truth undoubtedly lies somewhere in between these extremes.

Live cell therapy was begun in Europe in 1931 by Paul Niehans, a Swiss physician, who treated a woman whose parathyroid had been accidentally removed surgically. Dr. Niehans, knowing that the woman would die untreated, went for broke by injecting whole diced parathyroid gland from a freshly slaughtered sheep. The woman survived and lived into her nineties. Dr. Niehans went on to develop "live cell therapy," which still thrives in Europe and is recognized by the medical community there as legitimate and effective.

So, you can spend about $5,000 and go to Europe for live cell therapy or you can treat yourself with oral glandulars for about $10. Most people knowledgeable about glandulars believe that oral glandulars work on the same principles as live cell therapy, namely by providing the body not only the major hormone associated with a gland, but all the trace elements as well. Oral glandulars are certainly safer than intravenous cells from other species, which have the possibility of stimulating severe anaphylactic reaction and shock. Before you scoff at live cell therapy and glandulars, consider the fact that the well-acccepted practice of bone marrow transplant is the cousin of live cell therapy, in that live cells are injected into the patient. The major difference is that the cells in a bone marrow transplant are of the human variety. The same holds true of the new technique of injecting live fetal brain and adrenal cells into the brains of Parkinson's disease patients. Both these procedures are on the forefront of accepted medical research.

The objective in glandular therapy is to stimulate renewed, vigorous and healthy activity of aged or diseased cells by supplying natural cell stimulators found in the tissue of the corresponding organ of an animal. Even trace amounts of these cell stimulators are sufficient to do the job, so it is irrelevant that most of them are destroyed by stomach acid. Because of the action of stomach acid, most glandulars are enteric coated. There is no doubt that glandulars make a difference. These are powerful preparations, which should be used carefully.

Following is a list of glandulars with their therapeutic effects. Pancreatic Concentrate supplies digestive enzymes which not only aid in the digestion of food but also stimulate the pancreas to increase its own production of enzymes. It also stabilizes blood sugar and, before the isolation of insulin, was the treatment of choice for diabetes. Heart Tissue Extract has been shown to stimulate the regeneration of diseased heart muscle in animal experiments. Raw Liver Concentrate boosts resistance to disease, endurance, performance and strength over and above the effect of the vitamins and minerals contained. Testicular Concentrate and Prostate Extract stimulate the regeneration of these organs and enhance sexual performance in the male. Stomach Concentrate aids in the healing of ulcers both of the stomach and duodenum as well as enhances the absorption of vitamin B_{12}. Duodenal Concentrate enhances digestion, heals and protects the digestive tract from ulcers and enhances the absorption of B_{12}. Thymus Extract boosts the immune power of individuals with compromised immunity. Spleen Extract stimulates the immune system, especially in people with Hodgkin's disease. Adrenal Extract boosts the body's ability to deal with stresses such as infections, physical challenge, allergens and sexual stimulation. Lung Concentrate is recommended for all types of lung disease.

GLUCOSAMINE

Specific soft tissue structures in the body, such as cartilage, tendon, ligament, joint fluid, heart valves, blood vessels and several structures in the eye, are all dependent upon a substance called "glucosamine" for normal maintenance. Glucosamine is an amine group (nitrogen surrounded by three atoms of hydrogen, i.e., $-NH_3$) attached to a glucose molecule. The sulfate form is this molecule balanced electrolytically by two sulfate radicals (a sulfate atom attached to four oxygen atoms ($-SO_4$). Glucose itself is five carbons held together in a ring structure by an oxygen atom, with a hydroxylated carbon atom ($-CH_2OH$) attached as a kind of tail.

The body makes a sufficient amount of glucosamine to handle normal repair needs. However, if there is an injury to the body combined with a degenerative process — for example, damage to the intervertebral discs from years of regular jogging; basketball, with all the vertical jumping (and landing) and many other sports along with arthritis — the normal production of glucosamine may be insufficient to allow complete healing. Many of these chronic injuries may never heal without nutritional help.

Medical students are taught in medical school that arthritis is irreversible. With great diligence, they are told, we might be able to slow down the progression of arthritis, but we can never stop or reverse it. A lot of being a good doc is unlearning what was taught in medical school.

Because glucosamine is the major component of the synovial fluid (the fluid which lubricates joints), its deficiency leads to a thin watery condition of the synovial fluid — thus predisposing the joints to injury through poor lubrication. Each set of adjacent vertebrae is cushioned by synovial fluid. As the body ages, it produces less glucosamine, predisposing all joints to injury and arthritis. Arthritis may be nothing more than an accumulation of small injuries.

The intervertebral discs, which serve as cushions between vertebrae, are made of cartilage. With aging (and thus lower levels of glucosamine) and accelerated by lifting and running, the intervertebral discs degenerate. When something "degenerates" in the body, that simply means that it cannot repair itself as fast as it is being injured. It needs help from the outside. In the case of the intervertebral discs, this causes the loss of a few inches of height over the years. If you are over thirty and go measure your height now, you will find that you are shorter than you once were.

In contrast to the nonsteroidal anti-inflammatory drugs (NSAIDS) — some people say this stands for "new sorts of aspirin in disguise" — which suppress pain in the short run, and may accelerate joint destruction in the long run, glucosamine supplies what is most needed to help the body repair itself. Although there is no immediate pain relief (and we do live in a society addicted to instant results), the fact is that six to ten weeks after initiating therapy with glucosamine the pain does recede, and it stays gone without the need for synthetic drugs to suppress it. In addition, when taken in proper doses, glucosamine is free of side effects — which is to be expected since it is a substance natural to the body.

The treatment of osteoarthritis with pain and inflammation suppressors, including steroids (which cause further joint degeneration), is a classic example of societal addiction to instant results at any costs, an addiction all too willingly supported by allopathic medicine. The use of glucosamine sulfate, on the other hand, is an example of the application of modern nutritional medicine to handle a health problem at its root.

Sources

Kaufman, W. The use of vitamin therapy to reverse certain concomitants of aging. J. Am. Geriatr Soc;11:927-936, 1955

MacHaty, I. Ouaknina, L. Tocopherol in osteoarthritis; a controlled pilot study. J. Am. Geriatr Soc; 323-330, 1976

O'Ambrosia, E. et al. Glucosamine sulfate; a controlled clinical investigation in arthritis Pharmatherapeutica; 2:504-508, 1991

Pujalta, J. M. et al. Double blind clinical evaluation of glucosamine sulfate in the basic treatment of osteoarthritis Curr. Med. Res. Opin.; 7:110-114, 1980

Ronnigen, H. and Langeland, N. Indomethacine treatment in osteoarthritis of the hip joint. Acta. Orthop. Scan., 50; 169-174, 1979

Setnikar, I., Pacini, A., and Revel L., Antiarthritis effects of glucosamine sulfate studies in animal models Arzneim-Forsch, 41:542-545, 1991

Val A. L., Double blind clinical evaluation of the relative efficacy of ibuprofen and glucosamine sulfate in the management of osteoarthritis of the knee in outpatients. Curr. Med. Res. Opin., 8: 145-149, 1982

PERSPECTIVES ON NUTRITION IN RELATED SPECIES

Throughout this book, I will be recommending a no-meat, no-dairy diet balanced in respect to complex carbohydrate and protein. This diet should be high in fiber and feature organically grown food. I could recommend this sort of diet for nutritional reasons, without reference to spiritual and environmental considerations, which also have merit. Healing happens faster for a person on this type of diet. Speed of healing reflects overall health and is of great interest to most doctors.

I believe there is, for each species, a natural, ideal type of food which leads to maximum vitality for that species. I believe that the type of food on which any particular species thrives best is determined by the adaptation that species has made to the available food over the past few million years.

We are primates, and we are descended from a common ancestor with other primates. Darwin was right. God created life through evolution. Our closest living relative is the chimpanzee, and the most primitive living primate is the lemur, a small nocturnal animal with big eyes, which would fit in the palm of your hand, found in Madagascar, an island off the southeast coast of Africa. Madagascar separated from the African continent in the Age of the Dinosaurs, and the species there have not had to compete with new varieties for a hundred million years. Therefore, evolution slowed on Madagascar, and the lemur has been almost completely unchanged all these years. The interesting thing about the lemur is that it is not a meat-eater. However, it has recently been discovered that chimpanzees in the wild do eat meat when they can. Somewhere along the evolutionary line, things changed.

Man and chimpanzee split off from the same ancestor somewhere around six to seven million years ago. Other mammals, notably the canines and the felines, were developing themselves into strictly meat eaters. They came to have teeth specialized for tearing meat, with claws capable of ripping prey to bits. They also developed short intestinal tracts for quick processing and elimination of meat, because meat rots faster than plant food. Also, they became swift and able to chase down breakfast, lunch and dinner. Primates share none of these characteristics.

Man, in the meantime, came to eat meat. Why? This, indeed, is a good question. If you were an alien from another planet trying to classify the animals according to what they eat by looking at their anatomy, man would certainly be classified as a vegetarian. He has relatively benign-looking teeth, best adapted to grinding vegetable fiber. He has no claws but rather fingers and fingernails well-adapted to dissecting plants. He is not particularly fast; in fact, even slower than the bear and thus unable to run down a meal. He has a 28-foot-long intestinal tract! This long intestinal tract is designed for dealing with the more complex nature of plant digestion. All these characteristics indicate that, by nature, man's ancestors on the simian tree were vegetarians. This design apparently is rather ancient. In the meantime, man's digestive physiology has changed to that of an omnivore, also able to handle meats, preferably, from a digestive point of view, raw meats.

Fifteen million years ago, Africa was a land of dense jungle, beginning to give way to open plains and broken forests known as "savannas." In the forest was a species of ape which had developed the ability to walk on two, as well as four limbs. Around six to seven million years ago, one venturesome band of these apes came out of the forest to live part of the time on the savanna. The savanna was populated with large carnivores. Those ape-men/women who dared to walk more frequently on two legs were able to better see approaching danger by looking over the vegetation. They survived to reproduce, and thus did this band of ape-men/women become able, through natural selection, to walk exclusively upright. With their upper limbs freed, they found many interesting and useful things to do with them.

They became handy with sticks and stones, and because they stuck and stoned together, they survived without a lot of change in their anatomy. This all happened about five million years ago. This prehuman creature developed into several different varieties of human-like creatures: *Australopithicus robustus* (a giant who remained a vegetarian), *Australopithicus africanus* (a smallish creature) and *Homo habilis*, your direct ancestor. (This is the short course in paleoanthropology and human evolution.)

As his name implies, *Homo habilis* was very good with his hands. *Handyman* was so skilled with his hands that he eventually killed off the other two species of proto-humans. *Handyman* perfected his upright posture (paying a certain price in the form of lower back pain) and doubled the size of his brain; and by 1.5 million years ago became *Homo erectus*: the first fully upright man.

During all this time, "socialization" was proceeding — which means that man and woman were coming to depend on each other for survival. Man, always looking for a shortcut, took to killing other animals for food, while woman stayed closer to home and continued to gather plants. *Homo erectus*, as part of his newly developed hunting habit, completed the extermination of *Australopithicus africanus* and probably also the giant vegetarian *Australopithicus robustus* — unless a few of the later survived to become Sasquatch (this remains to be proven).

Around 200,000 years ago, *Handyman*'s brain case again expanded, and this led to the development of *Homo sapiens* or "thinking man." Fifty thousand years ago there appeared a new variety of Thinking Man, *Homo sapien sapien*, "wise thinking man," with a high forehead and a new kind of vocal apparatus, allowing the sophisticated kind of speech to which we are accustomed, an audible representation of the hand sign language which it replaced. These people are called the "Cro-magnons," and they are " us."

This new kind of man then managed to kill off, or breed and blend with, another strain of wise thinking man, who we now call Neanderthal after the valley in Germany where their remains were first discovered. There evolution stood until the about four thousand years ago. The next step in evolution did not occur with an anatomical change, but probably with a neuro-chemical change. Humans began to appear on the earth, aware of themselves as more than animals, but also possessed of a soul. This evolution was a transformation, and we are still in the midst of it right now. I interpret your participation with this book to represent your stand for forwarding this stage of evolution. Part of the transformative process is a heightened awareness of the importance of our physical nature and the value of attending diligently to the well-being of our bodies.

Human beings have always eaten what is easiest to obtain. For thousands of millennia, the diet was balanced between food of plant and animal origin. Then came agriculture, and the balance swung toward food of plant origin, principally cereals and grains. Only recently has modern animal husbandry made it easy to obtain meat again. We are now eating levels of meat probably unheard of in hunter/gatherer times.

So, why are we eating so much meat? The answer is: because we can. We are so absolutely able, we can manage to do things which are not in our own best interests. We also can smoke tobacco and drink alcohol. This fact does not make tobacco or alcohol in our best interests.

Human physiology and biochemistry is designed for a certain type of diet. Thanks to agriculture and animal husbandry, we have strayed so far from that diet that we no longer even know what that certain type of diet may be. Achieving optimal health means, for one thing, discovering and following that diet for which our evolution prepared us.

or "dieticians" know next to nothing about the effects of foods on the body, yet they are allowed to create the menus for sick people! Those good nutritionists who do understand these things are instructed, by profit-conscious hospital administrators, to toe the budget line or else. The big problem is that almost no one thinks for him/herself or bothers to find out the truth of the matter about food. Even vegetarians, who believe their choice to be the right choice, do not know why.

Our Pathetic Diet is Something New

Prior to 1900, the type of diet now prevalent in the West was unavailable throughout the world except to the very rich. High-protein, cooked foods, such as red meats, cheeses, eggs, as well as refined sugar and flour, etc., were rarely eaten by the average person, and when they were, they were considered delicacies. The exception was the classical fat monarch consuming an almost exclusively fat and protein diet and suffering gout for his reward.

Degenerative disease is not programmed into the genes. It is meant for a human being to be healthy, thin, attractive and full of life for at least 95 years, longer for some people. Few people realize this potential because of disease derived from contact with the environment. We contact the environment through food, water and air. Air is the most important in terms of volume, food and water are tied for second.

If you want to live a long, healthy life, free from degenerative diseases ordinarily associated with aging, you must adopt a health-supporting diet. The diet which best supports health is a balanced diet of ten parts carbohydrates to seven parts protein, on a caloric, weight, or volume (all the same) basis. Where fat is concerned, it will take care of itself, as it will come associated with healthy sources of protein. You can resign from the American Fat Phobia Club (also known as the Fat American Club) and be healthy.

Proper sources of carbohydrates are vegetables, the kind with color, not the white stuff like potatoes and rice. The stuff without color is relatively empty of vitamins. The healthiest source of protein is soy bean. If you must eat meat, stick with fish and skinless poultry only occasionally.

You may ask why these particular percentages. The answer is that these percentages have been demonstrated to balance a hormonal system in the body called the "eicosanoids." The eicosanoid system senses an imbalance of your diet through insulin and glucagon output from the pancreas. These hormones alter your fatty acid metabolism to produce aracidonic acid which leads to the "Series Two Eicosanoids." These are the so-called "bad" eicosanoids which make you feel ill and which cause degenerative disease.

When the eicosanoids are out of balance, your immune system is depressed, resulting in fatigue and more frequent infections. You have headaches, you need more sleep, have less physical strength and energy, and your digestion is off.

In a certain sense, people of the third world are more fortunate than you, because they cannot afford a diet of processed foods, low in fiber and laced with pesticides and herbicides. They exist on the likes of vegetables, corn, and soy which they grow for themselves. These people are not afflicted with degenerative diseases although they are, unfortunately, exposed to poor sanitation and thus infective and parasitic diseases you are less likely to encounter (although thirty percent of Americans are infected with parasites).

People of the third world also experience famine, with hunger and starvation, from time to time. It is true that longevity is greater in developed countries; however, this is not because of diet but rather because of better sanitation and an abundance of food.

People eat primarily to satisfy hunger. Hunger is tricky business. You may not be hungry until certain foods become available. A dish of ice cream can transform a state of satisfaction into ravaging hunger. The presence of tasty carbohydrates and the over-reliance on complex carbohydrates as a food source result in rampant obesity in America. People also eat to gain the nutrients needed by the body. Fast foods, processed foods and high-cereal-and-grain-content foods, such as pasta and bread, are lacking in many of the nutrients needed by the body.

Between craving for rich foods and this state of overconsumptive malnutrition, lies the explanation for the high incidence of obesity in developed countries like Germany, England and especially the U.S. People eat a load of rich food, which inspires hunger by its mere richness but lacks basic nutrients. Trying to get the needed nutrients, the body signals you to eat more through the mechanism of hunger. Soon the stomach is stretched to a size much larger than nature intended. Because a full stomach is then harder to achieve, the sensation of emptiness and hunger is reinforced.

Diets Don't Work

Dieting, in the sense of restricting calories, does not work to stay slim, because you are asked to limit the amount of food you eat in order to limit the number of calories which enter your body. You should be able to rely on hunger as an effective tool to lose weight, but you cannot, if you eat a diet of addictive, carbohydrate-rich foods. If you eat a balanced diet, you feel filled, and you can rely on your hunger to tell you how much food you need. This will lead to weight loss without dieting, if you are overweight — but not overnight.

Meat Contains Toxins

If you eat meat, you are eating the muscle tissue of dead animals — which is made of protein, fat and a small amount of carbohydrate. Unfortunately, you also are eating a number of other items. These animals are fed artificially, in most cases, and the foods they are fed have been grown using herbicides and pesticides. These environmental contaminants are fat soluble and become concentrated in the fatty tissue of these animals. When you eat their flesh, you get these environmental contaminants in concentrated form. You also receive a stiff dose of the hormones, stimulants and antibiotics fed to these animals to make them produce the most meat possible in the shortest time possible.

kilogram man, this amounts to 70 x 1.6 = 112 grams. I understand that this is more than the officially recommended amount, however I believe the official recommendation to be low.

Exceptions

People who are highly active in sports are breaking down muscle through exercise and should eat more protein than the average person. If you are not highly active, and you think you simply feel better on a very high protein diet, you may have an enzymatic condition in which protein and fat is metabolized especially well in your body. I suggest that you consult your nutritional medicine doctor to determine the perfect type of diet for you.

The liver breaks excess protein down into urea which is excreted through the kidneys. In circumstances of excessive protein intake, excessive quantities of urea pass through the kidneys. Urea is a diuretic, which means that water is made to exit along with urea, and this water loss means the simultaneous loss of minerals. The most important mineral lost is calcium.

A typical western diet of excessive meat, eggs, milk, fish and poultry throws the body into a negative calcium balance with more calcium lost each day than is gained. This lost calcium must come from somewhere in the body, and the largest store of calcium is in the bones. The bones are slowly decalcified, and the result is osteoporosis, one of the most serious health problems of elderly people in developed countries.

If you are wondering if you have osteoporosis, an accurate and economical osteoporosis test is the measurement of bone specific collagen, a urinary assay test, called the "NTx," offered by Meridian Valley Labs at (800) 234-6825. I suggest you stay away from x-ray and other radioactive tests for osteoporosis.

The high purine content of a high-protein diet leads to gout and kidney stones in some people, as purine breaks down to uric acid, which crystallizes in the kidneys and joints. A diet with a sensible amount of protein is highly beneficial for these conditions. This sensible diet is achieved through vegetables high in fiber (nondigestible forms of complex carbs) with a sensible amount of protein and whatever fat comes with that protein.

To make this simple, all you need to remember is to consume, three times each day, about the amount of protein source which could be held in the palm of your hand — about the size of a chicken breast — constituting about thirty percent of your calories. With that, have whatever fat comes associated with that protein. Add high-fiber vegetables, the equivalent of three handfuls.

Carbohydrates

Carbohydrates come in two basic forms: complex and simple. Simple carbs are one, two, or at most three units of sugar linked together in single molecules. Complex carbs are hundreds or thousands of sugar units linked together in single molecules. Simple sugars are easily identified by their taste: sweet. Complex carbs, such as potatoes, are pleasant to the taste buds, but not sweet.

There are two goups of complex carbs: high fiber and low fiber. High-fiber, complex carbs are not digestible, at least not by human beings, because we do not have the enzyme to do the job. Cows have that enzyme; that is why they can get calories out of grass, and we cannot. The main stuff in high-fiber, complex carbs which is indigestible by humans is called "cellulose."

High-fiber (high-cellulose) vegetable foods are the healthiest choices for human nutrition, and the ingestion is associated with lowered incidences of hypertension, cancer, arthritis, diabetes, etc. Examples are lettuce and broccoli. Examples of low-fiber, complex carbs are banana, tomato, squash and all cereals and grains (therefore bread and pasta), potatoes and rice.

It matters not if a carb is simple or complex. After digestion, it appears in the circulatory system in the simple form, as glucose, on its way to the cells where it is used for energy. To be transformed into simple sugars, complex carbs must be digested by the enzyme amylase. Amylase is secreted by the salivary glands, which empty into the mouth, and by the pancreas, which empties into the head of the duodenum.

Simple sugars and low-fiber, complex carbs represent a threat to health when they are consumed in inappropriate amounts such as may occur in low-soy, vegetarian diets where they are being eaten to replace the calories which would ordinarily come from protein.

Processing of plant food strips away its fiber and/or vitamin content. A simple example of processing is cutting an orange in two pieces, pressing the juice into a glass and discarding the fiber.

While it is true that fiber is an important part of your diet, even necessary to protect you from some diseases, carbohydrates themselves are not necessary. There are "essential" fatty acids and "essential" amino acids (from protein), however there are no known essential carbohydrates.

Most of our carbohydrates come from cereals and grains, both products of the agricultural revolution. Our bodies are not genetically designed to thrive on large amounts of these fiberless complex carbs. With the popularity of cereal- and grain-based "health diets," carbohydrate metabolism has been upset in approximately 3/4 of the population which simply cannot handle this large load of carbs. Increased insulin output from the pancreas, over the years, results in hyperinsulinism, insulin resistance and the resulting diseases mentioned above: hypertension, dyslipidemia, atherosclerosis and heart disease.

Complex carbs with lots of fiber should be consumed in proper proportion for maximum health and vitality. Complex carbs with lots of fiber are rich sources of necessary vitamins and minerals as well as enzymes when in the raw state. The problem happens when carbohydrates are altered by processes which provide empty calories stripped of much of their original food value.

I should also mention the relationship between simple sugars and mucus formation. The biochemical name for mucus is mucopolysaccharide. This literally means "mucus of many sugars," and it tells us how mucus is formed through the linking together of sugar molecules. If you have a condition, such as asthma or emphysema, in which mucus is part of the problem, you can do yourself a lot of good by stopping your intake of simple sugars and lowering your intake of complex carbohydrates (which convert to simple sugars upon digeston). Unfortunately, this means such wonderful sweet fruits as plums, peaches, apples, etc., must go along with breads, pastas and pastries.

The most healthy form of sugar is the complex carbohydrates present in high-fiber vegetables; however, it is certainly acceptable to spice up your diet in moderation with simple sugars in the form of whole fruits — unless, of course, you are trying to avoid mucus formation. Eat your fruits, do not juice them and drink them, unless you are on a juice fast as described earlier in this book. Eating the whole fruit results in the inclusion of natural fiber, which allows proper absorption of sugars. If you must have juice, dilute it with twice the recommended amount of water, so as to get the taste without overdosing on simple sugars.

Fiber

You can think of fiber as the skeleton of a plant. It is more difficult for your body to digest and usually passes through you without being 100% digested, thus adding bulk to the food you eat. Some digestion of fiber by bacteria occurs in your colon. You do not have the enzymes to digest cellulose yourself. The digestion of fiber by friendly bacteria in the colon supplies short chain fatty acids, including butyric acid, which are the major source of energy for the cells lining the colon.

The digestive value of fiber cannot be overemphasized. For approximately the past sixty years, the major thrust in the processed food industry has been to reduce or eliminate the amount of fiber left in food. Flour has been "purified" and comes from the wheat kernel stripped of the fiber-containing shell or chafe. Rice has been treated in an identical fashion. The result is that the average diet has had fiber largely replaced by fat, protein and simple carbs.

Constipation has become a common complaint, and the incidence of gastrointestinal disorders of many different varieties — for example, hiatal hernia, diverticulitis, appendicitis, gallbladder disease, irritable bowel syndrome, hypoglycemia and intestinal cancers — has shot up to unprecedented levels.

The processed food industry has made a lot of money in this transformation of food and so have physicians and surgeons! The losers have been the millions of people who trust the food industry to deliver healthy products for their consumption and who trust their doctors to know how to advise them to prevent illness.

The advantage of bringing fiber into your diet is that it moves food through your digestive system quickly, it protects you from absorbing toxins, which may be associated with your food (pesticides, for example), it modulates the absorption of simple carbs, and it keeps the walls of the intestine clean by removing toxins which are believed to cause cancer. Fiber also modulates the amount of salt you consume, containing just the right amount, and thus works to prevent hypertension and the results of hypertension: kidney and heart disease. Fiber is good stuff! You can get some at your local vegetable store.

The choice to be vegetarian, in my opinion, is a spiritual choice. Our ancestors were omnivores, eating food from both meat and plant sources. It is clear that our physiology is not prepared for large amounts of cereals and grains, made available only in the last ten to fifteen thousand years through agriculture.

On the other hand, we are quite well-prepared to consume a portion of our calories in the form of dead animals but only in the raw state, because fire was mastered by man only 80,000 years ago, and it takes 200,000 years for genes to transform themselves and fully adapt to such a change. Nevertheless, one can add enzymes to cooked flesh, and providing there is nothing in the flesh other than flesh, such as pesticides, herbicides, antibiotics and synthetic hormones, it makes a pretty healthy meal when combined with the proper portions of vegetables and fat.

One must ask oneself if it is right to take the lives of sentient beings to satisfy one's hunger when there is a viable choice to handle it another way. If the answer is yes, be a meat eater. If the answer is no, make yourself a vegetarian. I suppose it has to do with the ability, or lack of ability, to feel compassion for other creatures.

Reorganizing The Way You Eat

How does it look to handle nutrition unconsciously? Go to any grocery store, and you can find out for yourself. Watch people as they make their food purchases. Well over 95% of them are choosing unconsciously. They have commercials from mass media humming around in their brains as they select the foods they will eat. Make no mistake about it, if you buy it, you are much more likely to eat it than if you do not buy it. So, unconsciousness in nutrition begins and almost ends, with the purchasing process.

Why do people buy what they buy? Besides, the hypnotic effect of commercials, which create the favorite brands of food people like to buy, they are looking for what "tastes good."

What does taste good, and why does it taste good? As it turns out, tasting also is an unconscious process. Few people actually taste the foods they eat. What we "taste," instead, is the associations we have to a particular food. Those foods which, throughout our childhood, were given to us with love and affection, tend to "taste good." Those "special treats" they gave us "taste good" for a lifetime.

Our parents and/or grandparents lived through the Great Depression. Sugar and candy were hard to get and expensive. To put psychological distance between themselves and that Depression they showered their children and grandchildren with sugar-candy: high-fat, high-calorie, expensive food products combined with much love and affection. Therefore, we developed an addiction for these foods.

People are addicted to foods. You are addicted — strongly habituated — to the foods you eat. It is very much like smoking. Before Native Americans contributed tobacco to Europeans, Europeans did not miss having a smoke. There is nothing natural about the craving for tobacco (and the 200 chemicals added by the tobacco industry for taste and addiction). It is a learned habit, and it is associated with much more than the way the tobacco "tastes."

The foods to which we are commonly addicted are those foods our parents gave us with love and affection. In some cases, you also are addicted to those foods you felt it necessary to use to rebel against your parents.

There is a class of foods called "comfort foods." When you eat them, you feel more comfortable. You associate them with memories of being safe. Typically, these are high-carbohydrate, high-fat, high-calorie products that tend to be derived from grains, cereals and cows: breads, pasta, cake, cookies, ice cream, milk, yogurt; also chocolate. These are addictions probably equally damaging to your health as tobacco is for most smokers, yet you think of it as a healthy diet, because that kind of belief is the condition of mass consciousness around food.

How does one interrupt these addictions? When you are ready to do it, here is the way, the truth and the light.

1. Throw out all foods which are not supportive of real vitality.

2. Do all your own grocery shopping.

3. Purchase only those foods which are supportive of real vitality.

4. Do all your own food preparation.

5. Eat only at home (for a period of several months at least).

6. Learn to appreciate the taste of these foods.

If you live with someone who does not choose your method of nutrition, separate your food purchase, storage, preparation and consumption.

(For a smoker who wants to stop smoking, a parallel method also is the way, the truth and the light.)

Let us face it: if it never enters your environment, you will not eat it. Then your hunger becomes your friend instead of your enemy. If you become hungry enough, and you have only health-supporting foods in your environment, eventually you will eat them and learn to enjoy them. Eventually, you will learn to prepare these foods in special ways, with spices and special cooking methods to make them even more tasty. Finally, you will lose your desire for those foods to which you have become addicted and which damage your vitality.

Sources

Burkitt D Some diseases characteristic of modern western civilization Br Med J;1973:274

Kliks M Paleodietetucs: A review of the role of dietary fiber in preagricultural human diets,Topics in Dietary Fiber Research, Plenum Press;1978:181

Commoner B Formation of mutagens in beef and beef extract during cooking Science;1978:201

Harty S Hucksters in the Classroom - A review of industry propaganda in schools, Washington DC Center for the Study of Responsive Law;1979:25

Hill D The spectrum of cow's milk allergy in childhood Acta Paediatr Scand 68;1979:847

Parish W Hypersensitivity to milk and sudden death in infancy Lancet 2;1960:1106

Truelove S Ulcerative colitis provoked by milk Br Med J;1961:154

Bayless J Lactose and milk intolerance N Engl J Med 292;1975:1156

Donham K Epidemiologic relationships of the bovine population and human leukemia in Iowa Am J Epidemiol 112;1980:80

O'Brien B Human plasma lipid reponse to red meat, poultry, fish, and eggs Amer J Clin Nut 33;1980:2573

Dwyer J Nutritional studies of vegetarian children Am J Clin Nutr 35;1982:204

Conner W The key role of nutritional factors in the prevention of coronary heart disease Prev Med 1;1972:49

Editorial: Regression of atherosclerosis Lancet 2;1976:614

Lee RB and DeVore *Man The Hunter* Chicago: Aldine.

Cohen MN and Armelagos GJ   Paleontology at the origins of agriculture   New York: Academic Press 1984

Cassidy CM Nutrition and health in agriculturalists and hunter-gatherers. A case study of two prehistoric populations Nutritional Anthropology;1980:117-144.

FOOD MYTHS

Western civilization has created a degree of affluence unmatched in human history. Although all of us must eat food to survive, fewer of us than ever before are close to the farm where food is produced. Most of us see food in the grocery store and restaurant and give very little thought to its source.

Capitalism has wonderful attributes; however, as a system for bringing to market the kinds of food which lead to maximum health and vitality, it fails miserably. The advent of advertising and the profit motive has led to a kind of mass hypnotism regarding food, of which you and I are part. When selecting food to eat, you have virtually no chance of thinking for yourself, unless you have gone to great pains to educate and reprogram yourself about food.

The purpose of this section of the book is to plant in your mind key concepts and bits of information, which will allow you to think for yourself. Here are common myths about food.

If it's in the store, it must be okay.
FALSE !

You have never heard a commercial about food which has represented food as bad for you. Each piece of programming you have received, regarding food, relates to its health-giving, life-giving properties. Even milk! Even fizzy soft drinks! Even beer! Even candy! As a result of a lifetime of listening, watching, and reading food commercials, you have a large store of attitudes toward food, programmed into your mind, which are unrelated to the facts about those foods.

Therefore, when you walk into a grocery you believe that you are not only safe, you believe that you are in a friendly place where your nutrition and well-being are important. Nothing could be further from the truth!

In the eyes of the grocer or restaurateur, you are a pocketbook with money in it. The objective is to have you leave the store with as little money in your pocketbook as possible. This is capitalism. The store or restaurant will display for you, in an attractive fashion, whatever will best separate you from your money. Your addictions and your programming will be catered to.

Therefore, the proper attitude in a grocery store or restaurant is the same attitude you should have if you are a soldier traversing a mine field. Make the right choices and you come out all right. Make mistakes and you die. In the case of a mine field, you die quickly. In the case of a grocery store or restaurant, you die slowly. **Shop with the idea that the food store is a mine field!**

Fast food is fun food.
FALSE !

I have an idea for a new fast-food chain. It is called "Dr. K.'s Feedbag Restaurants." When you go in, you pay your money, and a feedbag (like that for a horse) is strapped around your neck. It is flexible, so when you are ready to eat more, you simply squeeze the bag. You may go about your business as you eat, because your hands are free. The stuff in the feedbag is a mixture of textured fat with plenty of sugar and salt. You can have it with or without alcohol and with or without caffeine. When you come to Dr. K.'s Feedbag Restaurant you will be eating more or less the same nutrition people receive at other fast-food restaurants, only it will be much faster. (By the way your feedbag comes with a very large napkin.)

Not such a great idea is it? Neither is fast food. You can have no idea of the method of preparation of food which you have not prepared yourself or seen prepared. Fast food is loaded with the stuff which addicts you and which tastes good: fat, sugar and salt, which also, by the way, causes degenerative diseases. **Never eat in a fast-food restaurant!**

Eating processed food is convenient and makes good sense.
FALSE !

When you venture into the isles of a food store, you find processed food. Some of it doesn't even look like food anymore; for example, pre-made waffles and pancakes. Other processed foods look like the original food; however, read the label for contents and weep. When you eat processed foods, you eat not only the original food but also the stuff they added to it to make it taste better and last longer. The label also may say something like: "better if consumed before the year 2000," or some such drivel, revealing just how much preservative and chemical additives it contains. Sure, this kind of food is convenient in the short term, but how convenient is it to die young and suffer from degenerative diseases in your later years? *Caveat emptor*! **Never buy or consume processed foods!**

Cooking helps digest food.
FALSE !

You grew up in a culture where almost everything people eat is cooked. It is very hard to question the wisdom of cooking when it is almost all there is, except for salads. The common wisdom about cooking is that it increases digestibility and enhances flavor. The fact is, cooking, for most foods, causes them to be broken down, thus destroying many of the nutrients in the process, necessitating more frequent meals.

There are some foods which must be cooked to be eaten, because they simply are too hard to eat without cooking. This is a small minority of the foods you eat. Meat should certainly be well cooked before eating; however, meat is a slow poison anyway. As to flavor, this is a matter of habit. If you habituate yourself to cooked foods, naturally they will taste best to you. **If you can eat it raw, do so!**

Three meals a day are best.
FALSE !

Your mother always told you this one. Mothers are gullible to food propaganda, as we all have been, and besides, it was much more convenient for her if you ate your meals at three regular times each day. Believe it or not, your body, in the absence of food addiction, knows better than your mother about when you should eat and when not. However, beware of hunger, if it is specific for an addictive substance. If you are "hungry" but only for sugar-containing foods, beware — you are not really hungry but rather in a state of addictive craving. **Eat only when you are hungry**!

Dairy products are good for you.
FALSE !

This one is a corollary of the Meat Axiom: you have had a "balanced" diet only when you have had your daily milk, cheese, butter, yogurt, cream cheese, cottage cheese, etc. "Only milk supplies sufficient calcium for a healthy body." This is bull. Calcium is present in sufficient quantities in vegetables. This is true however: only milk and milk products supply you with calcium caseinate, the major ingredient in wood glue. **Consume no dairy**!

If the food is natural, it is fine to eat all you want.
FALSE !

This is a fairly advanced myth held by many people who have pursued a healthy diet for several years. The rap goes something like this, for example: because honey, or apples, or oranges (or whatever) come directly from nature, it is acceptable to eat them in any quantity to satisfy hunger. Not so. Honey is usually cooked before packaging and this product is 75% sugar with little redeeming extra nutrition, because it is destroyed in the cooking process. Apples are somewhat less sweet; nevertheless, it is possible to feed a sugar addiction with apples. Oranges are very high in fructose (which is no better for you than sucrose), and when juiced and consumed, deliver a high concentration of sugar without the fiber present in the unjuiced orange. Almost any food eaten in disproportionate quantity is unhealthy.

When you combine natural food in variety, eating only when you are hungry, with regular aerobic exercise and care for the colon, your appetite should handle itself, unless you are addicted to *quantity* of food. In that case, you will pig out on natural foods.

A person addicted to quantity of food has a stretched stomach several times larger than it should be. This stomach does not feel full until a large portion of food has been eaten. Therefore, moderation in quantity is an important ingredient in your armamentarium of techniques for healthy eating.

If this is a problem area for you, each morning set aside the food you will eat that day. This should total about 2000 to 3000 calories, depending on your activity level. A relatively sedentary person needs 2000 calories and an active person needs more like 3000. This is assuming that you are not training for the Iron Person Competition or something similar. If you will do this for a few weeks, your natural state of hunger should prevail as your stomach shrinks to its natural size, and you will not need to continue considering quantity of food. **Eat only natural, unprocessed foods in great variety, but not great quantity**!

The best way to lose weight is to diet.
FALSE !

Billions of dollars are being made every year from people who are hypnotized by this idea. Millions of tons of fat are being lost by this method even as you read this. However, millions more tons of fat are being regained, even as you read, by people who previously lost weight in crash diet programs. Dieting does nothing for the basic problems, which are: (1) poor quality food, (2) addiction to certain foods and (3) eating habits which do not work. Studies show that of those people who go on crash diets, more than 95% gain the weight back plus additional weight. **Never diet!**

It is important to always eat all the food on your plate.
FALSE !

This myth has been created by the mothers and fathers of the world who are, understandably, not excited about cleaning up after children who stop eating when they are full. It can be useful to stop eating for five minutes somewhere in the middle of your meal and then ask yourself, "Am I still hungry?" If the answer is "No," then stop eating and store or discard the rest of your food. There is no virtue in a clean plate! The single secret shared by all permanently thin people is the following. **Stop eating when you are satisfied, even if it means leaving food on your plate**!

Snacking between meals is fine if the food is healthy.
FALSE !

Many people "graze," they eat small portions many times throughout the day. When these same people learn a bit about nutrition, they try to continue grazing using only healthy foods. Digestion of food is a major project for your stomach and small intestine. The first step in digestion is the addition of ptyalin by the salivary glands of the mouth. This begins the digestion of starch. The next step is acidification of food in the stomach. This breaks down protein and readies it for further digestion in the small intestine. Food spends about two hours in the stomach undergoing acidic breakdown. After this, it is moved into the small intestine. The stomach is ready for more food, at the earliest, two hours after the last meal. If you eat before two hours have passed, the new meal mixes with the old, and either the old meal stays in the stomach too long, or the new meal is dumped into the small intestine too early. Either way you lose. In the first case, the food is over acidified and loses a lot of its nutritional value. In the second case, the second meal is incompletely digested, because it misses part of the acidification step. **Let at least three hours pass between meals!**

There is no harm in eating fast.
FALSE !

In a world in which the success you achieve is related to the speed with which you move, it has come to pass for many people that food is eaten in an unconscious and speedy manner. This would work well, if digestion were a process which happened only in the stomach and small intestine and required no chewing. The fact is, however, that digestion begins in the mouth in two ways. First starchy foods begin to be digested with ptyalin and amylase contained in the saliva secreted by the salivary glands located in the mouth. The tongue secretes lingual lipase which begins the digestion of fats. If you bolt your food down, there is insufficient time for these starches to be digested, and the first stage of starch digestion is missed. Second, and this is very important to realize, is that your teeth are your most important organs of digestion. They cut and grind the food, so that it can later come into contact with digestive enzymes in the stomach and small intestine. If you eat fast you end up swallowing food which is not thoroughly cut and ground. Some of this food will pass straight through you without contacting the appropriate digestive enzymes. The nutritional value of this food is wasted. You are left hungry, eating more than you really need and putting an additional burden on the digestive tract, not to mention your waistline. **In this case, follow your mother's advice — eat slowly!**

It is good to drink liberal amounts of fluid with your meal.
FALSE !

Most people do not consider their meal complete without something to drink. Many restaurant personnel expect you to order a drink and are disturbed if you do not. You are best advised to resist these pressures, because fluid dilutes all digestive enzymes, beginning with ptyalin in the mouth and continuing with hydrochloric acid in the stomach. Hydrochloric acid is responsible for beginning the breakdown of protein, so that proteinase can complete that job in the small intestine. Drinking large quantities of fluid with a meal dilutes these digestive juices, making it impossible to digest your food properly. The best practice is to do your drinking between meals, beginning no earlier than two hours after your last meal. Two hours is the time required for your stomach to empty into the small intestine. A great time to hydrate yourself is when you first arise in the morning. A tall glass or two of steam distilled water will not only hydrate you but also may awaken your colon, so that you begin the day free from a powerful source of intoxication. The only good purpose served by fluid with meals is lubrication for swallowing. The need for fluid for this purpose may indicate that you are eating too fast — but not always, depending on the type of food you are eating. Very dry foods may require extra lubrication beyond the saliva you produce even after thorough chewing. **Drink the minimum amount necessary to swallow your food!**

It is natural to eat more as you grow older and to weigh more as well.
FALSE !

Many people accept increased weight with age as the price of aging. A teenager has no excuse for a big belly and thunder thighs; however, a forty-year-old person has a commonly accepted excuse. What really happens with age is that the digestive system is abused with sugar (which causes degeneration of the digestive organs, as well as other organs of the body) and other addictive substances, which are poison to the body (nicotine, alcohol, caffeine, for example), which cause degeneration of the digestive system. The result is that the digestive system is less and less able to extract needed nutrition from the foods presented to it. The result is a compromised, inefficient digestive system with an increased appetite as the body asks vainly for more nutrition through the mechanism of increased hunger.

When a large volume of food is consumed, often of the fatty variety, the colon, which is affected by these degenerative processes as well, requires more time to do its job. There is a kind of log jam in the colon, and this shows up as a belly somewhat larger than the natural state. Sometimes this process manifests in the teenage years or even earlier. Not knowing what to do with all the empty calories, the body stores them as fat, saying, in effect, "I'll figure this out later."

Most people can recall themselves as slim and trim as teenagers, and for these people the natural weight also is the weight of the body in late teens, seventeen to eighteen or so. You are not complete with your reeducation about nutrition until you are at that weight, using only natural changes without starving yourself. This does not mean you should panic about being overweight, but simply keep learning, and apply what you learn using your weight as one of your gauges. You do not have to settle for being overweight, nor should you have to suffer to come back to your ideal weight, unless you just want to. **Settle for nothing less than your ideal weight!**

Eating should be an orgasmic experience.
FALSE !

This belief has it that if it doesn't somehow feel like an orgasm to eat a particular food, that food should be avoided. Orgasm foods tend to be slick (laden with fat) and thus slide down the esophagus, and also tasty — which usually means salt and/or sugar. These are comfort foods, because they provide a pleasurable experience in an otherwise pleasureless life. Examples are ice cream, candy, chips, yogurt, cheeses, fried foods, and you can finish this long list. If it tastes and feels good, you put it in your mouth without further consideration! Comfort foods universally are foods which slice years off your life and rob you of vitality and alertness. They contain seriously addicting ingredients. **Avoid comfort foods!**

So, why should modern people fast? What is in it for us? Can there be a scientific validity to this ancient custom? Can it be that so many cultures have been mistaken in their practice of fasting, or is there some seriously positive benefit, which we also can reap? Can it be that a person who fasts on a regular basis can achieve a decidedly superior state of health? What about the spiritual benefits? Given that so many people have fasted through the ages for spiritual purposes, can it be possible that there is some spiritual value still available in the practice? We think of fasting as painful, but does it have to be painful?

This section of the book is about exploring your attitudes regarding fasting, not about actually doing a fast. Once you see the general sense of the matter, you may see the sense in it for your health. Despite the fact that fasting is an ancient practice promoted by religious practitioners through the ages, there also is a solid scientific basis for the practice of fasting. This scientific basis for fasting began to take shape in 1665 when the English scientist Robert Hooke discovered that cork is made of cells. In 1670 living cells (single cell, water dwellers) were described by the Dutch scientist Anton van Leeuwenhoek who invented the microscope.

However, it was not until 1839 that basic cell theory, as we know it today, was formulated. In that year the German botanist Matthias Schlieden and the German zoologist Theodor Schwann proposed that all living organisms, plant and animal, were made of cells and cell products. Thus, the biology of a whole organism could be understood through a study of its cells. The German pathologist Rudolf Virchow completed cell theory nineteen years later by proposing that the entire body is composed of cells and cell products. This led to an understanding of cell division and differentiation.

On a parallel track, a literal explosion of knowledge occurred in physiology in the seventeenth century, beginning with the discovery of circulation of the blood, in 1616, by the English physician William Harvey. This was followed by rapid advances in the understanding of the functions of the various body organs. Knowledge which we take for granted, for example, the purpose of the liver, the kidneys and the pancreas, was unknown before physiologists Marcello Malpighi of Italy and Regnier de Graaf of Holland illuminated the scientific world with their pioneering research. The existence of oxygen and the utility it has for living organisms simply was unknown before the work of John Mayow. The average man on the street today knows more about cellular physiology than the greatest scientist living in the sixteenth century.

Let me refresh your memory and perhaps add some new facts to what you know. The physiology of any living organism — your body, for example — is a dynamic interplay between anabolism (buildup) and catabolism (breakdown). Your body requires constant sources of fuel: oxygen and food. While oxygen is obtained through the lungs and taken in directly, food is broken down into the simple building blocks of life: single molecules of fat, sugar and protein. These simple building blocks are called fatty acids, sugars (also called the -oses — glucose, fructose, maltose, etc.) — and amino acids.

This job is done by your digestive system, which includes your stomach, small intestine, large intestine, liver and pancreas. These single molecules enter your body by passing through the single layer of cells which lines your intestinal tract. This single layer of cells is designed to prevent the entry of anything more complex than a single molecule. Even sucrose, a simple combination of two simpler sugars, must be broken into its individual components before entry can be made into your body. The exceptions to these comments are some small polypeptides (two and three amino acids each) and a small amount of emulsified fat, which enter the body without complete breakdown.

Until molecules cross the single layer of cells which line the gut, they are outside your body, even though they are inside your intestinal tract.

Once access is gained to the body, these molecules are whisked around your body through your cardiovascular system by the action of your heart, and through the lymphatic system in the case of incompletely digested fat. The lymphatic system empties into the vascular system at the aorta, the large vessel coming out of the heart. Each living cell in your body is in direct contact with the cardiovascular system by circulation through the capillaries, so that these nutritive molecules can be collected by each cell on an as-need basis.

The real action is happening inside your cells. This is where the process happens which can most accurately be described as "life." Thanks to Schlieden and Schwann, we know that who we are at the biological level is a collection of individual cells. These cells are incredibly different from each other, specialized for particular jobs. However, they all have one thing in common: if they are alive, they are engaged in anabolism and catabolism — they are building up and breaking down — both processes at the same time.

The most important thing to know about a cell is that it wears a coat. This coat is known as the "plasma membrane." The plasma membrane is a continuous double layer of phospholipid molecules 75 to 100 angstroms thick. What makes life possible is that the plasma membrane is selectively permeable. It permits the exchange of molecules and atoms in and out of the cell, but on a selective basis. No molecule can come in or out without permission from the plasma membrane. This allows the cell to regulate its metabolism for its own purposes.

The most amazing thing about any cell in your body is that it works for the good of the entire organism. If it must lay down its life and die, so that the whole organism can live, it will. Your white blood cells are willing kamikaze warriors to combat any threat of infection by invading organisms. This characteristic of cells hints at the presence of an organizing intelligence living in the blood and sinews of your body, a soul.

There is much to be said about cells. I could tell you about the nucleus, the nucleolus, the nuclear envelope, the smooth endoplasmic reticulum, mitochondria, centrioles, Golgi bodies, liposomes, ribosomes and on and on. Perhaps I don't need to. You are cells. Your health depends on how well you take care of your cells.

Here is what you need to know regarding fasting. Catabolism creates waste products. These waste products are mixed into the cell soup, the cytoplasm, of the cell. For life to go on and vital health to happen, these waste products must be transported out of the body. The plasma membrane has the task of allowing these substances — principally carbon dioxide, urea and uric acid — to leave the cell, so that they can be picked up by the circulatory system and transported to the lungs (in the case of carbon dioxide), and to the skin, kidneys and intestines (in the case of urea and uric acid), where they leave the body.

Here resides the problem. The plasma membrane of each cell can somehow sense the concentration of toxic wastes in the circulatory system. If this concentration is above legal limit, the plasma membrane denies an exit visa for toxic wastes inside the cell until conditions outside the cell improve. When we overload our bodies with food, even if we are able to burn it up without gaining weight, we create a chronic condition of low grade toxemia.

Each cell becomes a storage unit for unusable, toxic molecules. This is not what a doctor would call "toxemia," because it is not life-threatening. However, if what you are interested in is the most health and vitality possible for you, this is definitely a chronic condition of low grade toxemia. Only children who are on a health supporting diet as defined later in this book are immune from a chronic condition of low grade toxemia. **All adults are suffering from this condition in some degree**. The result is chronic, intermittent headache (look at the sales figures for over-the-counter headache remedies), or fatigue (take some No Doz, drink some tea or coffee), or arthritis (not natural to old age, but have a drug anyway), or irritability of the nervous system (have a tranquilizer), or insomnia (take a sleeping pill or drink some special herb tea — more enlightened)...and so on. Each pill you take adds to the total load of toxic wastes your cells must bear, and compounds the problem in the long run. Even people who have regular colon irrigation, as discussed later in this book, and eat the right foods can still be full of, well, toxic wastes.

Now the stage is set for fasting, for when we admit to the possibility that we may be in a condition of chronic low grade toxemia, the next question is "What can we do about it?" The answer: fast. Only when this state of knowledge is reached can we rationally consider the benefits of fasting from a scientific point of view.

Notice I said scientific, not medical. The mind set which doctors live in is: treatment of illness, once it is firmly established and obvious. Your doctor is the wrong person to talk to regarding a condition of maximum vitality or even regarding prevention of illness. Blue Cross cannot be billed for that, not yet anyway. Therefore, your physician is unlikely to know anything about the benefits of fasting, and when physicians find themselves not knowing about something (which is intolerable to a doctor's ego), you can be sure they will make up an opinion, usually a negative one.

Fasting creates a condition of low concentration of toxic wastes in the circulatory system. This is sensed by the plasma membrane of each cell and each cell will then let go of its load of toxic wastes. When this happens suddenly, as it does with fasting, the result can be a sudden case of mild systemic toxemia as the system cleanses itself. Those who fast must be prepared for a phase of headache, irritability, insomnia and fatigue. This is a natural part of the healing process and should be welcomed. How long a person should fast is an individual matter. A thorough cleansing will require at least a few days. A week-long fast will get the job done for most people. The fast should not end until the symptomatic phase (headache, fatigue, etc.) is finished by at least two days. **I recommend only juice fasting unless your fast is supervised by a person experienced in fasting.**

Any degree of overloading your body with food results in the intracellular collection of waste products. Fasting allows you to tip the scales in the other direction, so that your body can release itself from this condition of autointoxication.

Let me underline one point: the addiction to quantity of food as measured in calories. This is the item which creates the conditions which make fasting a useful tool. Addiction to quantity of food, as measured in calories, is the condition in which we live, it is almost the air we breathe, certainly it is the paradigm with which we unconsciously think about and experience hunger. You may not think you are addicted. You may be slim and exercise regularly, and yet you are addicted to quantity of food as measured in calories. Try making it on 2000 calories per day, and you will discover an awareness of your addiction.

Being grounded in knowledge relating to fasting is useless unless you apply that knowledge and actually fast. Fasting combined with colon cleansing (see section on the colon) is the fastest route to enlightenment I know of. I do it for spiritual and for health reasons which, if you think about it, are not entirely separate. I find myself much more productive when I am clear in mind and body.

I recommend juice fasting. I do not feel comfortable with you water fasting while not under my, or some professional's, direct supervision. Also, you can achieve the same results by juice fasting, although perhaps not as quickly.

If you are going to fast, the first thing you need is a juicer. I recommend either the Acme juicer or the Champion juicer. I have both and each does a fabulous job. The Acme juicer is better for citrus fruits (the juice of which you should not drink if you have arthritis), and the Champion juicer is best for making juice from "solid" plants such as carrots, apples, celery, etc. You can find these juicers at most large department stores. They also can be purchased through health food stores. Call around and find out locations and prices of these products. Expect to spend about $200-250 for a good juicer. This may seem like a lot of money, but it will pay for itself in thousands of dollars in saved medical bills over the years.

Once you have your juicer, the next thing you need, obviously, is something to juice. I recommend that you locate a source of organically grown fruits and vegetables. Exactly which items you choose from which to make juice is up to you. The key word here is **variety**. If you make a variety of juices, you will be less likely to become bored with your juice fast, and much more likely to receive a completely balanced complement of vitamins and minerals. No vitamin supplements will be necessary during your fast as you will be loaded with fresh natural vitamins and your need for co-enzymes of metabolic catalysts (vitamins) will be greatly reduced.

You should dilute all your juices with one part steam distilled water to three parts pure freshly made juice. Do not substitute bottled juice or juice made from concentrate, as these juices are robbed of most of their natural nutrition when they are prepared for market. There should be no "middle-men" between the farmer and you except perhaps the grocer.

Drink at least eight 8 oz. glasses (large table glasses) of **steam distilled water** every day, spread out evenly over the day. It is important that this be *steam* distilled water, preferably double steam distilled water, which has then been filtered using carbon filtration. It would be absurd to fast for the purpose of cleansing your body and simultaneously pour in the pollutants or anti-pollutants, chlorine and who-knows-what minerals from spring water or river water. Stay away from bottled water which does not say "steam distilled" on the label.

How about quantity of juice? Drink as much as you like as long as you dilute it three parts juice to one part steam distilled water and as long as you are drinking a great variety of juices. Do not go on a "citrus fast" or a "carrot juice fast." These sorts of fad "diets" are not good for you. Your body needs well-rounded nutrition. You should be drinking at least five different types of juices each day. This is not a diet. The objective is not to lose weight (although you will lose weight, if you are over your ideal weight) or to deprive you of calories. The objective is **cleansing**.

Drink your juice as soon after you make it as possible, since the freshly liberated enzymes of the plant cells begin autodigestion of the nutrients in your juice immediately after the cell plasma membranes are ruptured by your juicer. You want to digest the juice before the juice digests the juice.

With this much fluid intake you will find yourself with a full bladder most of the time, so remain close to the proper facilities and do not be alarmed. At some time during your fast, your body will release both fluids and toxins. You will be voiding even greater quantities of fluid than you are drinking in, and you will lose weight rapidly as you shed this excess fluid. This happens when the cells release their stores of sodium chloride, ordinary table salt, which is added for taste to almost all prepared foods off the grocery store shelf and out of the restaurateurs' kitchens. You have been collecting excess salt in your cells for many years.

An important part of your fast is cleansing of the colon. When you stop taking in solid food there is nothing to push out the food which is already in your colon. It therefore putrefies and adds even more toxicity to your system. The best way to accomplish this is to make an appointment with your colon therapist for the second day of your fast and have a thorough cleansing.

If this is not possible for you, the next best choice is to give yourself a daily enema for three days in a row. The problem with the enema route is that an ordinary enema bag contains only about half the volume of the average colon. So a good enema for these purposes consists of two bags instead of one, given one after the other before the first emptying of the colon. You should use steam distilled water only, and it should be heated to that temperature between the temperature easy for you to put your hand into and the temperature which is not quite possible to leave your hand in for more than a few seconds. This heat allows the wall of the colon to relax and accept the volume of water.

When infusing the water, keep your hand on the valve, and slow the flow if it becomes painful. An enema should not be a painful experience, but rather a pleasurable experience once you overcome the mental barriers to it. After the enema is in, you will know what to do next. When you pass the water out, try different alternate sitting positions and include pressing your thighs into your abdomen for complete evacuation of your caecum and your sigmoid colon. You will need a six-inch elevated foot rest for this maneuver. Do not do a fast without colon cleansing.

Between the second to fifth day of your fast, you will encounter a number of disagreeable symptoms such as headache, fatigue, dizziness, nausea, etc. This represents the release of stored toxins from their intracellular storage space. This is a good, although unpleasant, sign. When it passes, cleansing is almost complete. You may stop your fast on the second day after this event.

The largest problem you will encounter during your fast will be your addictions to chewing, tasting and the experience of being full of solid food. You will miss these items as an alcoholic misses the bottle. The best way to handle this situation is to have cleared your living space of solid food and always have on hand a plentiful supply of fresh fruits and vegetables from which to make juice.

When it comes time to break your fast, it is important that you do so with what usually is considered "bland" food. Fresh made tomato soup is ideal. Eat slowly, and pause frequently. When you feel full, stop eating. You will feel full on much less food than you think.

When you follow a juice fast as outlined, there is no way you will become malnourished. On the contrary, you will never have been so well nourished. What you can expect from your fast is a new relationship with food. You will be satisfied with smaller quantities of healthier foods. Your craving for salt, sugar, fat and calories will disappear. You will be able to taste food again, and you will be amazed how good food can taste. Your mind will be sharper, you will be more alert and awake and functionally more intelligent.

Here are some miscellaneous helpful hints. If you live with someone, see if you can enroll that person or those people in going on the fast with you. If they are agreeable, they need access to all the information you now have. If they do not care to participate, see if you can remove yourself when they are engaged in meals. If you live alone, empty the house of solid food at the beginning of your fast, so as not to tempt yourself to give in to your addictions.

If you have other major addictions, give them up during the fast; certainly give up tobacco, alcohol and drugs if any of these are in your life. You will be amazed at how high you can get without chemicals — much higher than with.

Maintain yourself in the condition of the least possible excitement and stimulation. The ideal situation would be to go to a nunnery or a monastery for reading and meditation. Barring that, create the most similar condition possible for you.

You should add to your juice a vegetable broth spiked with liquid amino acids. Make the broth by slicing up a pot-full of variegated organically grown veggies, and bring them to a boil in steam distilled water. Then allow them to cool. When you are ready to drink your broth, add up to one tablespoon of liquid amino acids per large cup of broth. I recommend Bragg Liquid Amino Acids. Your organic grocer or health food store should stock this item. All this nutrition will enter your body directly from the stomach, and give your digestive tract a time to rest. A lot of energy is consumed in digestion, so you will experience this surge of energy. Don't be alarmed. Have fun with it. However, do no heavy exercise until after your fast is broken. Competitive sports, hard running and weight lifting are not recommended during a fast. I recommend long walks to handle this surge of energy. Sex also is fine, in fact, recommended. On the other hand, you may experience a temporary quiescence of your sex drive. This also is fine. Do not worry. Your sex drive will come back multiplied after your fast.

Finally, I must tell you that a fast is not designed to replace treatment of diseases by a doctor. It is not a cancer cure or a replacement for surgery if surgery is needed. Naturally, a vitally healthy person can heal from illness faster, and properly conducted periodic juice fasting does produce great vitality. However, I do not want you to become irrational about the effects of fasting. What fasting is good for is cleansing and, in my opinion, cleansing is the single most potent way of preventing illness from beginning in the first place.

See page 358 for instructions on contacting my office for a referral to a doctor experienced in juice fasting.

ENZYME NUTRITION

The energy of life is expressed through DNA, desoxyribonucleic acid. These magnificent, complex molecules reside in the genetic material located in the nucleus of each living cell. DNA contains both the program to create the body and the ability to mobilize the energy to carry out the job. The first order of creation by DNA in the daily process of living is the production of more DNA (when the cell divides), and the second order of creation by DNA is the production of RNA.

RNA stands for ribonucleic acid and this molecule is made by DNA (and sometimes by other RNA) through DNA's ability to copy amino acid sequences in a selective fashion. Whereas there is only one structure for DNA, there are many RNA structures depending on the job assignment of a particular molecule of RNA. While many molecules in the body can be considered essentially dead when measured alone, RNA inherits a full complement of the vital life force contained in DNA.

The job of RNA is to make proteins (and other RNA). Proteins serve as building blocks of the body, as well as many other functions. A large percentage of lean muscle tissue, for example, is made of protein. Connective tissue, including fascia, tendon and bone also is made largely of protein.

Enzymes

A specialized type of protein is called an "enzyme." Enzymes are protein molecules made by RNA and other enzymes with the ability to facilitate and speed up chemical reactions throughout the body. In the haphazard process, thought to have been the beginning of biochemistry in nature which eventually gave birth to life, amino acids formed and strung themselves together by chance into polypeptide chains some of which became enzymes quite by accident.

These structures, which had the ability to speed up reactions between the molecules around them, made life possible. The reactions they facilitated otherwise took so long to happen as to put off the development of life to the infinite future. Enzymes are thought to have conspired with each other to create the first nucleic acids, very large structures which eventually evolved into RNA and DNA.

There now are around 3000 known enzymes in the body and probably several thousand more as yet undiscovered, one for each kind of biochemical reaction which occurs there. Enzymes inherit from RNA a full measure of the vital life force originally given to RNA by DNA. Enzymes are both the parents and grandchildren of DNA, the source of our vital life force. In the context of the living body, enzymes are living molecular entities.

Enzymes work by virtue of their shape. An enzyme molecule can be compared, in shape at least, to many short strings of pearls (amino acids) strung together. This long string folds in on itself as certain sequences of amino acids (pearls) are more attracted to each other than to other sequences, thus giving the enzymes a specific shape.

At one point on the surface of this string of pearls, there exists something which looks like a keyhole. This is called the "active site" on the enzyme. When matched with its specific coenzyme (a vitamin, or mineral, or trace element) this "lock" has the exact inverse contour of the "key" which is contained in the molecule of the enzyme's "substrate," the molecule the enzyme wants to transform into a different molecule. When the substrate appears, it inserts the "key" into the "lock." The molecular structure of the substrate is transformed into a different molecular structure, and both enzyme and the newly transformed molecule go on their merry ways.

The slowest known enzyme (lysozyme) processes one substrate every two seconds. The fastest known enzyme (carbonic anhydrase) processes a phenomenal 36 million substrate molecules per minute. The shortest lived enzymes function for twenty minutes, and the longest are around and doing their jobs for several weeks. When an enzyme is worn out, it is broken down and disposed of by other enzymes, its component amino acids and polypeptide chains used to make new enzymes.

Dr. Edward Howell

Every area of knowledge in progressive medicine has its early champion, Broda Barnes in the study of hypothyroidism, Jens Moeller in the therapeutic uses of testosterone, for example. The study of enzymes is no exception. Dr. Edward Howell has clarified enzymes and enzyme therapy for us. We owe Dr. Howell a debt of gratitude for his pioneering work. In helping us understand the role of enzymes, Dr. Howell studied man, animals and plants with equal curiosity and scientific acumen. By comparative studies of disease states in man and in animals, Dr. Howell clearly demonstrated the disastrous nutritional effect of cooking food — more about that later.

A Classification of Digestive Enzymes

Particular types of enzymes have digestive functions. The job of a digestive enzyme is to break down food during the digestive process. The intestine is more able to absorb food which is thus broken down into smaller units, and the rest of the body is more easily able to utilize food which is in this form. There are three basic types of digestive enzymes, one type for each class of food: lipase for fat, proteinase for protein and amylase for carbohydrate.

Enzymes which drive the other processes of living are called "metabolic enzymes." There is one enzyme for each type of biochemical reaction which happens in the body. Metabolic enzymes are by far the most numerous of all enzymes.

Enzymes which are present in raw, uncooked food are called food enzymes to indicate where they come from: the food itself. They also are called "exogenous" enzymes, because they come from outside your body.

Enzymes which are made in the body are called "endogenous" (meaning "inside-created") and include both metabolic and digestive enzymes. Enzymes which are eaten with your food and are made by other animals or plants, are exogenous (outside-created). Food enzymes are exogenous enzymes. Exogenous enzymes have two origins: animal enzymes from animal food (raw meat, raw eggs, raw milk, etc.) and phytoenzymes, which come from plants (*phyto* = plant).

Autolytic (meaning "self-digesting") enzymes, which are very important in this discussion, are endogenous enzymes contained inside cells. The purpose of an autolytic enzyme is to break down the cell in which it is contained after that cell dies. Autolytic enzymes are contained in little bag-like structures which rupture upon death of the cell, releasing the autolytic enzymes to do their jobs. Because the body is made of fat, protein and carbohydrate, these enzymes are lipases, proteinases and amylase.

It is important that you understand the above terminology for purposes of this discussion. I suggest you make a note card for each type of enzyme with a definition on the reverse side of the card. This terminology may seem confusing at first but as you study it, it begins to make an elegant kind of sense. The following flow chart will help you get all this straight.

Flow Chart of Enzymes

I. Endogenous Enzymes: (from inside the consumer or predator, i.e., you)
  A. Human enzymes
      1.   Endogenous metabolic enzymes (made throughout the body)
      2.   Endogenous digestive enzymes (made only in the digestive tract)
        a. Endogenous lipases
        b. Endogenous proteinases
        c. Endogenous amylase
      3.   Endogenous autolytic enzymes (also lipase, proteinase and amylase)
II. Exogenous Enzymes:
  A. Animal enzymes
      1. Exogenous metabolic animal enzymes
      2. Exogenous autolytic animal enzymes
        a. Exogenous animal lipases
        b. Exogenous animal proteinases
        c. Exogenous animal amylase
  B. Phytoenzymes (of plant origin)
      1. <u>Exogenous metabolic plant</u> enzymes
      2. Exogenous autolytic plant enzymes
        a. <u>Exogenous plant lipases</u>
        b. <u>Exogenous plant proteinases</u>
        c. <u>Exogenous plant amylase</u>

I have underlined the enzymes in which we have the most interest in this discussion. These enzymes can do a lot of work for us and save us a lot of energy. They are what this discussion is about.

Enzyme Activators and Inhibitors

Enzymes in the activated state are very busy little guys. They must spend most of their lives inactivated, otherwise they would digest their host organism in a few minutes. The body has elaborate mechanisms to keep enzymes inactive until they are needed. The usual condition of an enzyme circulating throughout the body is that it is held in check by an amino acid chain, which is part of the enzyme — a kind of safety latch similar to the safety latch on a gun or the lock on a door.

When the action of the enzyme is needed, an associated activating enzyme is released, for example, from an area of thrombosis (a clot — inside an important artery, let us say) or, to use another example, from an area of inflammation. This activating enzyme turns off the safety latch or, in the other analogy, unlocks the door, allowing the enzyme to go to work, causing a breakdown of the blood clot or cleaning up the inflammatory debris.

Another safety system is that of enzyme inhibitors. These are proteins, which fit into the active site of the enzyme molecule, thus preventing the admission of substrate (the stuff the enzyme is designed to break down). When the enzyme is needed , these proteins are signaled to release themselves from the enzyme thus freeing the enzyme to do its assigned task.

Examples of exogenous enzyme inhibitors include many antibiotics, which kill bacteria by inhibiting key enzyme systems. Unfortunately, they also inhibit the identical metabolic enzyme systems in the body and thus are toxic to both bacteria and host. (You are the host.) This is one more reason I prefer to avoid the use of antibiotics, if at all possible.

Another example of exogenous enzyme inhibitors are those contained in seeds and nuts (which are also seeds). From seeds (nuts are seeds) entire plants grow with only the addition of water, soil, sunshine and the right temperature. From these facts, you can guess that seeds are loaded with enzymes. However, they must be held in the inactive state until water is present.

Nature has loaded seeds with enzyme inhibitors, which are deactivated by the addition of water. This process is called "germination." Therefore, when you chow down on your favorite seeds and/or nuts, you are loading your stomach with enzyme inhibitors. These enzyme inhibitors slow down or stop the action of whatever digestive enzymes may be present with your food, whether from an endogenous or exogenous source. Therefore, either avoid seeds and nuts unless (1) you germinate them first by letting them soak in water for a few days or (2) you consume them along with sufficient extra enzyme powder to neutralize the enzyme inhibitors.

Misconceptions About Enzymes

Professor B. P. Babkin wrote, in 1935, that when the pancreas is stimulated to secrete enzymes for digestion, it secretes equal amounts of proteinase, lipase and amylase. This was known as the "Theory of Parallel Secretion of Enzymes." (These three enzymes are responsible for digesting protein, fat and carbohydrate respectively.) Babkin's theory held that if you ate a meal of almost all protein, for example, your pancreas would pour out enzymes to digest not only protein but also fat and carbohydrate as well, and that these latter two enzymes would simply go to waste. The Theory of Parallel Secretion implied that enzymes are so easy for the body to manufacture, it can afford the luxury to make some and then throw them away!

Regardless of how little sense this made, the theory was accepted and taught in medical schools because of the reputation of the eminent Dr. Babkin. This is an example of the operation of dogma in medical thought. The eating and digestion of dogma in medical schools is identical to the same process in theology and law schools. No enzymes are required, only lame brains.

It is now known that the pancreas exhibits "selective secretion," meaning that the organ is signaled as to what sort of food is present and needing digestion, so it can then secrete the enzymes which are specifically needed for that kind of food. This is not only experimentally true, but it also makes sense! Given how complex and specific enzymes are, obviously a lot of energy is required to create them, and it makes no sense that the body would then waste them. No intelligent being would create such a mechanism in the human body, or any other body for that matter.

Nevertheless, many doctors have not reconsidered what they were taught in medical school and find the idea of "enzyme therapy" to be absurd because, as they think they know: enzymes are so easy to make, the body is willing to waste them and, being so insignificant, they could not possibly constitute a valuable therapy.

For many years it was taught in medical school biochemistry classes that an enzyme was not changed in any way when it performed its function of facilitating and speeding up a reaction. Enzymes were thought to act as true "catalysts," just as some metal ions do in purely non-biochemical chemical reactions. This is now known not to be the case. Enzymes are used up and destroyed in the process of doing their jobs, and the remains must be disposed. They are broken down by other enzymes and new enzymes are made to replace them.

Enzymes do last a long time: from twenty minutes to a few weeks, doing the same job many times before wearing out. Enzyme creation and destruction is happening throughout the body at all times. It only stops when the organism dies and actually not even then as we will now see.

It was also once taught in medical schools that enzymes could not pass through the gut wall and, therefore, any exogenous enzyme would have to first be digested, i.e., broken down to its component amino acids like any other protein, before it could be absorbed and used by the body. It is now known that both enzymes and ordinary proteins can be absorbed whole without being fully digested. The fact of antibody (which is protein) absorption directly through the gut wall is the basis for the transmission of immunity from mother to child through breast feeding.

This has enormous therapeutic implications where enzymes are concerned, because once in the body an exogenous enzyme identical in structure to an endogenous enzyme can be used as though it were an endogenous enzyme — the body has no way to distinguish it from an enzyme made inside the body.

Comment on Medical Politics and Dogma

The medical dogma that proteins could not be absorbed without being broken down to the component amino acids died hard in standardized medical circles and medical schools, and this delayed the popular perception of the value of oral enzyme therapy immeasurably. The heyday of enzyme therapy has not yet come in the United States, although it certainly has arrive in other countries, notably Europe and Japan. It is truly unfortunate that the medical establishment in the U.S. is so intensely nationalistic as to believe that if a therapy has not been proven inside the boundaries of the U.S.A., then it is worthless until proven otherwise.

Autolysis

All animals and plants contain the enzymes to "autolyze" themselves when they die. "Autolysis" literally means "self breaking" and refers to the fact that plant and animal tissues digest themselves after they die. Nature, folks, has thought of everything.

The Egyptians developed a process to prevent bacterial breakdown of the body after death; however, they could not solve the problem of enzymatic autolysis. Therefore, a mummy, while it retains the essential form of the original body, is not exactly ready for a hot date. This fact, autolysis, leads us into the field of enzyme therapy.

Unfortunately for humans, we have discovered how to cook our food. Cooking destroys the autolytic enzymes contained in food! All enzymes are extremely heat sensitive. If you cook them, they die! While pre-fire man received all the benefits of exogenous enzymes, post-fire man is starved for exogenous enzymes and must rely almost entirely on endogenous digestive enzymes, those he makes for himself.

The Function of Fever

If you raise temperature a few degrees above normal body temperature, enzymes become hyperactive. The enzymes in the immune system are activated and powered up to fight infection by acceleration of the activity of certain white cells which literally eat and digest bacteria. This process is called "phagocytosis," which means literally "eating cells." At 104 degrees Fahrenheit, enzymes and phagocytic cells are at their maximum state of activation.

Therefore, a fever should not be artificially brought down unless it exceeds 104 degrees Fahrenheit. At 106 degrees, brain damage (i.e., enzyme destruction) begins. When there is a fever it should be monitored every thirty minutes and treated if it exceeds 104.

Cooking: The Great Nutritional Disaster

If you raise the temperature to 118 degrees for a few minutes enzymes are completely destroyed. It is practically impossible for the body to create such an intense fever; however, cooking can easily exceed this temperature. Therefore, cooking, even at low temperatures, is the death of enzymes.

Since man mastered the use of fire, the practice of cooking food has been with us. From a nutritional standpoint, this was a great disaster. Let me explain that. Enzyme production is so labor-intensive that the eating habits of animals in nature are designed to take advantage of the presence of living enzymes in food. Fortunately for animals, they have not discovered how to cook their food.

The Overgrown Pancreas

Because of cooking, our digestive organs, especially the pancreas, are called upon to do the job of enzyme production alone. In a person who eats even a moderate percentage of cooked food, the pancreas is hypertrophied (overgrown) to two or three times its normal size (that size found in people who eat only raw food).

Animals in the wild eat raw food and their pancreases are approximately 1/3 the size of the typical human pancreas when corrected for body weight. Those animals are busy taking advantage of exogenous digestive enzymes contained in the raw food they eat.

"So what?" you ask. So what, is that you have an organ (the pancreas) which is hypertrophied and is begging, borrowing and stealing from the rest of the body, so that enough enzymes can be produced to digest the food you eat. The precursors of **metabolic** enzymes, the amino acids and polypeptides, which are needed in the rest of the body are being hogged up by the pancreas to produce **digestive** enzymes because the pancreas is getting no help from the enzymes contained in raw food. Cooking has destroyed them.

It is this simple: if living enzymes can be derived from food sources, the body does not have to expend its precious energy making digestive enzymes in large quantity. It can utilize that energy in the process of living healthier and longer by concentrating its ability to make enzymes on the production of metabolic enzymes. This is important. If you do not understand this, read it again until you do.

Cooking Milk

Pasteurization — the heating of milk to 145 degrees centigrade for thirty minutes — totally destroys not only bacteria from sick cows but all enzymes as well. There was a time, before the turn of the nineteenth into the twentieth century, when doctors recommended a raw milk diet for the cure of many diseases. This was before cows were locked up, pumped up (on drugs and enzymeless feed) and sucked out, but rather were allowed to roam freely, foraging for raw plant food and came in every morning to be milked by hand.

Unpasteurized and unhomogenized milk, made in this fashion, is loaded with valuable enzymes and, if you can find it, will serve as a therapy for a number of diseases. Given what has happened to milk in this century, *informed* doctors recommend that you avoid milk like the plague rather than drink it as a treatment for illness. It was inevitable, I guess, that man would finally think of cooking (pasteurizing) milk also. This avoids the necessity to monitor the milk cows to insure that they are free of disease.

Eat Raw Meat? Thanks, But No Thanks

While it is true that raw meat contains loads of living enzymes, I am not suggesting that you eat raw meat. Given how animals are treated in modern animal husbandry, you cannot count on raw meat for being only raw meat. It also will contain hormones, antibiotics, herbicides and pesticides before and after cooking. Also, there is the matter of how it tastes.

But The Eskimos Did!

For primitive, fireless man and for Eskimos, before acculturating to white man ways, raw meat was a great source of energy which kept these people free from degenerative diseases. The name "Eskimo" is an Indian term meaning "he eats it raw." Alas, it is no longer so. Most Eskimos now are eating potato chips and hamburgers, having adopted the white man's habits.

Eskimo forebears knew empirically (simply by observation) that raw food, even raw meat, is healthy food. Nature has designed a process of assisted autolysis using both cathepsin made in your stomach and cathepsin contained in the raw meat. Cathepsin is a proteinase enzyme, able to break down protein, including meat.

Eskimos did not know this explanation, but they knew they felt good and stayed healthy when they ate raw meat. Besides, that was almost all that was available to them. Vegetables do not grow so well in snow and ice. The only choice the Eskimos had was to cook their meat or not. Empirically, by the way they felt after eating raw meat, they chose not to cook it.

The problem with raw meat is, of course, the possibility of infection with parasites living in the meat. However, in the colder climates meat-borne parasites are non-considerations. Because the life cycles of most parasites involve an out of body experience (out of the body of the host, that is), usually at the egg or larval stage, they are not able to survive in cold weather — they bite the ice, usually by having their eggs or larvae frozen solid. They do thrive, on the other hand, in warm tropical climes, and they do well in temperate climes. Eskimos did not have the parasite problem.

The point of this discussion about Eskimos is that the phobia of meat and fat is not justified. We should focus our attention where it belongs: the fact that cooking is the real culprit. If you are a vegetarian and you cook your vegetables, guess what? You would be better off not doing that.

Stomach Physiology

The first part of the stomach, called the "antrum" or "cardia," or as Dr. Howell named it: the "food enzyme stomach," is similar in function to the "extra" stomach(s) in ruminants (cattle, deer, elk, moose, etc), in cetacea (whales, porpoises and dolphins) and in seed-eating birds such as chickens and pigeons.

In all of these animals, the first stomach (or stomachs in some cases) and the food enzyme stomach in man, are where, together with cathepsin contained in raw meat, protein is partially digested. Of course, if you cook the meat, that portion of exogenous cathepsin is destroyed. In the food enzyme stomach, fats and carbohydrates eaten from raw sources (and thus containing lipases and amylase for autolysis), proceed to autolyze (predigest) themselves. In the food enzyme stomach, food is allowed to autolyze as much as it will for a period up to one hour.

In humans, the food enzyme stomach functions as a separate organ by virtue of the fact that the lower stomach, also called the "fundus" or "pyloric stomach" (it could also be called the "endogenous enzyme stomach"), remains shut, the potential space closed by forcible opposition of the anterior and posterior walls of the stomach against each other. After autolysis the fundus opens, receiving the food, making a load of hydrochloric acid and pepsin and proceeding with digestion.

Under "normal" circumstances of raw sources of protein, about half the stomach digestion of protein is achieved in the antrum or food enzyme stomach with cathepsin and other autolytic enzymes and the other half in the fundus with pepsin and hydrochloric acid.

The typical doctor might disagree with this description and cite "barium swallow" fluoroscopy studies which show the entire stomach frantically contracting and relaxing after a barium swallow. This may be how the stomach behaves when insulted with a solution of barium, but barium is not food! The stomach behaves differently when engaged in digestion and is not being assaulted by a barium swallow. If your stomach contracted frantically after a meal you would know it, you would not need a barium assault to prove it.

The point is: we can see by the behavior of the stomach during digestion that it is designed to take advantage of the enzymes which are contained in raw foods, so that we do not have to expend the large amounts of energy and resources necessary to make a huge load of endogenous digestive enzymes to do it on our own.

Exogenous Enzymes and Longevity

Lest you still are not taking this discussion seriously, let us consider some research relating to enzymes, health and longevity. Because insects are cold-blooded and short-lived, it is easy to demonstrate the value of enzymes to their longevity. A study done with *Daphnia magna*, the water flea, demonstrated that raising its environmental temperature from 46 degrees to 82 degrees Fahrenheit cuts its life-span to 1/4 of that at 46 degrees. Increased temperature raises enzyme activity, and when enzyme vitality is used up, life is over.

The same can be said for you, not because of increased temperature — because you are a warm-blooded animal, able to regulate your temperature — but because you deplete your enzyme stores in another way: by eating cooked food and requiring your body to divert precious resources to making digestive enzymes. This shortens your life span and robs you of your natural state of health.

Many people, even people otherwise well-educated in nutrition, do not take the idea of enzyme support seriously. Many seem to think that enzyme support should be done only if the pancreas is weak, while the truth is that it should also be done if it is strong. If the pancreas is strong — enlarged and producing triple doses of enzymes, thus robbing the rest of the body, including the immune system, of precious enzyme precursors — we would do well to supplement endogenous enzyme production with exogenous food enzymes contained in raw foods. People who eat lots of raw food live longer and feel better.

If you are interested in living long and remaining healthy, perhaps I can get your attention with the fact that enzyme production, both digestive and metabolic, decreases with age. When the enzymes finally check out, so do you.

Maybe Methuselah really did live a long time, if he ate pure raw food as the Bible assures us that he did. However, if he lived in excess of 900 years, we still need to know more about how he did that! Most scientists consider this account fiction; however, I prefer to keep an open mind about things outside my personal experience.

Enzymes and Obesity

Still don't have your attention? Let us talk about being fat. Have you noticed how many people are overweight, I mean, uh, fat? You may be one of them.

If the body is starved for the vital energy of enzymes which have been depleted in the cause of digestion, that body craves more energy. The only way the body knows to get more energy is to eat, and the only way to insure that you eat is to create the experience of hunger. So you eat and eat and eat, trying to get satisfied. What is missing is not calories but vital life energy, which has been robbed from your enzyme system.

So you eat more dead, enzyme-free food, the calories are stored as fat, and the craving goes on. You can eat more calories and lose weight, if your source of calories is raw food because you are consuming vital life energy, i.e., enzymes, with your food, and this energy will convert more food to motion and thought and less to fat. When the body is presented with exogenous food-derived enzymes, it is able to make more endogenous enzymes for metabolism.

One class of endogenous enzymes is lipase. The job of lipase is to break down fat. Got a fat problem? Get some lipase. Lipases are contained in all raw, uncooked food containing fat. Do not be afraid of fat, be afraid of fatty food which has been *cooked* and stripped of its autolytic lipases.

Remember what Einstein taught us: mass and energy are interchangeable. With exogenous, food-derived enzymes, you can convert some of your mass to energy, maybe not at the speed of light squared, but fast enough. That is not absolutely correct physics, but it is darn good physiology.

Too Skinny?

Some people weigh much less than they want to weigh because their pancreas has been exhausted by a lifetime of no support from exogenous enzymes. This person may eat loads of food and yet remain underweight. The solution for such an underweight individual is not to eat more but to digest better. If pancreatic exhaustion is the problem, digestive enzyme supplementation is the solution and will produce better digestion and dramatic weight gain.

Fasting and Enzymes

It has long been known by practitioners of fasting that health can be restored by this ancient practice. Water fasting — no food consumed, only pure water — relieves the body of the necessity of producing enzymes for digestion. The enzyme precursors can therefore be used for metabolic enzyme production. The same is true in juice fasting, which requires that only freshly prepared vegetable juices, and sometimes a smaller quantity of freshly prepared fruit juices, be consumed along with pure water. In this kind of fasting, fresh enzymes are given to the body in concentrated form in the juice.

If illness is present, it may be helped through fasting. The immune system is given what it needs to correct illness — enzymes — and thus a sufficient supply of enzyme precursors. There may be a "healing crisis," or detoxification stage, which is uncomfortable to go through but which leads to a new level of vital health. Fasting can be considered a form of enzyme therapy.

Enzymatic Therapy For Arthritis

Still not convinced? Lets talk about treating and avoiding disease. In the 1940s, Dr. Arnold Renshaw of Manchester, England suspected rheumatoid arthritis to be a digestive disease.

He based his suspicions, published in the Annals of Rheumatic Disease in 1947, on many observations at autopsy of the small intestines of people who had rheumatoid arthritis at the time of death. He found the small intestines to be consistently atrophied. Dr. Renshaw tested his hypothesis by having an enzyme preparation made for oral administration. He found that rheumatoid arthritis patients improved dramatically in just over one half of 556 patients. Another 219 of these 556 patients were improved to a lesser extent.

He also discovered that the pain of osteoarthritis could be helped with enzyme therapy. The time required for improvement in these illnesses varied from two months to two years, so persistence is the key in this type of therapy. Similar results can be obtained with raw diets. It may be a long time to wait for results, but for most people it is worth waiting for and easier to confront knowing that this type of therapy benefits the rest of the body as well.

Enzyme Therapy For Cancer

You may have heard of cases of cancer cured using only raw foods. If this happens, one of the explanations is clear: the immune system is powered up by a surge of enzyme precursors available when exogenous food enzymes are added to the diet, thus allowing the immune system to defeat (eat? digest?) the cancer. Enzyme treatment is the most exciting and promising approach to cancer. It attempts to duplicate the spontaneous cancer cures which are sometimes seen in oncology.

Some doctors, including Dr. Howell, offer enzyme therapy for treatment of cancer. It stands to reason that if a prolonged fast or a diet of only raw vegetables can help some cases of cancer, massive doses of enzymes should also be able to help. This kind of therapy is done in a hospital and involves frequent small meals and doses of enzymes every thirty minutes. The need for careful supervision is obvious. I do not offer such a therapy, however, the folks at the Bradford Research Institute in Tijuana, Mexico offer this therapy along with others.

Enzymes and Allergy

It is undeniable that some people react to certain foods. The explanation is that digestion is proceeding badly due to poor enzyme and/or stomach acid production. This causes food to arrive in the lower small intestine and colon relatively undigested. This upsets the normal flora of bacteria found there by favoring those bacteria able to digest that food. These bacteria replace so-called friendly species of bacteria which normally live symbiotically with us. The overall result is a condition called "dysbiosis" and malabsorption. The body forms antibodies to foods and bacterial breakdown products in the lower gut. These antibodies also attack, as if to neutralize, normal tissue of the body such as joint and skin tissue. Arthritis and skin disease are only two examples of diseases which have their origin in disordered digestion, diseases which have long been considered incurable in medical circles.

Lipase and Atherosclerosis

As we grow older, the supply of all endogenous enzymes decreases. This includes lipase. It may be that the decrease in lipase as a function of aging has a lot to do with fatty deposits on the walls of arteries and the acceleration of atherosclerosis. Decreased supplies of lipase occurs in the intestines and in the serum (the noncellular part of blood). Therefore, as we grow older, it becomes increasingly important to either cut fat intake or to ingest exogenous lipase along with fat to help prevent atherosclerosis. This means raw food or supplementation with enzyme powder.

Elsewhere, I have expressed the opinion that fat is not so disagreeable to the human body (provided there are plenty of antioxidants on board), rather what is in the fat constitutes the problem: herbicides, pesticides, synthetic hormones, antibiotics, etc., all fed to cattle to increase production. For an older person, it also may be that it is what is *not* in the fat: lipase is not in the fat if the fat is heated to 118 degrees Fahrenheit for only a few minutes.

A rational approach to vascular disease is to load up on lipase with each meal containing fat. If you cannot bear to eat raw meat and you have no access to raw dairy products, buy some enzyme powder from your friendly health food store or organic grocery. In this manner, you can obtain the nutrition contained in the fat (the most powerful source of calories available) and not have to be concerned with the consequences. Nevertheless, it is not wise to unbalance your food intake in any direction, including excess fat.

Comparative Pathology

Let us see how can we be relatively sure of the importance of ingesting exogenous enzymes. Domesticated animals suffer the same degenerative diseases which humans are subject to: cancer, arthritis, atherosclerosis; whereas this does not happen with animals in the wild. Animals procured from the jungle, when dissected, show no evidence of arthritis, cancer, or atherosclerosis, unless they live close to human pollution. But pity the health of the animal in captivity which is fed processed food.

The explanation which makes the most sense to me is that domesticated animals fed processed food, because they receive no exogenous enzymes, fall ill with the same diseases we have. Processed human food (heat is part of the "process") is stripped of its enzyme content. It is what some people call "dead food." The animal equivalent is dog and cat chow, as well as cattle and chicken feed, which has gone through heat processing. This stuff is the animal version of the dead food we eat ourselves. Animals in the wild must eat fresh raw food, because nothing else is available. Therefore, they receive liberal amounts of all enzymes.

The Point

The purpose of this discussion is to point out to you the importance of enzymes. Enzymes are not yet in the consciousness of the public, whereas the importance of vitamins and minerals is firmly entrenched. Your nutritional regime is not complete until cooked-food-induced enzyme starvation is corrected.

The best solution, of course, would be to revert to raw food exclusively. The next best solution would be to revert to eighty percent raw food. A salad with your meal is a nice gesture, but it is not enough, although every little bit helps, I suppose.

If you are not able or, more likely, not willing to make the change to exclusively raw food, the next best solution is to supplement your diet with enzymes. These should be taken just as you begin to eat, and they should be in powder form. If you have the type which is powder in a capsule, separate the capsule, and pour the powder on your first bite of cooked food after it has cooled to around body temperature (otherwise, the enzyme is destroyed by the heat of the food). Do not use the tablet form of enzymes unless you chew it up.

The best choice of enzyme is the plain powder (not in a capsule) made from plant sources. Simply add a half teaspoon to the average size meal, and you are set. The brand I like best is called "N-zimes."

Unless chewed up or presented to the stomach as powder, enzymes will not dissolve in time to help your (pre)digestion in the food enzyme stomach. Rather, they will dissolve some time later after your pancreas is already powered up to douse your food with a load of enzymes derived by hogging enzyme precursors which are needed for the metabolic enzyme production trying to happen in the rest of your body.

See page 358 for instructions on contacting my office for a referral to a doctor familiar with enzyme nutrition.

Sources

Ambrus JL et al. Absorption of exogenous and endogenous proteolytic enzymes Clin. Pharmacol. Ther. 8:362;1967

Barrett AJ Proteinases in mammalian cells and tissues Elsevier, North Holland Biomedical Press; 1967.

Baumueller M XXIV FMS World congress of sport medicine Symposium on enzyme therapy in sports injuries May 29, 1990, p. 9 Elsevier Science Publishers, Amsterdam 1990.

Beard J Enzyme therapy of cancer. In: Wolf, M. (Hrsg.) Maudrich-Verlag, Vienna;1971.

Blonstein JL Oral enzyme tablets in the treatment of boxing injuries Practitioner 198: 547; 1967.

Bramwell FWR The transmission of passive immunity from mother to young Frontiers of Biology, Vol. 18, North-Holland, Amsterdam;1970.

Ekerot LK, Ohlsson K, Necking L Elimination of protease-inhibitor complexes from the arthritic joint Int. J.Tissue Reac. VII:391;1985.

Emele JF, Shanaman J, Winbury MM The analgesic-anti-inflammatory activity of papain Arch Int Pharmacyn Ther 159:126;1966.

Gardner MLG Intestinal assimilation of intact peptides and proteins from diet — a neglected field? Biol Rev 59:289-331;1984.

Jaeger H Hydrolytic enzymes in the treatment of HIV disease General Medicine (Allgemeinmedizin) 19(4):160-164;1990.

Layer P, et. al Fate of pancreatic intestinal enzymes during small intestinal aboral transit in humans Am J Physiol Gastrointest Liver Physiol 251:475;1986.

Neuhofer C Enzyme therapy in multiple sclerosis Hufeland Journal 2:47-50;1986.

Lopez DA, Williams RM, Miehlke M *Enzymes, The Fountain of Life* The Neville Press Inc. 1994 ISBN 1-884303-00-5.

Howell E *Enzyme Nutrition, The Food Enzyme Concept* Avery Publishing Group Inc., Wayne, New Jersey 1985 ISBN 0-89529-221-1.

ORGAN

HEALTH

THE BACK

The back is the most sensitive part of the human body. It is often the first part of the body to detect disease and the first to alert its owner to the presence of a problem in the body. This is why backache is the most common presenting complaint in medicine.

Despite the commonness of back problems, they are also the problems for which you are least likely to receive help from your doctor. Many doctors do not appreciate the complex and varied causation of back problems. Many doctors will treat the pain of a back syndrome and never understand the origin of the back pain itself.

Of course, doctors think about such things as cancer, and cancer can certainly be a cause of backache. It is important to consider the possibility of cancer and either make the diagnosis or rule the diagnosis out of the list of possibilities. While it is true that a backache, especially one of recent onset, may indicate a cancerous or ulcerative condition of the internal organs, it is not likely. When a backache has been present for years, it becomes very unlikely that the origin is from a life-threatening disease.

I want to talk to you here about the common and yet unappreciated causes of back syndromes. Most chronic back problems have several origins, and only if all the contributing factors are eliminated will the backache clear up completely. The most common initiating cause of a chronic back problem is chronic injury.

Larry Bird, the great professional basketball player, had his career ended with a back problem from chronic injury. Every time a basketball player leaps for the ball, he comes down to a small, perhaps only microscopic, injury on impact. Although each injury is almost insignificant in itself, when you add up thousands and tens of thousands of small injuries, the effect becomes noticeable.

I know a guy who thought he was taking great care of his health by running five times every week, three miles each time. He did this from age eighteen until age 36 before his back finally complained at the end of a marathon. Despite this warning signal from his back, he continued to run regularly until age 48 when he was forced by back pain to put an end to his running career. This fellow especially enjoyed fast running, in which the speed involved required that he raise his knees and pound the ground. He usually ran on sidewalks and streets, sometimes on tracks and occasionally through wooded areas. He finally went for an evaluation and was amazed to see on his x-ray that he had destroyed two intervertebral discs in his lower back.

Years later, this guy went to his friend, an orthopedic surgeon, finally ready for surgery. His surgeon friend was honest and told him that surgery probably would not help. His friend said these words: "There is nothing I can do to help. You will always have this problem. You had better just learn to live with it!"

In desperation, he tried one thing after another to cure his aching back. During this period he pushed his stiff back to the sitting position with his good right arm every morning and waited for his wife to tie his shoes, because he could not reach his feet due to back pain. That was four years ago. Today this person is completely pain free, can lift anything he wishes without fear of injury and has earned a blue belt in Tang So Do Karate. I know this fellow very well. I am this fellow. From this intimate case study of myself, I learned most of what I know about curing back problems. Let me tell you what I have learned about back problems.

Lesson 1: Never give up.

Do not lose hope for a normal back. If an authority figure tells you to learn to accept your back problem, excuse yourself and leave. Do not return. This person does not know much. Never accept your back problem as the way it must be for the rest of your life. Do not "learn to live with it." If you do, you will cease your search for a cure, and you will therefore not find a cure.

Lesson 2: Make lifestyle changes.

The low back is the most sensitive organ in the body. If you are stressing your body with a lousy diet, tobacco use, alcohol consumption, lack of exercise, poor sleep habits, poor relationships, then change all that. Start eating right, drop tobacco and alcohol, exercise regularly, assign the proper hours for sleep, clean up your relationships, take your vitamins — especially take liberal amounts of vitamin C. You may be surprised to discover that these actions alone will eradicate your back problem and if not completely eradicate them, you can certainly expect changes for the better.

Lesson 3: Colon cleansing

You may be one of those people who, despite a healthy diet of vegetables, including lots of fiber, still has a sluggish colon. I suggest going on a juice fast of seven days (see the section on juice fasting) and having a few visits to a colon therapist (see section on the colon). You will be amazed at the difference a clean colon will make to your back. After your colon is cleansed, work out a dietary and herbal program with your colon therapist to keep it clean. This will involve eating right: low fat, no chocolate, plenty of fiber, no coffee. (I didn't say no caffeine, I said no coffee. Coffee is loaded with toxins other than caffeine, and some of them, notably tannic acid, help degenerate both the back and the adrenal glands — therefore, no decaf either.)

Lesson 4: Do daily specific exercises for the muscles of your back.

Part of the problem in most backaches is poor tone in the muscles of the back. This comes from lack of the right kind of exercise. When pain builds up in the back, the structures of the back reflexly try to hold motion to a minimum. This results in degeneration of the muscle tissue of the back. You need to build up the strength of both the flexors and extensors of the back.

The flexors are made stronger by doing what are called "crunchies." Lie flat on your back, put your hands behind your head, and flex your abdomen, bringing your chin a few inches closer to your pelvis, touching your chest with the point of your chin. As you do this, your shoulders and shoulder blades should come off the floor about two inches. Relax and repeat. Find your tolerance level, and build from there. A good routine is 100 crunchies every day. If you can do them all at one time, great, do it. If you cannot, keep working at it every day, doing 100 per day divided into several sessions until you can do 100 at one session.

Avoid full sit ups. Full set ups put an unnatural strain on your lower back and can result in back problems, even if you have none now.

After your abdominal muscles are strong, you are ready to start on your back extensors. Lie face down and bow your back bringing your head a few inches closer to your ankles and your chest, toes and knees off the floor. Now, swim, with one hand in front and the other behind; reverse and repeat. Build up to maintaining this position with this action for at least three minutes.

An even better exercise, once you have advanced your strength to the task, is done with a Roman hyperextension machine. This device makes it possible to lie face down, with a couple of stable pads at your anterior hip level and your ankles held in place from behind with a bar. With your hands behind your head in this position, allow your head to drop down forming a reverse, up-side-down L-shape with your body as viewed from your right side. Straighten your back bringing your body into a straight line again. Repeat this exercise until exhaustion.

You can find a Roman hyperextension machine at almost any health club and, if your back problem is helped by this exercise, you might be wise to purchase one for your own private use at home. I use mine every day — 40 hyperextensions per session.

Lesson 5: Chelation Therapy with AMP

If you have done all of the above and your back still hurts, it is time to take the next step. Chelation therapy is a potent treatment of the arthritic component of your back problem and is dealt with in great specificity in pages 14-24.

The addition of AMP (adenosine monophosphate) to the chelation mixture addresses a poorly appreciated problem of back disorders: the degenerated condition of the muscles of the back. When the back is in pain for protracted periods of time, the muscles do a thing called "splinting." When a muscle splints, it is straining to hold the joint structures in place. Splinting occurs when the other structures of the back (bones, joints and ligaments) are damaged and cannot hold the back in proper alignment. This happens, for example, when an intervertebral disc collapses and brings the vertebrae closer together than they were meant to be. It also happens when there is ligament damage.

Ligaments are the cables, so to speak, in the back structure, which can be compared to a suspension bridge. When they break or become stretched out of shape, the vertebrae go out of alignment. Then the paraspinal muscles try to fill in for the damaged ligaments by holding (splinting) the spine in a rigid alignment. Muscles are not made for constant strain, and they eventually degenerate from this activity.

AMP is the first step in the biochemistry of building the substance the body itself manufactures to store energy (ATP - adenosine triphosphate) which is used by muscles in movement. When there is a lot of splinting, the muscle becomes exhausted. Supplying new AMP for the muscles is like fueling up a car. Muscle tissue is given a new lease on life.

Another item (you can take orally), which is a precursor of ATP, is creatine. I recommend five grams per day. This is especially useful when taken before exercise to increase the muscular strength of the back. However, the problem of splinting may still be present, therefore...

Lesson 6: Prolotherapy

Prolotherapy is discussed at length on pages 33-35. I refer you to those pages for a more thorough discussion. When ligaments are severely damaged, they are not going to repair themselves on their own and no amount of chiropractic work is going to repair them. They need the help of prolotherapy, which involves the injection of a proliferative solution into the back. The presence of this proliferative solution attracts macrophages and fibroblasts, cells whose job it is to move in, clean up and repair a damaged area of the body. The prolotherapy solution mimics an acute injury, calling these cells to move in and repair damaged ligaments. If you have damaged ligaments, only prolotherapy is going to restore your back to health. The other things you can do will not cure it. However, even prolotherapy cannot do the job unless you make those lifestyle changes listed above. Until that happens, your ability to heal is impaired, and prolotherapy depends upon your ability to heal.

Lesson 7: Use Glucosamine

Glucosamine is the substance the body makes to repair cartilage, tendon, ligament, joint fluid, heart valves, eyes and blood vessels. In the face of chronic injury, the body simply cannot make enough glucosamine to make this major repair possible. A degenerated disc in the back is a classic example. Taking glucosamine as a supplement makes possible the repair of joints, which were once thought to be beyond repair. See pages 142-143 for more information.

Lesson 8: Avoid vigorous manipulation of joints.

Chiropractic manipulation of joints can help you feel better, no doubt about it, especially early in the disease process. It is important for you to know that such manipulation is not curative of the disease process. No number of manipulations will make your collapsed disc become normal again and no amount of manipulation will make your ligaments repair themselves.

If your chiropractor performs dramatic, vigorous manipulation, while this may feel better in the short-run, in the long-run this type of spinal manipulation will damage your back by further ripping already torn and degenerated ligaments. Therefore, the alignment will not hold, and you will soon be back for another adjustment.

If you do have chiropractic manipulation, go to a chiropractor who appreciates the value of gentle manipulation over dramatic, vigorous manipulations. Determine this by interviewing the chiropractor by phone before you make an appointment. If you do go in for treatment, and you find the adjustment to be too vigorous, do not hesitate to say so. Say this word: "STOP!" It is your body, and it is your right to stop anyone from damaging your body.

Lesson 9: Avoid back surgery.

The rationale for back surgery is to stabilize the vertebrae by fusing unstable vertebrae together (spinal fusion) after removing diseased discs (laminectomy). Hopefully, the vertebrae grow together and become one unit.

This may or may not stabilize the spine. If it does, it does so at the expense of mobility. Two, three, four, or five vertebrae, fused together as one, also move as one. This makes for an unnatural stiffness. If stability is not attained through fusion, pain continues, and you have lost time and money having surgery, and you still have a painful back. Also, you have risked your life by going under anesthesia.

It is very possible to achieve stability through fusion surgery and still have the same old back pain. The reason for this is that there is more involved in back pain than unstable joints. The degeneration of muscle tissue from months and perhaps years of splinting must be corrected, or pain will persist. Removing discs stands a good chance of making the problem worse, because with each disc removed, the vertebral column becomes shorter. The muscle and ligament structures of the back are made for a certain length in the vertebral column. When you shorten that length, the structures which attach to the vertebrae become less functional.

Also avoid back surgery because there are far better ways to handle your back or neck problem, as we already have seen. If you already have had back surgery and still have a back problem (as usually is the case) do not despair. Follow this program, and it should work for you as well as if you had never consented to surgery.

Lesson 10: Do not take anti-inflammatory drugs, prescription or over-the-counter.

The pharmaceutical industry is up to its old tricks: profits by whatever means necessary. Several new (therefore patentable) anti-inflammatory medications have been developed which are a lot like aspirin in effect, except that they cost a fortune. The effect usually is dramatic for the first few days, and then the effect is no better than normal aspirin.

All anti-inflammatory agents retard healing and healing is, in the long run, the most important aspect in your recovery of normal function. Avoid all drugs in treating a back problem. This applies especially to steroids. This class of drugs, which includes cortisone, hydrocortisone and prednisone, has a dramatic pain-relieving effect and powerful anti-inflammatory effects, but these effects wear off after a week or so. The down side of steroids is that they do more than simply retard healing, they actually promote degeneration of tissues. In the long run, your back problem will be much worse for having used steroids — as will your immune system.

Although the effect is not so quick and dramatic, I believe that in the long run the best medicine for a spinal problem includes a clean diet with vigorous vitamin, amino acid and essential fatty acid therapy. I refer you to the section on vitamins and supplements for a more complete discussion of this type of therapy. What is optimal for your overall health also is best for your back. The rule of thumb here is that if you need a prescription for it, it is no good for your back! Crazy world, is it not?

Lesson 11: Remember the adrenal gland.

Adrenal dysfunction is the most common and yet most undiagnosed organ dysfunction in the body. The adrenal gland is by far the most sensitive of the organs to the daily assault of the 500-plus synthetic chemicals the average person is exposed to during the average day in America. Future research may illuminate which of these chemicals do the most damage, but at this time all we can say for sure is that the adrenal glands take a beating. It is very common for them to wear out in middle age as measured by DHEA (dihydroepiandosterone) levels. (I refer you to the chapter on DHEA for details.)

The point is that the effect on the body from a pair of exhausted adrenal glands includes an aching back. DHEA therapy turns out to be an important element which leads many people out of Backache Woods.

Lesson 12: Remember the thyroid gland.

The hormonal secretions of the thyroid gland control the basal metabolic rate — the speed with which the body carries out all of the chemical processes of life. Included in these processes is healing. If you are trying to persuade a part of your body to heal itself, and there exists a thyroid imbalance, that healing will progress more slowly than normal.

In the case of a back which is already diseased with damaged cartilage and weakened ligaments, the rate of healing in the presence of thyroid dysfunction may not be fast enough to keep pace with the rate of breakdown. Normal use of the back induces microscopic injuries, which must be repaired in a timely fashion if they are not to accumulate and present themselves as a painful back condition.

The ability to repair tissue quickly declines with age, and an important component of this decline is not only the occasional falling off of thyroid hormone but also the increased resistance of tissue to respond to the thyroid hormone which is present. See the chapter on thyroid replacement therapy for more information.

Lesson 13: Remember the importance of digestion.

Good food and vitamins cannot make a difference in the process of healing, even in the presence of a strong thyroid, if the food you eat and the vitamins you take do not absorb well. If they remain in the gut and are therefore eliminated without entering your body, you have gained nothing from them. As surprising as it may seem, many people suffer from the inability to make sufficient stomach acid to initiate proper digestion. This condition is called "achlorhydria," if there is no ability to make stomach acid. It is called "hypochlorhydria" if there is reduced ability to make stomach acid. Hypochlorhydria is present in fifteen percent of people who go to a doctor's office for evaluation at age thirty, thirty percent at age forty and fifty percent over sixty! See pages 200-208 for more information.

Lesson 14: Maintain a good attitude.

Having a bad back is no fun and the discomfort is magnified by the attitude of resignation you may encounter in the medical establishment. Many people with lumbago and neck problems simply give up and accept the life of an invalid. To handle your back problem, you must educate yourself and practice what you learn. The good news is that if you do this, your overall health will improve, you will feel much better and probably live a longer, happier, healthier life.

To get through the back problem to a restoration of full function requires that you educate yourself and think for yourself. The medical establishment does not know what to do for you as evidenced by the millions of people whose backs and necks are in pain at this very moment even after seeing their doctors and following their medical advice to the letter. Among these people are many doctors, some of them the same doctors you went to for your backache!

Lesson 15: Sleep on a supportive surface.

The surface you sleep on makes an enormous difference to your spine. It should be a solid surface but not rock hard. There should be no sway to it. The worst possible choice would be a hammock. The best choice, it my opinion, is a six inch thick layer of egg crate foam on top of a solid surface such as board. The foam provides comfort, and the hard surface under the foam provides support. If it is possible to sleep on your back, do so. If not, an extra pillow for support placed to the side of your abdomen as you lie in the prone position turned slightly to one side is very helpful. Experiment to find the best arrangement to fit your body.

Lesson 16: Colchicine

Intravenous and oral colchicine (an extract of the *Autumn crocus* plant) is a powerful anti-inflammatory agent for the spinal nerve root and the intervertebral discs. It also washes out uric acid and calcium pyrophosphate dihydrate crystals which are found in degenerated discs. Intravenous colchicine gives major relief of symptoms in 91% of patients with slipped disc syndrome, far better than the 50% offered by surgery and without the possibility of surgical or anaesthetic damage. No one should have disc surgery without first having a trial of colchicine.

Lesson 17: Be patient, and never give up.

I believe you can have confidence in the accuracy of the information I have given you. This information is derived from my own personal experience, and backed up with scientific studies. We live in a time when people want a quick-fix, an instant cure. While this is occasionally available, there may be no quick-fix, miracle cure to your back problem.

As for myself, I had to use every element in the above discussion for over one year before I could honestly pronounce myself completely recovered. My wife is now married to a man who not only does not need his shoes tied for him but who also can carry his bride from one room to the next with ease, and without any pain.

So, never give up, and do not expect an instant cure. The process which got your back in trouble spanned years, and the recovery may not come instantly. Be that person who insists on a complete restoration and does not settle for half-way measures which leave the problem persisting. You deserve a normally functioning back!

See page 358 for instructions on contacting my office for a referral to a doctor experienced in using the above approaches for the treatment of back and neck problems.

THE STOMACH: HYPOCHLORHYDRIA

Why is it some people age faster, require more medical attention and die earlier in life than others? The medical answer has always been that it is because of "constitution," or in the most modern mythological jargon, "It's in your genes." All this is another way of saying "We don't know." (Medical jargon has a lot of ways of saying "We don't know.") I know. Let me tell you about it.

One branch of progressive medicine is nutritional medicine. There is no category of disease which cannot be helped by the nutritional approach. By the term "nutritional approach" I mean the use of oral and intravenous nutrients, as well as the institution of dietary changes. There is no such thing as a person who is ill from a degenerative disease process (breakdown of joints, sclerosis of arteries, cancer, etc.) who also has been optimally nourished his or her entire life. All degenerative disease has its origin in malnutrition.

"But, how can people in America be malnourished?" you may ask. Easily. Eat the typical American diet, and you become borderline nourished. Do worse than that, and malnutrition appears in the form of degenerative disease. Many people who eat a perfectly nourishing diet also are malnourished and end up with degenerative disease. How can that be?

If the proper food is eaten and the proper nutrient supplements taken, that is one thing. It is quite another for that food and those nutrients to be absorbed into the body. Just because something goes down your esophagus does not mean that it will make it to the cells of your body. First, it must penetrate the wall of your intestines. If it does not encounter the proper acid and enzymes, it will not digest and absorb properly, and you will become malnourished, making your body fertile ground for the development of infectious and degenerative diseases.

Normal digestion is a complex cascade of events beginning when food is placed in the mouth and ending with elimination about 24 hours later. Normal digestion requires thorough chewing, mixing of food with enzymes, efficient swallowing, followed by exposure to a large quantity of acid and enzyme in the stomach. About two hours later, the chyme (food in the process of digestion) is moved on to the small intestine where it is bathed in bile, bile salts and more enzymes. More absorption occurs, and the chyme is mixed with bacteria to aid in digestion. After being moved to the colon, water is reabsorbed, and vitamin E is manufactured by "friendly" bacteria.

Digestive disturbance can happen anywhere along the intestinal tract resulting in less than optimal digestion and a state of relative malnutrition. Many of these conditions are rare, and it is unlikely that you or your loved ones are suffering from them. It is possible, however, and if they are present, your doctor should be able to diagnose and treat them. While each disease is important, especially to the well-being of the person who has the disease, my purpose here is to alert you to a condition which is both common, frequently undiagnosed and usually untreated: hypochlorhydria.

Hypochlorhydria is the underproduction of hydrochloric acid by the stomach. Hydrochloric acid, or HCL as it is called, is responsible for two important functions: (1) it begins the breakdown of protein by simply frying it in acid, and (2) in the presence of food it activates an enzyme called "pepsin," which further breaks down protein.

For many years, hypochlorhydria was a condition doctors could only suspect but not diagnose — except with lab tests so difficult to administer, it was easier to rationalize not making the diagnosis and not treating the illness. This test involved shoving a tube down the esophagus and periodically suctioning out the stomach contents after a meal, so the acidity of those contents could be measured.

So, doctors rationalized a point of view that the disorder is not worth treating. Therefore, medical students were taught to ignore symptoms of hypochlorhydria, because the necessary test to make the diagnosis was more difficult for the patient than the disorder itself. Medical students do believe what their med school professors tell them, and this led to a generation of doctors unwilling to further examine the problem of hypochlorhydria.

However, that situation began to change in the late 1960s with the invention of the Heidelberg Machine. This elegant (but expensive) device involves swallowing a capsule about the size of a vitamin capsule. This capsule is an acid-measuring radio telemetry device. It measures the acidity of the stomach and radios the results to an antenna which the patient wears like a large belt around the waist during this one- to two-hour test. While the telemetry capsule is in the stomach, we challenge the stomach's ability to make acid by having the subject swallow a teaspoon of water saturated with sodium bicarbonate. If the stomach is normal, we can see the acidity return to the stomach. If the stomach is unable to withstand five of these challenges, we know we are dealing with hypochlorhydria. The ability to diagnose hypochlorhydria is a wonderful advance in medicine, one which too few doctors are taking advantage of due to the party line that hypochlorhydria is not worth treating.

Many people who have too little stomach acid are being treated as if they have too much. The reason for this is that the symptoms are similar. Because ten to fifteen percent of the population is hypochlorhydric, there are many people out there who are being misdiagnosed and mistreated. A full fifty percent of people over age 60 are hypochlorhydric and, of all the patients coming to a doctor, up to fifty percent of these have underlying hypochlorhydria. The image of the *over*active stomach is so common, many people are treating themselves with antacids without even bothering to consults their physicians.

The view that the action of the stomach on digestion is so inconsequential as not to merit proper and concise diagnosis and treatment is, in my view, indefensible. Why would nature have given us the ability to concentrate HCL in the stomach one million times more than the surrounding tissues, if it were not needed?

Stomach acid serves many important functions, not only in digestion, but also in keeping the body free from disease. Many bacteria enter the body with food. Some of them are not friendly to human life. In a normal stomach, these bacteria are doused with acid and die. In a person with hypochlorhydria, these bacteria are escorted into the small intestine along with a generous food supply. It has been shown that people with hypochlorhydria have more than their share of infections. The ever present yeast organism makes its entrance via the mouth. Many people with the so-called "yeast syndrome" are unable to get rid of their yeast because the organism continues to reinfect the body through the mouth.

Frequently, stool analyses of people with hypochlorhydria reveal the presence of undigested protein fibers. While able to digest enough protein to live using their own pancreatic enzymes or enzyme supplements, these people are not getting the full benefit of the food they eat. The final result is that these people do not feel as good as they could and have no idea why.

Certain symptoms of hypochlorhydria make life very unpleasant for a person as well as for other people around. The collection of gas in the stomach results in frequent burping, a troublesome and embarrassing symptom. Unexplained bloating, belching and "heartburn" frequently are diagnosed as symptoms of *hyper*acidity and wrongly treated with antacids, when what is really going on is insufficient acid production. The resulting imbalanced bacterial flora further down the digestive tract produces a lot of hydrogen sulfide gas, and this does nothing for your social standing.

Some people have done all they can think of doing for their health: vitamins, exercise, etc., and still do not feel right due to the poor nutritional status of unrecognized hypochlorhydria, often combined with an underactive or overactive production of enzymes by the pancreas. See pages 178-192.

A voracious appetite may be related to hypochlorhydria simply because the person is not getting full nutritional value from food eaten. The body tries to solve this by demanding more food. "I am hungry all the time" should ring the hypochlorhydria bell.

The "big belly' is a common sight on the streets of America. In most cases, this is contributed to by hypochlorhydria and a relative absence of digestive enzymes, which should be derived from raw food. This combination of circumstances results in excessive eating and stasis of food in the colon. The excessive eating occurs because incomplete digestion causes a condition of undernourishment and hunger. When incompletely digested food reaches the colon, the colon reacts by slowing down, causing chronic congestion of food in the colon. After being stretched like this for a few years, the colon can hold several gallons of food. Many people are not "fat," nevertheless, their big bellies hang on their bodies like giant water balloons, except it is not water.

Some people with hypochlorhydria report that food seems to sit in the stomach far too long after a meal. Others say they can eat only a small amount of food before feeling full. Still others are constipated while others have diarrhea. Many have no symptoms referable to the digestive tract.

That is not to say that they have no symptoms, however, because the number of non-intestinal disorders which are associated with hypochlorhydria is truly astounding. Because these diseases can be helped by nutritional means, it is reasonable to consider them nutritional in origin. Here is a list of those diseases associated with hypochlorhydria:

Allergies	Chronic fatigue
Autoimmune Diseases	Weak nails
Thyroid disorders	Dry skin
Diabetes mellitus	Poor night vision
Gallbladder disease	Hypoglycemia
Asthma	Weak Adrenals
Vitiligo	Rheumatic arthritis
Acne rosacea	Lupus erythematosis
Chronic hepatitis	

Given the commonness of the problem, I believe anyone with any of the symptoms or conditions above should have a Heidelberg test or a test trial on hydrochloric acid supplementation. While the Heidelberg test is rather expensive (at present $175), it more than pays for itself when the proper diagnosis is made.

Alternatively, under your doctor's supervision, you may elect to take Betaine HCL with your meals. If you are able to do this without a burning sensation, and if your symptoms are alleviated, this is sufficient, in my opinion, to confirm a diagnosis of hypochlorhydria.

If the diagnosis is not hypochlorhydria, the Heidelberg test will pick up the problem if it exists in the stomach or first part of the small intestine. Hyperacidity, the "Dumping Syndrome" (in which food passes directly from the stomach into the small intestine), achlorhydria (the complete absence of stomach acid), gastritis, gastric ulcer and pyloric insufficiency are all easily seen on the graph drawn by the Heidelberg machine. Even if the test turns out to be perfectly normal, this information can be invaluable, because your doctor does not need to continue to look at your digestive tract for the cause of your problems.

The standard medical approach to hypochlorhydria has been to ignore it and say that it makes no difference. This movement in medicine was partially based on studies using HCL replacement alone. In fact, there is more missing than hydrochloric acid. The same cells (the parietal cells) which make HCL also make pepsinogen, which is converted to pepsin in an acid environment. Therefore, pepsin usually is also deficient and must be replaced for best results. Most Betaine HCL preparations come with 30 or 40 mg. pepsin.

An item called "intrinsic factor" may be in short supply, because it also is made by the parietal cells which produce acid and pepsinogen. Intrinsic factor makes the absorption of vitamin B_{12} possible, and without it B_{12} deficiency sets in. This disease is called pernicious anemia.

The hypochlorhydric stomach often makes insufficient amounts of intrinsic factor and, therefore, it is necessary to give a series of vitamin B_{12} injections to get the best result from treatment of hypochlorhydria.

The question is sometimes asked: what is the root cause of hypochlorhydria, and what can we do to restore function naturally so the stomach resumes its function of manufacturing acid? There probably is a root cause, although we are unaware of what it may be. I suspect it has something to do with an as yet unrecognized nutritional deficiency, although I have nothing to back up this hunch.

There also is the possibility that the parietal cells of the stomach simply die off before the rest of the organism. Perhaps each individual has certain cell lines which are destined to die before the entire organism bites the dust. It also may be that industrial pollution and the pollution of our food supply with pesticides, herbicides and preservatives contributes to the early demise of parietal cells.

Treatment of Hypochlorhydria

We do not yet know the true cause of hypochlorhydria. When we find it out, we may be unable to cure it, but at least we can now treat the condition and return the patient to normal functioning.

Once the diagnosis is certain, one of two items can be used: betaine hydrochloride or glutamic acid hydrochloride. These "carrier molecules" make it possible to introduce the HCL as a powder in a capsule and thus avoid damage to your teeth, which occurs with the liquid form of HCL. These preparations should always contain pepsin for best results.

The solid tablet form of HCL is to be avoided because it is not as effective as the powdered form. When you put the HCL into your stomach with a meal you want it to work then, not later when the tablet has finally dissolved.

The amount of HCL needed can vary from 30 to 100 grains. The largest capsules are ten grains, so this means three to ten caps with each meal. The number per meal can vary based on the quantity and type of food you are eating, but no exact guidelines can be stated. You should start with one cap with a meal, and if this is tolerated, build up with each successive normal meal (whatever is "normal" for you) until you experience a burning sensation. One cap less than that dose which produces a burning sensation is your proper dose for a normal meal. The dosages for smaller or larger meals are adjusted accordingly.

These may seem like large doses; however, they represent considerably less acid than a normally functioning stomach can make. I recommend no more than this, because this amount seems to work. I believe in using the lowest dose of anything which works.

The lab tests which will reveal the benefit of HCL supplementation are: (1) stool analysis to demonstrate complete protein digestion, (2) a blood count to demonstrate correction of pernicious anemia or a previously iron-resistant form of anemia (due to poor iron absorption) and (3) x-rays to demonstrate recalcification of certain types of osteoporosis caused by poor calcium absorption in turn due to low stomach acid.

In addition, a few weeks of supplementary vitamin B_{12} intramuscular injections twice each week usually produces marked improvement in well-being and a clearing of several symptoms. The B_{12} is given in combination with folate, so that folate deficiency is not masked and left untreated by the injections. B_{12} and folate together usually result in more sound sleep, more energy and less anxiety.

As you might suspect, B_{12} injections are out of vogue with the medical establishment because of the fact that a seven year supply of B_{12} can be stored in the liver. The fact that it can be stored does not mean that it *is* stored in this quantity in every individual, however. Even if B_{12} is stored in these quantities, this does not guarantee availability when needed in larger-than-usual quantities.

While it certainly is an inconvenience to supplement stomach acid with each meal for a lifetime it may be less inconvenient than the alternatives. It is well-known that hypochlorhydria is associated with increased risk of stomach cancer, and this may be due to the conversion of nitrites into cancer-inducing nitrosamines in an abnormally alkaline stomach. Also, intestinal overgrowth of bacteria and the incidence of parasitic infections is increased when stomach acid is low. Risk of cancer, risk of parasites, expected bacterial overgrowth and remember the always-present yeast organism, ever ready to become a problem — all adds up to a lot more inconvenience than popping a few betaine HCL caps with each meal.

The doctor who knows the most about diagnosis and treatment of hypochlorhydria is Dr. Jonathan Wright, M.D. of Tahoma, Washington. Dr. Wright is a folk hero among progressive physicians in the U.S. He has the distinction of his clinic having been raided by the FDA, with guns drawn, in 1992. In that raid, his female staff was pat-searched, and much of Dr. Wright's equipment was taken and impounded without cause. The raid came after Dr. Wright sued the FDA for return of his supply of tryptophan, which the FDA had illegally confiscated. Soon after he filed the suit, the FDA showed up with guns drawn to raid his clinic. Next, because he is a courageous doctor who wants the best for his patients, he ordered a supply of preservative-free vitamin B_{12} from Germany (because preservative-free B_{12} is not available in the U.S.). As of this writing his supplies have not been returned, and he has not had the privilege of being charged with any crime which would justify stealing his supplies.

Dr. Wright's response to this fascist tactic on the part of the FDA was to take out a loan, purchase new equipment and go on with his practice of medicine. He also began to offer seminars in nutritional medicine along with his friend and former student, Alan Gaby, M.D. These two physicians have trained thousands of other physicians in the practice of nutritional medicine — just what the FDA wanted to prevent!

The FDA has flatly stated that they intend to put him out of business. In a way, I hope they do, as this will give him more time to teach the rest of us docs how to practice medicine the way he does. If this is the result of FDA raids, I say let us have more of them! Perhaps the rest of us will get lucky, and the FDA will raid our offices also.

See page 358 for instructions on contacting my office for a referral to a doctor experienced in the diagnosis and treatment of hypochlorhydria.

Sources

Wright JV *Dr. Wright's Guide To Healing Nutrition* Keats Publishing Inc., New Canaan Connecticut;1990:31-41. ISBN 0-87983-530-3.

Hartfall SJ Achlorhydria: a review of 336 cases. Guy's Hospital Report, vol. 82;1932:13-39.

Oliver TH, Wilkinson JF Critical review achlorhydria Quarterly Journal of Medicine, vol. 2;1933: 431-455.

Schiff L, Tahl T The effects of dessicated hog's stomach in achlorhydria Amer J Diges Dis vol. 1;1934-35:543-548.

Williams RH The Adrenals in *Textbook of Endocrinology, 5th ed.*, WB Saunders;1974:271.

Dotevall G, Walan A Gastric secretion of acid and intrinsic factor in patients with hyper- and hypothyroidism Acta Med Scan, vol. 186;1969:529-533.

Matthews DM, linnell JC Vitamin B_{12}: an area of darkness Brit Med Jour, Sept. 1, 1979:533-535.

Jacobs A, Rhodes J, Eakins JD Gastric factors influencing iron absorption in anemic patients Scan Jour Haematology, vol. 4, 1967:105-110.

Gillespie M, Hypochlorhydria in asthma with special reference to the age incidence Quar Jour Med, vol. 4;1935:397-405.

Ruddell WSJ et.al. Gastric juice nitrite Lancet, Nov. 13;1976: 1037-1039.

Rabinowitch IM Achlorhydria and its clinical significance in diabetes mellitus Amer Jour of Diges Dis, Sept. 1949:322-332.

Gianelli RA Broitman SA Zamcheck N Influence of gastric acidity on bacterial, and parasitic enteric infections Ann of Int Med, vol. 78;1973:271-276.

DeWitte TJ et.al. Hypochlorhydria and Hypergastrinemia in rheumatoid arthritis Ann of the Rheu Dis, vol. 38;1979:14-17.

Ryel JA et.al. Gastric analysis in acne rosacea Lancet, Dec. 11, 1920:1195-1196.

THE COLON

With your car, you can rely on a mechanic to perform maintenance. With your body, you do it yourself or it goes undone. A thorough knowledge of the entire digestive tract is necessary to allow you to perform needed maintenance procedures for your digestive system. It is important to understand the three basic areas of digestion: the stomach, the small intestine and the large intestine.

Please consult an encyclopedia for a diagram of the digestive tract. Locate the structures on the diagram mentioned in this discussion.

The stomach and small intestine together are called the "upper intestine," or "upper GI." The colon and rectum are is known as the "lower intestine," or "lower GI." In the stomach, a load of hydrochloric acid is dumped on your food, transforming it into "chyme." After two hours of this kind of harsh treatment, chyme is moved into the small intestine where it is acted on by bile from the liver and digestive enzymes from the pancreas. Bile breaks down fat into fatty acids, so that lipases, the enzymes for fat from the pancreas, can break down the fatty acids. Proteinases breaks down proteins. Amylase breaks down carbohydrates and is secreted both in the small intestine and in the mouth.

Between hydrochloric acid, amylase, lipases and proteinases, the upper digestive tract breaks down the food you eat. When food has reached the end of the small intestine and is prepared to be pushed into the large intestine by peristalsis, a waving rhythmic contracture of the intestines, almost all of the nutrients have been extracted and absorbed.

The best way to take care of your upper intestine is to eat a lot of high-fiber foods. We will deal with that later in this book. The upper intestine is easy to take care of, just eat the right foods and make sure you have plenty of stomach acid and enzymes.

The colon is another matter. The entire digestive tract is, on average, 28 feet long, about nine meters. The last five of these 28 feet is the colon. The colon is the toxic waste dump of the body, and most people take care of it by ignoring it and pretending that it does not exist. We treat the body in a parallel fashion to the way we have treated waste disposal in society.

It is no secret that the world is an increasingly more toxic place in which to live. This began with the industrial revolution. We breath toxins, they contact our skin, we drink them, and we eat them. Pollutants are everywhere, beginning with our drinking water, which is treated with heavy doses of chlorine to kill the bacteria. If chlorine kills bacteria, by the way, how do you suppose it treats the cells of your body? The only solution to this problem is to drink only steam distilled water (see pages 165-167).

Where food is concerned, the typical western diet is loaded with pesticides, has been treated with artificial fertilizer and contains artificial preservatives. The usual human diet has been altered drastically in the last seven or eight generations. The best solution here is to eat only fresh, organically grown foods of plant origin.

How likely is it, however, that you will be able to drink only steam distilled water and eat only fresh, organically grown foods of plant origin? If you are able to stay at home all day and grow your own food, maybe you can. Not likely.

The situation described here leads us to a discussion of the colon, because it is the colon which must finally encounter all these toxins, and the usual result is an overwhelmed colon. The colon is not immune to all these toxins; the result is a sick colon, which, like any sick organ, slows down and retains these waste products longer than it otherwise would.

"Transit time" is the time it takes a meal to travel from the dinner table to elimination from the colon. A healthy transit time is twelve to eighteen hours. However, the usual transit time in western countries is 65-100 hours! Putrefaction happens when that which has been rejected for digestion by your body is broken down by bacteria. Bacteria extract the last possible food value from the contents of the colon, and the waste products from that process are reabsorbed back into the body. As mentioned in the chapter on fasting, this is called "autointoxication" or "self-poisoning."

If you handle your body any other way than by eating only fresh, organically grown foods of plant origin, with plenty of pure water (about eight large glasses per day), you suffer from some degree of autointoxication. Even if you do treat your body to fresh, organically grown foods of plant origin, and you are older than 21 years, your colon is slow with age, and you also experience some degree of autointoxication. The point here is that your colon is probably sick right now, to some degree, whether or not you know it.

The most common symptom of autointoxication is mental dullness and fatigue. Other common symptoms are headache, constipation, diarrhea, colds, general aches and pains, particularly up and down the spine and especially in the low back, skin problems, common infections (due to lowered immuno-competence), morning sluggishness, gas, bad breath, foul-smelling stool, allergies, intolerance to fatty foods, premenstrual tension, breast soreness and tendency to repeated vaginal infections.

Most colon therapists are convinced, as I certainly am, that the great increase in colon cancer over the past few generations is due to autointoxication in the colon. High-fiber foods change the bacterial flora of your colon to noncarcinogenic organisms and drastically reduce the possibility of colon cancer.

The big problem with becoming responsible for your colon is that no one wants to. Let's face it, this is not a nice area of the body to deal with. Nevertheless, it is necessary to deal with it, if you are to be fully responsible for your body. If you are not willing to handle the colon and keep it handled for the rest of your life, I assure you that you will pay a high price, much higher than any inconvenience you may experience in handling your colon now.

That said, what is to be done? There are two qualities you want to have in your colon. You want it to be (1) clean and (2) functional. If you are under 21 and eating only fresh, organically grown foods of plant origin, and your upper gastrointestinal tract is working well, relax. However, if you are not, you need to put some attention to this matter.

How does one cleanse one's colon? How do you even know if it needs cleansing? You cannot look inside it to see how dirty it is. However, if you have symptoms from it, you can be sure it is quite messed up. Pain, discomfort, swelling, gas, constipation, a big belly; all these symptoms should tip you off that your colon is in trouble.

When food putrefies, the colon secretes mucus to protect itself. This mucus then glues the putrefied food to the colon wall where it may remain for years. If this has happened, there is little likelihood that you will be able to handle this problem by yourself. If it hasn't happened, you have no way of knowing it hasn't happened. Either way, I recommend at least one visit to a colon therapist. Everyone should have a dentist, and everyone should have a colon therapist.

I recognize that this is a frightening prospect. However, an experienced colon therapist can put you at ease and teach you more about your colon in one hour than you can ever learn from reading about the subject and much more than the typical physician knows.

So, how do you cleanse your colon? To be certain of the result, see a colon therapist. How do your keep your colon clean? Eat only fresh, organically grown foods of plant origin for starters. Beyond that, follow the recommendations of your colon therapist. This may include taking an intestinal bulking agent like psyllium or guar and an herbal agent to stimulate the colon and bring it back to life.

"Clean" and "functional" are the key words. "Clean" means without putrefied material glued to the inside of your colon by mucus. "Functional" means a fast transit time, something like 8-24 hours. What you eat now should be out within 24 hours.

I am not laying out a generic program for everyone to follow, because I cannot know your particular situation. My task here is to make you aware of the possibilities and to mention a few good reasons for you to follow up on this area, learn more and take better care of your colon. After those tasks are accomplished the rest is your responsibility.

To locate a qualified colon therapist in your area, you should contact:

The International Association of Colon Therapists
11739 Washington Blvd.
Los Angeles, California 90066
(310) 390-5424

> **I do not have a comprehensive list of colon therapists, so please rely on the above information for a referral.**

KIDNEY FUNCTION AND CARE

The kidneys are twin organs with one on either side of the spine in the region of the mid-back (when reclining) to lower mid-back (when upright). They are bean shaped, and each one is about the size of your two fists together. Each is supplied with a renal artery and renal vein for delivery and removal of blood which is filtered and returned to the body. Each kidney is supplied with about one million glomeruli — microscopic tangles of capillaries — each surrounded by a capsule draining through the renal tubular system to the ureter and thence to the bladder.

Please consult an encyclopedia for a diagram of the kidneys. Locate the structures on the diagram mentioned in this discussion.

You can simulate the relationship between a glomerulus and its Bowman's capsule by making a fist with your left hand and holding it in your right hand. Your left hand represents the glomerulus and your right hand represents Bowman's capsule. In this model, blood is delivered and removed through the structure represented by your left hand and waste products are carried away by the structure represented by your right hand.

Each glomerulus contains a tiny network of capillaries through which blood flows and is cleansed. The healthy kidney very precisely removes exactly what needs to be removed for the body to stay in a vital state. The kidneys are miraculous, and their functions are only crudely duplicated by dialysis machines.

The job of the kidneys is to filter the blood and remove toxins and waste products. As with most other organs, nature has given you much more than you need to survive. You can donate or lose one of your kidneys and never miss it as long as the other kidney stays healthy. When the kidneys are diseased, it is possible to destroy up to 75% of the functioning glomeruli and still be healthy.

Nevertheless, the kidneys are a common source of illness due to mistreatment from negligence or ignorance. Infection is the most common form of disease to affect the kidneys. Usually bacteria reach the kidneys by ascending the urinary tract. Due to the obvious anatomical differences between men and women, kidney infections are more common in women. For a bacterium, the trip from outside of the body to the bladder is much shorter and easier to negotiate in a woman than in a man. Therefore, urethritis (infection of the ureters, the tiny tubes which bring urine into the bladder) may be followed by cystitis (*cyst* = bladder in latin). Infection of the kidney tissue itself is called "nephritis." Infection of the large collection system (the pelvis) leading to the ureter is called "pyelitis." A combined infection of the kidney and its pelvis is called "pyelonephritis."

If the infection ascends through the drainage structure, you will usually be aware of pain and burning on urination. If it appears first in the kidneys, you may become aware of pain in the back and tenderness over the area of the kidneys. When you bend forward you may experience pain up and down the back from stretching the inflamed tissues. You also may experience burning on urination (dysuria), the desire to urinate when you cannot (urgency), and you may note cloudy or foul urine (pyuria). **On the other hand, there may be no symptoms at all, a so-called "silent" infection**.

"Glomerulonephritis" is a primary inflammation of the kidney tissues, which does not involve the drainage structures (the glomeruli). It usually follows a streptococcal infection in the kidneys or in another part of the body, most commonly the throat, by three to six weeks. It is thought to be an autoimmune disease involving antibodies made in response to the streptococcal infection, which then attack the glomeruli of the kidneys. Usually a course of antibiotics handles this illness, although it makes no sense that it should, and no one knows why it does. A few people do progress to an asymptomatic condition known as "chronic nephritis" which progresses on to kidney failure within a few years.

Artery disease caused by a poor diet and low exercise level also can affect the arterial system supplying the kidneys. This illness is known as "nephrosclerosis" (literally kidney hardening), as the kidneys are noted to be hardened when examined at surgery or at autopsy. The kidneys feel hard because the arterioles are hardened and the kidney is made up in large part by the arteriolar system. (Arterioles are the small branches of arteries before they branch into tiny capillaries.)

Kidney stones ("renal calculi") may develop when the level of calcium and oxalate is abnormally high, as when the parathyroid gland becomes diseased or when there is excessive intake of dairy products. When the level of uric acid becomes abnormally high due to excessive intake of meat, gout can develop and cause the development of uric acid crystals in the drainage system of the kidneys. (Gout also can cause severe arthritis in the big toes, which is the classic picture of gout.) The most excruciating pain known to man is the movement of kidney stones down the ureter. If the stones are too large to pass, surgery may be required or lithotripsy may be employed, which uses focused shock waves originating from outside the body to break up the stones, so they are small enough to pass.

The purpose of giving you this information is to make you aware of your kidneys. The awareness of the individual has more to do with the prevention and early treatment of disease than any other factor. The astuteness of a good physician is useless unless you know when to make an appointment and show up in the office. Awareness of the structure and function of the kidney, along with the possibility of the various disease states, can go a long way toward preventing disease altogether.

Here are measures you can take to help prevent kidney disease:

1. Bathe each day, and use soap in the groin region, as this is the origin of ascending urinary tract infections. Women with UTI (urinary tract infection) problems should take only showers, because reflux of bath water up the urethra plays an important role in beginning UTIs in women.

2. In the case of streptococcal infections, the sooner they are treated the less is the possibility of progression into glomerulonephritis, which can turn into chronic glomerulitis and finally renal failure, a deadly condition requiring dialysis and/or kidney transplant. Prompt treatment of infection applies especially to sore throats, because this area of the body is more frequently infected with streptococcus than other areas.

3. Stay totally away from pasteurized, homogenized dairy products and excessively high protein diets. Eat complex carbohydrate foods (veggies) to balance protein intake on a ratio of ten grams carbs to each seven grams protein. This will tend to prevent kidney stones and, over the long term, will prevent or perhaps reverse hardening of the arteries and thus prevent or reverse nephrosclerosis.

4. Drink plenty of steam distilled or double-filtered/reverse osmosis water each day, at least six 8 oz. glasses, preferably eight. A plentiful supply of water makes transport of cellular waste products from the cells to the kidneys easier, as well as filtration of same much more efficient for your kidneys. Do not, for God's sake, drink tap water!

See page 358 for instructions on contacting my office for a referral to a doctor familiar with treatment of kidney conditions.

THE PANCREAS

Please consult an encyclopedia for a diagram of the pancreas and the surrounding organs. Locate the structures on the diagram mentioned in this discussion.

The pancreas is a small lumpy gland with a head and a tail with the head pointed to your right. The pancreas would fit easily in the palm of your hand, as it weighs only about 85 grams. It is located on the posterior wall of the abdominal cavity at the level of your belly button. It lies transversely across that wall and consists of two glands in one.

The larger gland is the so-called "exocrine" gland, which manufactures and supplies digestive enzymes to the small intestine. These enzymes include lipase, proteinase and amylase for the digestion of fat, protein and complex carbohydrates respectively. These enzymes are injected through the pancreatic duct into the head of the duodenum (the first part of the small intestine) about four centimeters from the pyloris, the valve that separates the stomach from the duodenum. The secretion of these enzymes is stimulated by the presence of food in the duodenum. Because enzymes are injected into the open space of the duodenum, this part of the pancreas is called *exo*crine (exo = outside).

The smaller gland in the pancreas is made of many anatomically separated glands called the "Islets of Langerhans," after the person who first described them. They are seen, by microscopic section of the pancreas, to be clumps of cells isolated from each other and embedded in the exocrine tissue of the pancreas. The Islets of Langerhans secrete their products directly into the blood stream, thus earning the name *endo*crine ("endo" = inside) gland. These products are called "insulin" and "glucagon," and they have the function of regulating the metabolism of sugar in the body.

The consumption of alcohol is very hard on the pancreas. It is even less able to withstand alcohol than the other organs of the body. There is a variety of toxic substances in coffee, some of which are thought to be damaging to the pancreas (and the adrenal glands), particularly caffeine and tannic acid.

Equally or even more toxic substances to the pancreas are the simple sugars. Ingestion of large amounts of sugar results in degeneration of the tissues in the body and sugar is hidden in almost all processed foods which are commonly eaten in the West.

When the pancreas degenerates, the result is a decreased ability to respond with the secretion of enzymes to the presence of food in the small intestine and an imbalanced ability to respond with insulin and glucagon to the presence of sugar in the blood. The final result is a lessened ability to carry on the vital functions of the body, because less nutrition is being delivered to the cells. When the body is receiving less nutrition, appetite is stimulated, and greater quantities of food are ingested — but to little avail, since the pancreas cannot respond adequately.

The overall result is a colon overworked by shear quantity of food. Under this circumstance the colon slows down, allowing food to collect and putrefy there. This releases toxins, which the body must deal with. This process accounts for premature aging so commonly seen and — combined with hyperinsulinism/insulin resistance disease — for the rather round figure commonly associated with middle age.

By age twenty, at least in people eating a typical Western diet, the pancreas is already seriously compromised. This shows up as increased appetite, slowed digestion with excess gas and loss of normal vitality.

The good news is that it is possible to provide the conditions for the pancreas to regenerate its normal capacity to handle food and sugar. The first step is to stop the ingestion of alcohol, coffee and all other forms of caffeine and excessive carbohydrates and then balance your diet in relationship to protein and carbohydrate in a ratio of 7:10. This allows the pancreas an opportunity to heal in the absence of further insult. This is the first and most important condition for regeneration of function. It is possible to do even more by using oral pancreatic enzymes. These are available off the shelf of your organic grocer, health food or vitamin store. Simply buy a supply, and take them within the dose range recommended on the label at every meal.

It is possible to have assays done to determine if you need enzyme replacement or not. However, in my opinion, the best test available is to use a good enzyme replacement for a period of ten days and see if you notice a difference. The evidence that this therapy for the pancreas is making a difference is better digestion and greater vitality.

You may or may not need this therapy for the rest of your life. As your pancreas regenerates its abilities, you may be able to come off enzyme replacement without a noticeable difference. My experience is that one to two years are necessary to see full regeneration of the pancreas to a youthful condition. For other reasons, discussed on pages 178-192, you may elect to continue to supplement with enzymes, even after your pancreas is up to the job again.

See page 358 for instructions on contacting my office for a referral to a doctor experienced in the treatment of pancreatic diseases.

THE LIVER AND GALLBLADDER

Please consult an encyclopedia for a diagram of the liver and gallbladder. Locate the structures on the diagram mentioned in this discussion.

The liver is derived embryologically from the gastrointestinal tract, budding off that part of the GI tract which will become the duodenum in the first trimester (first third) of pregnancy. The liver is located in the right upper quadrant (quarter) of the abdomen directly below the diaphragm. It is the largest organ in the human body.

Unlike any other organ, the liver has a dual blood supply, one arterial and the other venous. The arterial blood supply comes from the hepatic artery which is a branch off of the aorta (the great vessel coming from the heart) and brings fresh, oxygenated blood. The other blood supply comes through the hepatic portal system and brings nutrient rich "venous" (i.e., already having passed through a capillary bed and on its way back to the heart) blood from the small and large intestines, the pancreas and the spleen.

Blood coming directly from the digestive tract requires immediate attention and processing. Not only is it rich in nutrients, which need to be stored in the liver, it also is rich in toxic material derived from the digestive process. It may also have a load of toxins usually present in the colon of a person eating a typical Western diet rich in cooked foods.

Blood leaving the liver is collected in the hepatic vein, and from there it goes to the inferior vena cava thence to the right side of the heart for a trip through the lungs and a bath in oxygen.

The liver is divided into hundreds of thousands of lobules, each one a storage and detoxification plant. Each lobule receives a dual blood supply, just like the liver as a whole, from the digestive tract (the portal system) and the hepatic artery. Each one drains into the hepatic vein. Each cell in the liver makes direct contact via capillaries with all three of these systems: portal vein, hepatic artery and hepatic vein. The first two deliver nutrients and fresh blood respectively. The hepatic vein delivers deoxygenated blood, along with processed nutrients, back to the heart.

There is a second drainage system (besides the hepatic vein) to which each liver cell has direct access. This is called the "canalicular system." Each canaliculus drains into progressively larger ducts and culminates in the hepatic duct, which combines with the duct coming from the gallbladder to form the common bile duct. The common bile duct empties, in turn, into the duodenum. Most waste products formed by the liver exit the body through this system, and the rest is shunted via the blood stream to the kidneys, where it is excreted in the urine.

Notice on your diagram of the liver the position of the gallbladder and the bile duct. The gallbladder is a small sac, about the size of a golf ball, attached to the inferior surface of the liver. It stores the bile, a mixture of emulsifying agents, which are useful in the breakdown of fats for digestion by lipase from the pancreas. The gallbladder empties its contents through the common bile duct into the duodenum in response to the presence of fatty substances in that organ. There it emulsifies the fat into small globules, making it easier for lipase to make contact and do its job.

About 1.4 liters of blood pass through the liver every minute and, at any time, the liver contains ten percent of the blood volume of the entire body. The liver is capable of storing large quantities of glucose as glycogen, a starchy substance made of glucose molecules which allows the controlled release of glucose into the circulatory system on an as needed basis. The conversion of glycogen to glucose is controlled by the presence of insulin from the Islets of Langerhans in the pancreas.

It is this substance — glycogen — which endurance athletes try to build a large store of by eating lots of starchy foods the day before a contest. The liver also is responsible for storage of iron, copper, vitamins A, D and a large number of B vitamins. It also produces albumin, the major protein found in the blood, as well as prothrombin, fibrogen and heparin, all extremely important to the normal clotting and healing of wounds.

Amino acids are deaminated in the liver, and the nitrogen is made available for metabolism in the body as a whole. The liver also synthesizes cholesterol, which is necessary for construction and maintenance of cell walls and for the synthesis of many hormones. The liver can, to some degree, balance the proportion of carbohydrates, proteins and fats and make up for disproportionate intake in this way. This is achieved by the liver's ability to both break these substances down and reassemble them into different forms: fat to protein, protein to carbohydrate, carbohydrate to fat, carbohydrate to protein, etc.

Certain white blood cells (phagocytes), when they are in the liver, remove foreign substances and destroy bacteria. Drugs are detoxified in the liver, and cholesterol is excreted through the bile, which flows through the bile duct into the intestine. Also, hemoglobin breakdown — a natural outcome of aging of red blood cells — is accomplished in the liver and excreted as "bilirubin."

Naturally, all this metabolic activity produces a lot of heat, and together with the heart and skeletal muscles, the liver has a major role in maintaining normal body temperature.

This information is meant to assist you in placing the liver and its gallbladder in your awareness, so that you know you have them and so that you can live your life in a way that supports the health of these organs. It must be clear from the description above that the liver is "vital," i.e., necessary for life. You would die without your liver in a matter of days.

Because the liver has so much reserve capacity, it is possible to live with up to ninety percent of your liver function destroyed. However, when that line is crossed, deterioration of general health is rapid. Furthermore, you cannot enjoy all the vitality which is possible for you with less than 100% of your normal liver function.

The health of the liver is a reflection of the health of the rest of the body. There are do's and don'ts regarding the liver. Do enjoy a diet balanced in carbohydrates, proteins and fats; do achieve and maintain your ideal body weight; do not expose yourself to toxic chemicals such as alcohol. The most important thing you can do for the health and vitality of your liver is be aware that it exits; be aware of the jobs it does, and appreciate it. This will lead naturally to the desire to maintain excellent general health and therefore a very healthy liver.

The major diseases of the liver are cirrhosis and hepatitis. Cirrhosis is a scarring process combined with an attempt at regeneration. Liver cells can regenerate themselves but do a poor job of it, architecturally speaking. Regeneration of liver cells follows fatty degeneration caused by any prolonged toxic insult to the liver, the most common being ingestion of alcohol. Prevention lies in avoiding the ingestion of substances which damage the liver.

Hepatitis is caused by invasion of the liver tissues by an infective agent, sometimes a bacteria but most commonly a virus. Viral hepatitis is a serious, life-threatening disease. It is transmitted by fecal contamination of anything entering the body and through dirty needles. People who inject street drugs run a high risk of hepatitis and AIDS. While AIDS gets all the publicity, hepatitis kills many more people. Prevention lies in maintaining sanitary conditions and avoiding dirty needles.

The major diseases of the gallbladder are called "cholecystitis" (literally gallbladder inflammation) and cholelithiasis (literally gallbladder stones). These diseases are much more common in people who are overweight, in people over forty and especially in pregnant women. However, the most important factor in gallbladder disease often is overlooked — allergy. A gallbladder attack, with or without stones present, is often a manifestation of allergy. This should never be overlooked, and it should always be suspected. Many people have had unnecessary gallbladder surgery because the doctor was not informed, or simply forgot about this aspect of gallbladder problems.

See page 358 for instructions on contacting my office for a referral to a doctor experienced in the treatment of liver and gallbladder problems.

THE BRAIN AND SPINAL CORD

Consult your encyclopedia and locate a diagram of the brain and spinal cord.

The structure and function of the brain and spinal cord are so complex, we cannot cover what is known in this book, even in general terms. The purpose of this section of the book is to place the presence of the brain and spinal cord in your awareness, so that you appreciate having them.

The brain and spinal cord together are known as the "central nervous system" ("CNS"). They are derived, embryologically, from the same layer of cells that gives rise to the skin: the ectoderm. This seems appropriate, since the skin and CNS, together with the various sense organs, are derived from these two structures and deal with the task of sensing and interpreting the external world.

The brain is a biological computer of remarkable capacity to which the human spirit is fused in a poorly understood way. The brain is divided into three parts: the forebrain, the midbrain and the hindbrain. The forebrain is the thinking part of the brain: the cortex, with gray matter containing ten billion neurons — individual brain cells. This is the "hardware" of the system, the neural space in which information can reside.

As knowledge is gained, neurons develop more connections between each other and evidently exchange information through these new "hard wires." The midbrain is a relay station between the body and the cortex with its ten billion neurons. The hindbrain is made up of the pons and cerebellum, which are responsible for coordination of the musculoskeletal system and the medulla where breathing and heartbeat is regulated.

The CNS is divided into the motor system and the sensory system. These systems exist side by side. The motor system is designed to carry out movement of the body. The sensory system is designed to sense the reality around the body. Somewhere in between the motor and sensory systems cognition (thinking) occurs.

The automatic functions of the body such as digestion, heartbeat, breathing, etc., are handled by the Autonomic Nervous System, the ANS. The ANS is divided into the sympathetic and the parasympathetic systems. The Sympathetic Nervous System is designed to survive the body in emergency and is responsible for the fight or flight response in all its variations. The Parasympathetic Nervous System is designed to survive the body in nonemergency situations. It handles the so-called "vegetative functions," such as eating, digesting, pumping blood, sexing, etc.

Part of what you are conscious of, in any given moment, is a dynamic interplay between these various systems. Because survival of the species is dependent on the overall survival of consciousness, nature considers the safety of the CNS to be of paramount importance. Accordingly, nature has evolved a strong housing for the CNS, the skull and vertebral column. The brain and spinal cord are suspended in a liquid medium and surrounded by three layers of protective coating, the pia mater, the arachnoid and the dura mater. The latter is a tough, tear-resistant covering.

The brain requires a lot of energy and therefore receives fully 25% of the blood volume pumped by the heart at rest. It also requires constant cleansing and has its own unique system of cleansing itself, called the "ventricular system." Cerebrospinal fluid (CSF) is created by filtration of the blood in the lateral ventricles, cavities in the left and right hemispheres of the forebrain. The CSF flows through these ventricles and into the third ventricle, bathing and cleansing the midbrain, then to the fourth ventricle, bathing and cleansing the hindbrain and finally into the space surrounding the spinal cord, bathing and cleansing the spinal cord, where it is reabsorbed into the blood.

The fuel used for energy by the brain is limited to only two: glucose and oxygen. Although there are many nutrients necessary for proper brain function, only glucose and oxygen are use for energy. To many substances, especially those made up of large molecular size and weight, there is a barrier to admission, a kind of wrapping, around the blood vessels which supply the brain, called the "blood brain barrier." In a healthy condition, the blood brain barrier admits only those substances to the brain tissue, including glucose and oxygen, which the brain can utilize for its nutritional or energy needs.

The neurons of the brain are surrounded by helper cells, responsible for keeping them clean and well nourished. These are called "glial" cells. The brain of Einstein, although unremarkable in terms of numbers of neurons, was found to contain twice the usual number of glial cells, so they are apparently very important to clear thinking. These cells are, in turn, supported by the capillary bed through which the brain is perfused with blood.

The health of the arteriolar system supplying this capillary bed is the weak point in brain health. Along with the arteriolar system supplying the capillary bed, which supports the heart, this system in the brain is the most critically important capillary bed in the body. With age, poor diet and lack of regular exercise, this arteriolar system becomes blocked and susceptible to "infarction" (loss of blood supply). When this happens, it is called a "stroke" and, depending on the area or areas of the brain infarcted, one loses this or that mental function.

For example, there is an area on the left parietal lobe of the cortex called "Broca's Speech Area." If the vessel to this area is blocked, one losses one's ability to speak. Prevention of this kind of event lies in proper diet over a lifetime, a balanced diet of carbs, protein and fat, along with the liberal intake of antioxidants. Take care of it or lose it. A condition of atherosclerosis of the brain (or heart) also can be helped by a course of chelation therapy. See pages 14-24 for a more thorough discussion of chelation therapy.

The brain loses ten percent of its neurons every ten years, due to age. This can be more than made up for by increased interconnectivity between the remaining neurons. Mental capacity does not have to decrease with age, but it will unless these new interconnections are made. These connections are created by using the mind through learning. If you stop learning, you lose your mind with age, little by little. I recently read a study which followed a group of 100 very bright and inquisitive men from age seventy to age eighty. In this group of men, intelligence at eighty was measurably greater than it had been at seventy, evidently because these men pursued knowledge even in those advanced years. Use it or lose it.

A final word about the brain relates to illness. The brain is in charge of the body more than any other organ. It also houses at least part of the psyche. It is not surprising, therefore, that the brain can produce effects in the body which mimic physical illness for purposes known only to the unconscious reaches of the psyche — often to distract your attention away from emotions it wishes to repress and keep away from your awareness.

Making the distinction between a physically based illness and a psychosomatic illness is never complete until this possibility is carefully considered. Most backaches, stomachaches, headaches, etc., are, in part, psychosomatic illnesses. Treating them only physically misses the real opportunity..

See page 358 for instructions on contacting my office for a referral to a doctor experienced in the treatment of nervous system disorders.

THE JOINTS

The experience of youthfulness, at any age, is determined by the condition of your joints more than by any other system of the body. When joints are in a healthy condition, the body moves easily. This agility is characteristic of youth and of people who have maintained the health of their joints over their lifetimes.

A joint is present wherever two bones meet each other. There are movable and immovable joints. Immovable joints are not designed to move in relationship to each other. If they do, breakage occurs.

Immovable joints are divided into two categories. One is the rigid and absolutely immovable type of joints known as "synarthroses" (literally together joints). For example, the connection between the various bones of the skull and the attachment of the different bones of the pelvis. These bones are held together by actual intergrowth of the bones and by strong fibrous cartilage, which cannot be stretched.

The other kind of "immovable" joints are called "symphyses," an example of which is the pubic symphysis, the joint which binds the two pubic bones together in the pubic symphysis, the anterior center part of the pelvis. Symphyses are held together by elastic (stretchable) cartilage.

The rest of the joints are freely movable, according to their design, and are known as "diarthroses" (movable joints). They include the joints of the extremities (arms and legs) and the vertebral column. Diarthroses are lined with a very smooth, glass-like cartilage, which is lubricated by a thick fluid: the synovial fluid, which is produced by the synovial membrane — the lining of the joint. These joints make us what we are — without them we would be as statues.

There are several types of movable joints (diarthroses). One type of diarthrosis is called "ball and socket." These are found in the shoulders and hips where the arms and legs attach to the trunk. These joints allow free movement in all directions. Without them, we would walk and move as the robot C3PO of Star Wars.

Hinge joints allow movement in flexion and extension and are found in elbows, knees and fingers.

A pivot joint allows only for rotation, and there is only one in the human body: the junction between atlas and axis (the first and second vertebrae of the spinal column). In this joint rests your ability to rotate your head from side to side.

Gliding joints, in which the surfaces of the joints slide over each other for short distances, are found in the carpal and tarsal bones of the wrist and ankle respectively.

Diseases of Joints

The condition of inflammation in a joint is called "arthritis," literally joint inflammation. There are several varieties. Osteoarthritis is, by far, the most common, affecting one out of every fifteen people in the U.S. and Europe. It affects women more often than men and may advance to destructive changes in the joints.

The causes of this disorder are poor nutrition, poor digestion, and low levels of exercise over a long period of time. The best treatment is a diet balanced in protein and carbohydrate, relatively low in salt and sugar, and a regular program of exercise augmented with antioxidants. (More later on this.) It is critically important to evaluate digestion in a case of arthritis, because disordered digestion is probably the major cause of arthritis.

Contrary to popular myth, milk products are not good for the joints (or bones), only bad for the entire body. There is more than sufficient calcium in a vegetable oriented diet. A hypercalcific, milk-centered diet promotes arthritis. I suspect that the addition of pesticides to growing foods plays a role in osteoarthritis as well. I strongly suggest that you eat only organically grown foods.

Symptomatic treatment of osteoarthritis should be undertaken, in my opinion, only after all natural methods of treatment (diet, treatment of digestive disorders, exercise, stretching, antioxidants) have been used and found not to provide complete relief. The ingestion of drugs which inhibit prostaglandins synthesis provide some relief for the inflammation of osteoarthritis. It is possible to spend a fortune on some of these new drugs.

What the drug companies are trying to keep from public awareness, is that the best prostaglandins inhibitor is very inexpensive, very safe, protects against cancer and heart attack as well and has been around since 1899 — ordinary aspirin. There are no large profits for drug companies in trying to market a drug which has been around seventy years after its patent expired.

From a doctor's point of view, there is little to impress the patient by saying "Go take aspirin." Therefore, doctors prescribe drugs which are new, extremely expensive and do not work as well as aspirin. Children should not receive aspirin due to Reye's Syndrome (a type of encephalitis) which may be caused by aspirin. For adults, no problem at all except that it increases slightly the time required for blood clotting (this quality also provides protection from heart attacks). If you are scheduled for surgery, take no aspirin for three weeks before surgery.

Another type of arthritis is rheumatoid arthritis. This is a much more debilitating illness, although mercifully, a much more rare disease, affecting about one out of every 240 people in the U.S. and Europe. It can be extremely painful. The classic picture of rheumatoid arthritis is that of red swollen fingers held in an abnormally flexed position, the small fingers being the most flexed and the index finger being the least flexed. The wrist also is held in a flexed position.

However, rheumatoid arthritis is a systemic disease affecting much more than the hands. It causes inflammation in connective tissue throughout the body and is accompanied by fever, weakness and fatigue as well as the deformity already mentioned.

This disease affects women much more than men and also affects children. The cause is unknown. While there is a hereditary predisposition (if your parents have it, you are more likely to have it), the cause also may involve an as yet unidentified virus and repression of anger. It, too, has a strong relationship with digestive dysfunction, and a comprehensive digestive analysis should be part of every workup for rheumatoid arthritis.

Conservative treatment is the same as for osteoarthritis. Severe cases can be treated with gold compounds, hydroxychloroquinone, penicillamine, and/or surgery.

Arthritis also can be caused by gout. The classic picture is an obese person with a red, swollen, painful big toe, although gout also is a disease affecting connective tissue throughout the body. The treatment is a diet high in complex carbohydrates, relatively low in salt, sugar, fat and protein. Gout is caused by the deposition in the joints of the breakdown products of protein.

Rheumatic fever also can account for arthritis. The presentation is similar to osteoarthritis and the treatment is penicillin. Rheumatic fever is the body's own immune reaction to the streptococcus bacterium.

In addition to joint damage, rheumatic fever also can result in damage to the heart valves (particularly the mitral valve) and to the kidneys (glomerulonephritis). Prevention rests on the prompt treatment of streptococcal infections. Most strep infections occur in the throat, so while you may think of a throat infection as not so important, you could live to regret that point of view. Strep also is the most common cause of bacterial dermatitis.

Ankylosing spondylitis is a disease sharing many characteristics of rheumatoid arthritis. The cause is unknown although, like rheumatoid arthritis, it is thought to be related to a genetic predisposition, perhaps a virus, perhaps repressed anger or some combination of the three. The disease attacks the lower back, eventually fusing together the lumbar vertebrae. It may extend higher, in severe cases, to the thoracic or even cervical vertebrae. The treatment is the same as rheumatoid arthritis. This is an extremely painful and difficult to manage disease.

Doctors are just beginning to realize that all of the arthritides, except rheumatic arthritis, are related to digestive disorders. The importance of this aspect of the evaluation cannot be overemphasized. If you have an arthritis and your doctor has not evaluated you for digestive dysfunction, call this to his or her attention.

Prevention of Joint Disease

The best medicine for the joints is prevention, and prevention begins with a proper diet high in complex carbohydrates, relatively low in salt, sugar, fat and protein, combined with sensible exercise to keep the joints strong through use.

There is some debate about the long-term effect of jogging. Many feel that jogging, over a period of years, combines with any inherited weakness of the joints to produce arthritis. The most common joints affected are the knees and the lower back. The intervertebral discs may be most affected by the constant up and down jarring of running. I recommend against running on a regular long-term basis. Save running for the occasional game of basketball, football, tennis, handball, etc.

The best exercise is swimming and the second best is using a machine which works out the arms and shoulders, as well as the legs and heart — such as the Schwinn Aerodyne exercycle. Rowing machines also are excellent, and walking is better than nothing. Whatever you use, it should be used regularly, at least three times per week. This will handle your aerobic needs as well.

Where stretching is concerned, it is important to maintain the normal range of motion of all joints; however, it is possible to overdo it. Vigorous stretching, while it may feel good now, stresses the ligament structures around the joint and causes microscopic tearing of ligaments. Ligaments do not repair themselves. When enough fibers are broken, the adjacent joint will become unstable, and there will be movement in directions for which it was not made. If this happens, there is prolotherapy, but it is better to avoid the problem in the first place. If you practice stretching, take it easy, do not overdo it.

See page 358 for instructions on contacting my office for a referral to a doctor experienced in the treatment of joint disease.

THE SKIN

As you may have noticed, skin covers the entire exterior surface of the human body. Its functions are to (1) protect the deeper tissues from injury, (2) prevent the wholesale escape of fluids from the body, (3) help maintain body temperature within a constant range, (4) assist the kidneys in excreting salt and waste products, (5) sense the presence of dangerous, possibly injurious, conditions in the external world and (6) serve as an organ of sensual pleasure. Consult your encyclopedia under "skin" for a diagram of human skin.

The top layer of skin is called the "epidermis." It includes three layers. The topmost layer, which you can easily see with your eye, is the stratum corneum, or hardened layer of skin. This layer is composed of "cornified squamous epithelium," which is dead and soon to be sloughed off. Each time you rub against something or take a bath, you lose millions of these dead cells. This layer of skin contains no nerve cells. Sensations of hot and cold, sharp and dull are not perceived by this layer of skin, but rather through it. If this were not the case — if this layer did contain nerve cells — life would be a very painful situation indeed.

Below this layer lies the very thin, one cell layer thick, "stratum lucidum," or clear layer. This clear layer is nothing more than a layer of freshly made cornified squamous epithelial cells. If you burn yourself or sustain an injury to the stratum corneum and stratum lucidum, but not deeper than that, we say you have a "first degree" burn or injury.

Bacteria are found in the skin down to this level. These bacteria represent a variety of species, most of which are harmless and known as "normal flora." However, contained in these normal bacteria, there may be some which will cause disease if they gain access to deeper layers of skin as happens with burns, cuts, scrapes, etc. in which the skin is penetrated to deeper layers.

Streptococcus is the most common bacteria which causes skin infections. A strep skin infection is diffuse and without pus formation. *Staphylococcus*, skin infections, on the other hand, progress to pus-filled, discreet, walled-off carbuncles.

Below the stratum lucidum, but still part of the epidermis, is the "stratum germinativum," or germinative layer. This layer of skin is composed of living cells, which are destined to grow closer to the surface, die and transform into stratified squamous epithelium.

Skin originates at the bottom of the germinative layer and grows outward. Your skin is totally replaced over a period of approximately one month. Contained in the stratum germinativum are the sebaceous glands which secrete an oily substance serving to lubricate the skin. If you suffer a burn or injury as deep as this level, but no deeper we say you have a "second degree" burn or injury. You can have such an injury and still suffer no permanent scarring.

Below the stratum germinativum is the "dermis," which is made of connective tissue (proteins called "collagen" and "elastin") penetrated by nerves, veins, arteries, venules, arterioles, capillaries, lymph ducts and containing sweat glands and hair follicles.

As you age, the collagen strands form crosslinked bonds with each other, decreasing the elasticity of the skin, resulting in the wrinkles we associate with aging. The presence of free radicals speeds up this process, and the presence of antioxidants slows it down.

There are two kinds of sweat glands: "apocrine" and "eccrine." Apocrine sweat glands are concentrated under the arms, are larger than the eccrine glands, secrete a milky fluid and are responsible for body odor. Some fair-skinned individuals have few or no apocrine glands and have no need for deodorants. Darker skin is associated with large numbers of apocrine glands. Eccrine sweat glands are located throughout the body and secrete a thin, odorless liquid made mostly of salt water.

In order for a cut to bleed or a burn to hurt, the injury must penetrate at least as deep as the dermis. Above this level, there are no blood vessels or nerves. If you suffer a burn or injury as deep as this level, but no deeper, we say you have a "third degree" burn or injury. If you have an injury this deep or deeper, you will have some degree of scarring.

Cellular life must exist in a fluid environment in order for cellular reproduction to occur. The dead skin on the surface serves as a container for these deeper processes, and can be thought of as a protective device, just as a test tube is a protective devise allowing chemical reactions to happen in an environment undisturbed by the outer world. It is important that the fluids in this living test tube not escape — therefore, the stratum lucidum is impermeable (unpenetrable) to body fluids. Very few substances are able to penetrate in the opposite direction, so that the internal environment is not only held in but also is protected from the external environment.

Skin has the most important role of any organ in regulating body temperature. It does this by contracting and relaxing the capillary bed. There are approximately fifteen miles of capillaries for each square inch of skin, so any contraction of this capillary bed serves to hold a large volume of blood deep within the body, which otherwise would come close to the surface and lose its heat. This serves to retain heat within the body. Conversely, when the weather is hot, or with vigorous and/or sustained exercise, the capillary bed dilates bringing larger volumes of blood near to the surface, thus loosing heat.

The sweat glands assist in this process by placing water on the surface of the skin. The evaporation of water is an endothermic phenomenon; i.e., it requires heat for water to evaporate. Part of this heat is derived from the body (from the dilated capillary bed) and part from the environment. The part which is derived from the body is lost to the body, thus leaving the body cooler.

Central control of body temperature is located in the hypothalamus of the brain, which is connected by nerve cells to all the capillary beds and sweat glands throughout the body. Skin is useful for losing heat up to an ambient temperature of 115 degrees Fahrenheit. Above that it does not work, as the skin absorbs as much or more heat than it can dissipate by sweating and vascular perfusion.

Contained in sweat is salt in higher concentration than found in the body fluids and also waste products that also are excreted through the kidneys. Each sweat gland can be considered a tiny kidney-helper, and because there are hundreds for every square inch of skin, this represents a significant contribution to cleansing the body of excess salt and waste products.

An interesting sidelight is that fingernails and toenails are made of skin products. Nails are made hard by the same keratin contained in the stratum corneum, except even more concentrated. Hair also is derived from skin. The follicles from which hair grows out are made of modified skin cells. Even the covering of the cornea, the clear part of the eye, is made of layers of cells continuous with, and modified from, skin cells.

In embryonic development, skin is derived from the outermost of the three basic layers of cells, the ectoderm. The brain, spinal cord and all the nervous tissue of the body also are derived from the ectoderm. The ectoderm simply invaginates (turns inward into a tubular formation), which then meets in the middle of the back and seals itself off from the outside. There are two other layers of cells in the embryo, the mesoderm and the endoderm. The mesoderm forms all the connective tissue of the body along with the heart and blood vessels — as well as the lymph system, spleen and bones. The endoderm forms the liver, pancreas and digestive tract from the lips to the anal sphincter.

The neural sensors of the skin include specialized organs to sense hot/cold, others to sense pressure, others to sense light touch. Pain is the individual's interpretation of the sensation caused by the release of large numbers of neurotransmitters into the synapses between nerve cells in the skin. This happens in response to severe hot, cold, pressure or tissue injury, such as that caused by cutting or scraping. Pleasure is the individual's interpretation of the sensation caused by the release of smaller numbers of neurotransmitters into the synapses between nerve cells in the skin. Pleasure and pain are caused by the same process with pleasure transforming into pain at some point on a continuum of increasing intensity, according to the nature of the individual experiencer.

Sensual love probably would not be possible without the sensations derived by light touch of the skin. When administered by touch of a loved and loving person, these sensations add immeasurably to the pleasure of living.

Skin color is determined by the concentration of melanocytes in the skin. These cells contain melanosomes which produce the pigment melanin. Melanin serves the function of protection from ultraviolet rays of the sun. Usually, melanin is gathered together in clumps within the cell. Tanning represents the production and dispersion of melanin throughout the melano-cytes, and happens as a result of measured exposure to sunlight.

Over about eighty generations of people (2000 years), skin color will transform from light to dark by increasing the number of melanocytes, under the influence of levels of sun exposure common to the equatorial regions of the earth.

Exposure to massive doses of sunlight over a short period of time, allows UV rays to damage the capillary vessels in the dermis, causing them to swell, releasing fluid into the skin, resulting in the inflammation of the skin tissues. This is, of course, known as "sunburn." Ordinary, everyday exposure to sunlight, even indirect sunlight, has been shown to be the major cause of aging of the skin. It is also known to be strongly associated with the later development of skin cancer.

To prevent sunburn, and the changes of skin aging, requires protection from sunlight. This can be achieved by daily application of sunscreen containing both UVA and UVB blockers, in high concentration. However, I question the wisdom of putting these chemicals on the skin every day, many of which are suspected carcinogens. A better solution is to limit your exposure to the sun and load up on vitamins A, C and E. These antioxidants will slow down skin aging, sunburn, and also benefit the rest of your body.

Aspirin is also effective against sunburn. On that special vacation, when you feel that you must spend the entire day at the beach, okay, slop on the sunscreen (and take A, C, E and aspirin), but let this be the exception.

The relationship between sun exposure and the development of skin cancer is irrefutable. If you have now, or have in the future, any blemish on your skin such as a mole which is new and changing, see a dermatologist immediately.

Vitamin D is manufactured in the skin as a function of exposure to sunlight. However, ordinary exposure is more than enough to get the job done. Consuming dairy products is not necessary for adequate levels of vitamin D.

Health and youthful longevity of the skin is aided by low levels of exposure to sunlight. A few years of intense tanning, although cosmetically pleasing in the short run, will damage the proteins collagen and elastin of the dermis and result in premature wrinkling.

Diet plays an important role in skin health. High levels of free radicals, in the absence of antioxidants to neutralize them (as is caused by digestion of fatty substances in middle or old age), causes crosslinking (as mentioned above) and thus acceleration of the wrinkling phenomenon of aging. A diet high in fat is partially dealt with by the sebaceous glands, which attempt to rid the body of excess fats. This can lead to clogged pores and small fatty cysts, which can become infected, forming carbuncles.

Below the skin, there is a pad of fat (the subcutaneous fat pad) which varies in thickness depending on the area of the body under examination, and varies according to the percentage of body weight which is fat. The thickness of this fat pad can be measured by taking a pinch of skin and measuring it with a caliper. This represents a double thickness of skin plus fat pad. Divide this number by two and subtract a couple of millimeters for the skin itself, and you have the thickness of the fat pad. This measurement is used in nutrition surveys to estimate level of nutrition, undernutrition and overnutrition. If you sustain a burn or injury into this layer, which also may involve muscle and bone, it is said that you have a "fourth degree" burn or injury.

The skin is a vital organ contributing greatly to overall health and vitality. Care of your skin is an opportunity to increase your health and longevity, but for this to be the case requires knowledge and attention.

One way to revitalize the skin is to stimulate it each day, before bathing, with a skin brush. The proper technique is to begin at the hands and feet and brush the skin vigorously toward the heart, covering each square inch carefully. This awakens the skin, enlivening the lymph drainage, capillary circulation and the sweat glands, which cleanse the entire body.

Retin-A is a medication derived from vitamin A which revitalizes the skin by repairing sun damage done over the years. Regular use on the face typically results in rejuvenation of the skin by five to ten years. If you want to use it, consult your physician for a prescription. This is one of the few patented medications worth using.

See page 358 for instructions on contacting my office for a referral to a doctor experienced in the treatment of skin disease.

CANCER

The Fall 1994 Conference of the American College for the Advancement of Medicine convened in San Diego. Several hundred doctors were in attendance from all over the U.S. and the world. The keynote address was delivered by Dr. Samuel Epstein, an internationally recognized expert in toxicology and cancer prevention. He is the chairman of the Cancer Prevention Coalition, an activist group working to make the public aware of the presence of easily avoidable carcinogens in our environment. He is the author of the following books: *Mutagenicity of Pesticides, The Politics of Cancer, Hazardous Wastes in America, Cancer in Britain, The Politics of Prevention, The Safe Shopper's Bible* and *Breast Cancer Prevention.*

I found Dr. Epstein's address so informative and so useful that I am reproducing my edited notes from his lecture. Dr. Epstein...

DR. EPSTEIN'S LECTURE

A National Epidemic

The increased incidence of cancer in the past forty years represents a true epidemic. Let me explain that. Statistically speaking one-third of our population will get cancer in their lifetimes, more than one-quarter will die from it. Last year more than 500,000 people died of cancer in the U.S. This is a national epidemic!

In high-risk groups, the incidence is markedly higher. From 1950 to 1990, the incidence of cancer, age adjusted, has increased by 44%; breast cancer and male colon cancer has increased over 60%; prostate cancer, about 100%; malignant melanoma, malignant lymphoma, non-Hodgkin's lymphoma, 150%; testicular cancer for males between 28 and 35, 300%; childhood cancer, over 20%.

After one gets cancer, the ability to treat and cure the disease has not improved for the overwhelming majority of cancers. For whites, the five-year survival rate is around 50% and for blacks, 38%. This is unchanged since 1950. For epithelial cancers, for which most chemotherapy is given, there has been no improved survival rates demonstrated and no evidence of efficacy of chemotherapy for these cancers. Despite this lack of effectiveness, chemotherapy continues to be routinely given. Although leukemia and other blood and lymph cancers in childhood can have prolonged remissions with chemotherapy, ten or fifteen years later the incidence of second cancers in these children is ten times the average. This points to the fact that these drugs themselves cause cancer — they are carcinogens.

The cost of cancer to our nation is about two percent of our gross national product. The costs of cancer for Medicare exceed that of any other disease. According to the American Hospital Association, by the year 2000 cancer will be the dominant specialty in American medicine.

The Causes

What has happened to cause this enormous explosion in the incidence of cancer? From the 1890s until the 1940s, organic chemicals were produced by the fractional distillation of coal and tar. No new chemicals were produced, only those already present in coal and tar were isolated. The petrochemical era was born in the 1940s. In 1940, by using new technology, synthetic chemicals were created which had never existed before. With the advent of thermal cracking and catalytic cracking, it became possible to take petroleum, fractionate it, isolate particular chemicals and then, with a process of molecular splicing and recombination, to produce any chemical you wanted to produce.

In 1940, we produced about one billion pounds of new synthetic chemicals. By 1950, the figure had reached fifty billion pounds, and by the late 1980s, it became 500 billion pounds, including a wide range of toxic, carcinogenic, neurotoxic and other chemicals. Most of these chemicals have never been tested for toxic, carcinogenic or environmental effects.

We have been able to identify around 600 of these chemicals which are carcinogenic in animals and, although one can say that is just in animals, and they are not proven to be carcinogenic in humans, the fact is, without exception, all chemicals which are carcinogenic in humans are carcinogenic in animals. The probability of the reverse being true is extremely high. No exception has ever been proven. In cases of chemicals now known to be carcinogenic for humans, the carcinogenicity in animals was known as long as four decades prior to the establishment of proof of human carcinogenicity. We cannot afford the luxury of waiting for proof of human carcinogenicity after animal carcinogenicity has been proven, and yet that is what is happening. We are subjected daily to a host of chemicals of known carcinogenicity in animals.

It took over three decades and thirty million dollars in research to prove the relationship between smoking and lung cancer. This was a huge number of people, as high as fifty percent of the population at one time, exposed to the same source of carcinogens. When you are dealing with smaller numbers of people and large numbers of carcinogens, it becomes practically impossible to prove a human cancer linkage beyond a scientific doubt.

ACS, the American Cancer Society and NCI, the National Cancer Institute, imply in their literature and public statements that tobacco is the only cause of the increase in cancer. This is nonsense.

Since 1950, if you subtract lung cancer, the increase in overall cancer is more than seventy percent, and this in the face of the fact that smoking has decreased from around fifty percent to around twenty-five percent since 1950. The nonsmoking attributable lung cancers are about thirty percent, most due to occupational hazards and urban air pollution. For example, the incidence of lung cancers has more than doubled in recent decades despite the fact that people are smoking less, not more. These cancers must be caused by other factors.

Avoidable Causes of Lymphomas and Childhood Cancers

Non-Hodgkin's lymphoma has increased 150% since 1950. Prolonged use of black and dark brown hair dyes causes a major increase in blood-related diseases, particularly non-Hodgkin's lymphoma. Childhood cancers are associated with maternal and paternal occupational exposures, particularly in the petrochemical industry. Also, parental use of pesticides at about the time of pregnancy is strongly associated with childhood cancers.

Avoidable Causes of Breast Cancer

Pesticides

Breast cancer is associated with heredity (although this is disputed) and reproductive history (early menarche, no children, late menopause). The attempted association between breast cancer and a high-fat diet is now totally discredited by the Willits study at Harvard. However, there probably is a relationship with the contaminates concentrated in fats.

Organic chlorine pesticides are associated with breast cancers. These pesticides are specific for the location of the cancer on the breast, and they concentrate in breast fat. They also have an estrogenic effect, which is carcinogenic when in excess. DDT and PCB are present in increased levels in the blood of women with breast cancer. These data are not new; they have simply not been made available to the general public.

Meat Hormones

Now, to meat hormones. The great majority of cattle are raised in feed lots where they receive high doses of estrogens before slaughter, so that the meat will be tender for market. The levels of estrogenic hormones present in meat are terrifyingly high. There is no effective regulation of feed additives, including antibiotics and hormones in meat. Women who eat meat are exposed from birth to death to high levels of estrogenic hormones because of feed additives. This goes on with the tacit approval of The FDA and the silence of the American Cancer Society and the National Cancer Institute (abbreviated ACS and NCI from here on out).

Industrial Carcinogens

Polyvinyl chloride is manufactured from vinyl chloride. Women who work in factories where this is done have a greatly increased incidence of breast cancer. These studies have been "replicated." (That means they have been repeated and are considered reliable.) Despite the fact that over three million women are working in the petrochemical industry, there has been no serious attempt to look further into this matter. Electrical industry work also is an important risk factor in cancer.

Location

Where you live also affects the incidence of breast cancer. People living near hazardous waste dumps are at high risk for cancer. Living in proximity to a nuclear plant results in major excesses of breast cancer.

Mammography

There also are iatrogenic (doctor caused) breast cancers. In 1971, the National Academy of Science published a report revealing that for every rad of x-ray exposure, the risk of breast cancer increased by one percent. Nine months later the ACS and NCI promoted a mammography project in which 300,000 women were enrolled and were told that the dose of radiation would be perfectly safe, and that the procedure might pick up breast cancer and save their lives. The minimum dose women received in this procedure was two rads per mammogram. Some centers administered five rads and some ten rads. Think of that — an increase in cancer risk of two percent, five percent, or ten percent by a single test for cancer — without being informed of the risks!

The premenopausal breast is much more sensitive to radiation than the postmenopausal breast. If a premenopausal women gets an annual mammogram each year for five years, involving two rads each time, she will have an increased risk of breast cancer of ten percent! The NCI and ACS knew this. They chose to do it anyway for publicity and research money reasons. These women have never been followed up. Probably, part of the story in the increased incidence of breast cancer has been these studies back in the 1970s.

Even though in the 1980s the level of radiation given in mammography was lowered to the range of 200 millirads, there has never been a single published study showing the effectiveness of mammography in the premenopausal woman. There have been seven randomized, controlled trials showing no efficacy whatsoever. In contrast, these studies demonstrate increased mortality in premenopausal women for the three to five years after a mammogram. These data were presented to the ACS and NCI years ago, but they were dismissed and trivialized. Last year, however, the NCI reversed itself and stands against premenopausal mammography, but the ACS still persists, and they are supported by radiologists who fear losing their "premenopausal market." That is the language, the "premenopausal market!"

Breast Implants

There are two types of breast implants, a straight silicon gel and a silicone gel implant surrounded by an industrial polyurethane. The object of polyurethane was to reduce contractures and prevent scarring and hardening of the breasts. About two million women have been implanted. From 1960 to 1964, Wilhelm Huper at the NCI — the greatest cancer authority of the age — published a series of research papers revealing that injection of polyurethane into animals resulted in a wide range of sarcomas and carcinomas. He warned that polyurethane would degrade in the body and that its degradation would be accompanied by the appearance of these cancers. There was no question in his mind these cancers were caused by polyurethane, and under no circumstances should polyurethane ever be implanted in the human body.

The chemicals from which polyurethane is made were proven to cause cancer, and these chemicals appear in the breast milk and urine of women with breast implants. Their appearance in breast milk obviously puts the nursing baby at risk as well. The chemical industry was well aware of this. The plastic surgery industry was well aware of this. Nevertheless, 400,000 women were implanted with polyurethane — despite the fact that evidence of its carcinogenicity goes back to the 60s.

The evidence of carcinogenicity was just as clear for the silicone gel. The scientists who were aware of this pushed for a medical alert. The FDA responded by firing those scientists and burying the documentation for years. This information was available to plastic surgeons. We have records of a conference of plastic surgeons in 1985 where serious concern was expressed as to what might happen if the data became available to the general public. And yet they went on doing it! This is our profession. What should we do with these people? Do we dissociate ourselves? Do we condemn them?

Who is Responsible?

Now, let's turn to who is responsible. There is no question that the NCI and ACS bear the major responsibility, because they have failed to provide Congress with information about a wide range of avoidable carcinogens in air, water, food, cosmetics, and the workplace. The only voices lifted in protest have been those of independent scientific activists. Never has the cancer establishment gone to Congress and said "Here is the information, and we need to develop the appropriate responses."

The ACS has trivialized this information and worked with industry to suppress this information. The ACS refused to support the Clean Air Act, the Toxic Substances Act and even supported efforts to reverse the ban on saccharin. Every year the ACS comes out with a volume called *Facts and Figures*, which never includes a discussion of preventable causes of ovarian cancer, nothing on avoidable occupational causes of breast cancer, nothing on the risk factors of childhood cancers. The emphasis is, rather, "You drink too much, you smoke too much, you've chosen the wrong parents. These are the real reasons." The rest is glossed over. The cause for this is a mind set, because doctors are trained in diagnosis and treatment and generally are ignorant in matters of prevention.

Also, there are conflicts of interest. Of the 300 members of the Board of Directors of the ACS, there are 150 lay and 150 professional people. If you analyze who they are, it reads like the Fortune 500 Who's Who. The tie-in to banking, petrochemicals, pharmaceuticals and the cancer drug industry is overwhelming.

Every year, in April, there is a fund-raising drive by the ACS, and every year they tell us they can fund only ten percent of the research grants applied for. The budget of the ACS is

350 million dollars. There is a standard in philanthropic organizations that one should keep only 150% of the annual budget in reserve. Yet in cash, assets and real estate, the ACS is worth 1.2 billion dollars — yet every year they come out and say, "We need money for research."

The NCI has a two-billion-dollar annual budget. Less than 2.5% is used for primary prevention — informing the public about avoidable causes of cancer. Even though occupational hazards account for ten percent of cancers, the study of prevention and information distribution in this area account for only one percent of the NCI's budget.

In 1971, when President Nixon declared the "War on Cancer" and the NCI was given autonomy, two things happened: (1) a massive influx of money went into the NCI and (2) Beno Schmidt was appointed as chairman of the President's Cancer Panel and served ten years. He was a New York investment banker with close ties to the pharmaceutical industry, interested only in treatment of cancer with drugs — and for every cancer drug that was sold, he made a handsome profit. For the next ten years, Armand Hammer was chairman. He was the ex-CEO of Occidental Petroleum, one of the nation's major polluters, who gave us Love Canal among other things. So, for over twenty years, the NCI was in the hands of people from the pharmaceutical and petroleum industries.

A detailed analysis of the results of drug therapy for cancer by the GAO (the U.S. General Accounting Office) has shown us that there is not a shred of evidence for the efficacy of drug treatment in epithelial cancers (cancers involving the linings of the body — lung cancer, colon cancer, skin cancer, etc.). Here we have clear-cut data on the lack of efficacy of a multibillion dollar industry, and yet this is the very argument standardized medicine raises against progressive methods of treatment of cancer. Of course, progressive methods should be scrutinized, but so should standard methods. This is a double standard, and it is unjust. The fact is, standard medical treatment does not face that kind of scrutiny — thanks to a lapse in consciousness, to this date, of watchdog groups and to the general lack of integrity of the cancer/pharmaceutical industry. The same goes for Congress, which does nothing other than listen to platitudes from the NCI and ACS about smoking, drinking and fat being the only causes of cancer. Unwillingness to confront and challenge authority and accept activist positions lies behind this deadly sin of omission.

What Can We Do?

First we must inform ourselves. In the area of iatrogenic cancer, we must accept responsibility. For example, DES, diethylstilbesterol, has been shown to cause adenocarcinoma in the daughters of women who were given this drug in the 1950s. These women were told that the drug was totally safe, just a vitamin, no problem. The evidence was clear, and yet these women were subjected to a carcinogen and, not only that, but without being informed of the data regarding DES, which had been available since the 1930s. We are certainly doing similar things today. Let me explain.

Commonly Used Carcinogens

Flagyl, the most common drug used for trichomonas infections, is a carcinogen. The evidence is unequivocable. The animal data has been replicated. Lindane is a pesticide we use for not only bugs, but also for head lice in a preparation called "Quell." Up to ten percent of children are treated with Lindane. Lindane is a highly potent animal carcinogen, and in the last few years we have seen data incriminating the use of Quell as a cause of brain cancer in children, and also Lindane as a pesticide as a cause of brain cancer in children. Clomathin (which is used as a fertility drug) is related to excess ovarian cancer.

Tamoxifen is touted as something that will reduce the chances of breast cancer. There is no solid evidence for this point of view — you can see claims of such evidence as wildly optimistic or non-existent. However, the evidence of the carcinogenicity of Tamoxifen is overwhelming. It induces uterine cancer in people who are treated with Tamoxifen for breast cancer. When I mentioned this in an article for the L.A. Times a few years ago, the leader of the trial commented "Well, no big deal, you can always do a hysterectomy for uterine cancer." Quote: "No big deal." Tamoxifen also is a potent liver carcinogen. Its molecular structure is similar to DES. And women are not informed about this. The consent form trivializes the risks.

The interface between science and one's responsibility to speak out as an informed doctor demands that we take a stand to inform people of these things. (The author agrees, emphatically.)

The breast implant situation is even more shocking, because two million women are involved. The best FDA scientists recommended a medical alert to go out to these women in 1987. The recent 4.52 billion dollar settlement relates to autoimmune disease without a word regarding breast cancer.

Cosmetics

Let us talk about cosmetics. The cosmetics industry is in a state of regulatory anarchy. Cosmetics are laden with a plethora of unlabeled carcinogens. Let me give you a few examples.

Hair dyes contain phenylenediamines and various coloring agents, which are proven carcinogens, documented to relate to non-Hodgkin's lymphoma, chronic lymphocytic leukemia and multiple myeloma. Lotions and creams contain diethanolamine and triethanolamine. These react with nitrites added as preservatives or as contaminants to produce nitrosamines which are extremely potent carcinogens.

In the average cosmetic or cream, you find highly potent carcinogens. In others, you find agents which release formaldehyde (from polyethylene glycol, bronopal, quaternium 15). Several of them contain dioxane. Others contain artificial colors, including arsenic and lead.

The use of talc has been shown to be related to ovarian cancer. However, the ACS "Facts and Figures" mentions nothing about this.

The average farmer uses one and a half to two pounds of pesticides per acre. Home lawns take ten pounds per acre. Golf courses take fifteen pounds per acre. Up to thirty different pesticides are used, ten of which have been shown to be carcinogenic: such as 2-4-D, related to lymphomas; Atrazine related to ovarian cancer; DDT related to pancreatic cancer. Golf course superintendents have excesses of non-Hodgkin's lymphoma, brain cancer, prostate and lung cancer. Dogs living where lawns are repeatedly treated have a five fold excess of non-Hodgkin's lymphoma. Children also get lymphomas and leukemia and these are in excess in children living in houses where lawns are repeatedly doused with pesticides.

Clothing is dry-cleaned with perchlorethylene (or tetrachlorethylene). When you put it in a cedar closet, the levels of perchlorethylene in that closet become greater than that permitted to a trained worker with protective gear.

Many domestic aerosols have as the propellant dichlormethane, a carcinogenic chemical related to breast cancer. Furniture polishes contain formaldehyde. Cat litter contains crystalline silica, another potent carcinogen.

Food

Xeronol is a nonsteroidal estrogenic compound. It is broken down to xerolenone, a carcinogen. The levels are very high in meats, fantastically high. The hormones are implanted in cattle ears, one allowed per cow. However, to save money and get the cow to market faster, many are implanted and the FDA does not enforce the regulations. There is no requirement for a withdrawal period. This is regulatory anarchy.

We use nearly sixty carcinogenic pesticides in the growth and production of food crops, and instead of the NCI and ACS going to Congress and making the problem clear, they are totally silent. In fact, the ACS has performed damage control in one case. When the TV program "Front Line" was to present a program on the dangers of pesticides in foods, ACS put out a media blitz trivializing the risk of pesticides in foods before the Front Line show was aired. It was subsequently canceled.

Industrial contaminants, PCBs, dioxans, food coloring agents, etc., and now we come to nitrite preservatives. Nitrites react with amines in cosmetics and in meat and fish, producing nitrosamines. We knew in the seventies of the high content of nitrosamines in hot dogs. The FDA tried to bury the data. In the last few years, we have clear proof of increased brain cancers and leukemia in children eating hot dogs, 5-10 per day.

What Can We Do?

How can we, as clinicians, deal with this? We must first inform ourselves, so that we can counsel our patients. We must remember an important part of our sacred Hippocratic oath:

"First, do no harm." The Cancer Prevention Coalition takes initiatives on labeling at a national level. Every citizen has the right to know if there are carcinogens in his household products and his food. This is unarguable. You can argue about the science or the economics, but it is unassailable to say that people have the right to know the truth. This also provides a powerful incentive to responsible and responsive industry to phase out carcinogens and replace them with safer alternatives.

The German government has taken steps to phase out diethanolamine and triethanolamine from cosmetics, because they produce nitrosamines. There has been no such attempt in this country. Nor has there been any such attempt to label this information on hot dogs. This is outrageous, scientifically and constitutionally outrageous. More important is the realization that we are in the middle of an avoidable cancer epidemic. It is untenable to say "I am just a doctor, and I have nothing to do with this."

Who should be telling doctors and citizens about these things? The NCI and ACS, of course. However, the NCI and ACS are part of the cancer/pharmaceutical industrial complex and, as such, are unlikely to change.

I feel that you all have the right to demand documentation and proof of the assertions I have made today. For that purpose, I refer you to the article I wrote for The American Journal of Industrial Medicine, June 1993 which has detailed citations to verify all the information given in this lecture.

This is the end of my notes from Dr. Epstein's lecture. Next I will be examining various treatments for cancer with an emphasis on the progressive methods. Whether or not one is concerned with the problem of cancer, these will be valuable inquiries because of two reasons: (1) cancer may appear in one's life at any time, and it is prudent to have sufficient knowledge to make informed choices if and when that happens, and (2) what we learn about cancer treatment can be applied to cancer prevention. Cancer is much easier to prevent than it is to treat.

PROGRESSIVE APPROACHES TO THE TREATMENT OF CANCER

If you have cancer, it is time to prepare — prepare to die, and prepare to live. It is a transforming experience to prepare to die. Few people ever have that opportunity. It is radically transforming to prepare to live. That is practically unheard of — almost no one ever prepares to live. It is important that you make out your will and make your peace with life and the people who love you. It is equally important that you prepare for a long life because, unless you simply want to die from this cancer, you may yet live a longer life.

If you have cancer, are possibilities of which you may be unaware. It is important that you know that and that you not lose hope, unless, of course, you simply want to die. This does not mean that you will have a cure, it simply means that there is no type of cancer which has not been cured many times. Let me repeat: there is no type of cancer which has not been cured many times.

The Positive Value of Your Cancer

If you want to live, it is important that you take heart, have hope, and beyond that, a certain attitude toward your cancer. It is important that you see the value of the cancer in your life. If you are unwilling to see the value it has for you, you probably will fight it vainly and give up in a condition of lost hope.

Perhaps your cancer has made you glad for the life that you have; perhaps every moment seems precious, whereas before life did not seem to have a particular value and each moment was like all the others. Perhaps the cancer has revealed, or may yet reveal, the true nature of your relationship with loved ones. Perhaps through confronting death you can see the purpose for your living. Many people report coming face to face with God's love during their struggle with cancer.

Above all, you must give up the attitude of feeling sorry for yourself. Pity instead the poor bloke who dies never having awakened to the value of life, to the preciousness of each moment, to the absolute beauty of love, to the purpose for living. Count yourself as lucky for having the opportunity to wake up to life, and in that spirit of gratitude, get on with the business of learning about what cancer is and how you can become one of the survivors of cancer.

There is ample reason for you to have this healthy attitude. The world is full of people who have been cured from the same type of cancer you have, whatever it is. Adopting this healthy attitude makes you a healthier person. There are even a few people around who cured themselves through the use of mind-body techniques alone. I believe your attitude makes a everything possible, probably by strengthening your immune system, as the scientific literature suggests.

Your approach to your cancer will be determined by your personality. You may be that person who rigidly believes in authority. In that case, you go to your doctor and do whatever that person tells you to do. You may be that person with a good intellect and a natural curiosity, gifted with the ability to think for yourself. If this is so, you will want to know everything about cancer, so that you can think critically about the treatment of your cancer. Whatever your personality, if you are going to have a successful relationship with your cancer, you must have the experience of responsibility for treatment of your cancer and responsibility for your destiny. In this context, your doctor becomes your partner in the project of making your body well. **Take charge of your situation.**

If you find yourself in bad shape mentally and emotionally, an act of responsibility is to place yourself in that condition from whence you are able to recover. If you need psychotherapy, find a good therapist. If you need to discover and express negative emotions, do that. If you need to make amends with people in your life, do so. If you need to acknowledge people who have loved you, do so without delay.

I have written a one year correspondence/telephone course for people who want to complete all the uncompleted issues in their lives. I have given this course to over 100 people since 1990. Taking this course creates possibilities which cannot exist in the presence of a life cluttered with incompletions, and this, in itself, handles the psychological and spiritual components of illness. Handling this aspect of your illness frees you to fully pursue a physical cure without the drag of incomplete life situations. The name of this course is *Ready To Live!* If you want to know more details about this course to evaluate its use for you, write or e-mail for further information.

Ron Kennedy, M.D.   e-mail address: *nexus@sonic.net*
P.O. Box 2909
Rohnert Park, CA 94927

An Open Mind

The most important attitude for you to have is that of an open mind. If your doctor tells you that you can be cured with his treatment, that there is no room for doubt of that and when he can back up his talk with proof, then you may close your mind to all else. Until then, having a closed mind is definitely dangerous to your health. There may be more things in heaven and earth than are contained in your philosophy, but a closed mind makes them impossible for you.

I do not want to make your decisions for you. I do want to inform you of what is available for the treatment of your cancer. I want to tell you what a mainstream doctor practicing standardized medicine will not tell you — for lack of knowing or for fear of condemnation by his peers.

A lot of this information you can put into effect yourself without consulting a doctor. If you do choose to consult a doctor, you will be armed with information and able to converse intelligently. This information may make it possible to make your choice of a doctor wisely, based on the quality of that doctor's approach to cancer and not just because you know him or her, or he/she has a "reputation," or she/he wears the $2000 suit and belongs to the country club. The object is to become a cancer survivor, not be impressed by your doctor. There are plenty of impressed former cancer patients in the local cemetery.

It is important for you to be in charge of your treatment. Your best chance of surviving lies in becoming an equal partner with your doctor. For this, you need knowledge. You need the full story about the approaches to cancer treatment. This introduction to the various treatment approaches will get you started. In reading this introduction, you may find that you want to know more about one or more approaches. For this purpose I have listed, at the end of the discussion of each discipline, the sources to whom you may write or call for more information. At the end of this section I have prepared for you a sheet of addresses, which you may simply cut into mailing labels. Write a letter of inquiry to the places from which you want further information.

Sadly, the treatments for cancer acceptable to the U. S. medical establishment are: surgery, chemotherapy and radiation. Other forms of treatment, if given specifically for cancer, can, in many states, result in the loss of one's medical license. If a doctor loses his or her license, it becomes much more difficult to help people. Therefore, the competition to standardized cancer care, as offered by the medical monopoly, has been almost eliminated by this threat. The sad fact is that to treat cancer as I would like to treat cancer, I would have to move to another country — Mexico, for example. Many good doctors have done exactly that.

Many progressive medicine doctors do treat cancer patients for such things as bolstering their immune systems; however, we cannot tell them that this is for the purpose of treating cancer itself. If you go to one of those doctors, you may be asked to sign a waiver recognizing this fact. Please understand that the doctor will help you, but that his or her hands are tied in what can be said to you. Because the medical establishment in the state of California has succeeded in persuading the state legislature to outlaw cancer treatments which do not fall into the pigeonholes of surgery, radiation, or chemotherapy, you must understand that any other treatment is not for your cancer.

As far as I know, an absolute cure for cancer has not been discovered. What I mean is that a single cure, which works on every cancer, every time, has not been discovered. I may be wrong, and the cure or cures may be known but suppressed as many people claim. What we can say and be certain about is that an absolute cure for cancer has not been discovered and universally agreed upon.

However, if ever there is such a discovery, unless it is made by the mainstream medical establishment, and unless it yields a huge profit in which a large portion of the cancer industry and the cancer establishment can share, the arrival of this discovery will not be greeted with open arms by those who are making a fortune on ineffective cancer treatments at present.

Realizing this state of affairs — the reality of the perversion of medical truth by the profit motive, which is inherent in capitalism — I find it easy to believe that one, or several, or many cancer cures may already have been discovered and then discredited and suppressed by the cancer industry.

The argument a mainstream medical doctor would make to this is, "Yea, but all you have to do is perform the necessary double-blind, placebo controlled studies, prove the statistical validity of the findings and publish in a 'respected, peer-reviewed journal.' " The problem with this argument is twofold.

First, if a cure for cancer is discovered, is it ethical to withhold it from half of the people in a large study — to simply allow them to die to prove a point? This is exactly what a "double-blind placebo controlled study" does. Second, if one looks at the financial contributors to, and the advertisers in, these so-called "respected" medical journals, one finds a list of the major moneymakers in the medical industry. Without these advertising dollars, "respected peer-reviewed medical journals" would go broke almost immediately. These businesses have no interest in funding the publication of reports which undermine their profits.

The fact is, that the major medical journals have been bought by vested interests who pressure the publishers to consider not publishing such things as studies showing the efficacy of EDTA, hydrogen peroxide therapy, DMSO and progressive treatments for cancer. If you have performed a study in one of these areas, you will have your paper rejected by these "respected" journals, prima facie, simply because it is about a subject about which it is forbidden to publish.

If one has cancer, or if one is the relative or friend of a person who has cancer, these considerations are important to understand when selecting a treatment program. Most people who receive a diagnosis of cancer will go to the doctor they know best and receive from that doctor (or perhaps a doctor to which that doctor refers them) advice and treatment about how to handle that cancer. This is understandable, given a state of fear, alarm, panic and desperation to cling to some stable system of authority.

At this point, if one is intent on being free of cancer, rather than merely lining the pockets of the cancer industry before dying, it becomes important to inform oneself quickly. This is where it pays off to have developed an intellect, the capacity to think clearly and the intuitive ability to separate truth from hype, even if the hype is commonly accepted.

After the shock of the cancer diagnosis wears off, it is important to ask critical questions. Here are those questions:

1.   Is there an absolute cure for my type of cancer?

2.   If there is not an absolute cure for my type of cancer, what is the percentage of people who are cured of this cancer when it is at this stage?

3.   What is a "cure?" Does this word mean free of this cancer forever, or does it merely mean survived for five years but still sick?

4.   Can you give me a copy of the studies from which your answer is derived?

5.   Will the therapy you recommend damage my body, perhaps my immune system?

6.   If it is damaging to my immune system, and it does not cure my cancer, will this damage to my immune system make it less likely that subsequent progressive therapies will work?

7.   Does this therapy make it more likely that I will develop another cancer later; i.e., is the therapy itself carcinogenic?

These are critically important questions not only to ask but to which one should insist on receiving thorough answers. If your doctor balks at supplying the answers, or is irritated that you asked these questions, the chances are good that he does not have the answers, that is to say, the doctor does not know!

This is an unimaginable circumstance to some people — the doctor does not know! We believe that doctors know everything, but the fact is that a large portion of medicine is practiced based on what the doctor's medical school professors believed.

It is important to know that doctors were educated in medical schools and that medical schools have been purchased for the most part, by "grants" from the medical industry and from the government, which exists in a "good old boy" network with the medical industry, wherein favors are granted as rewards for "correct" opinions. Medical school professors are like anyone else, they want to keep the money flowing, and they want to be in sync with their superiors — and their superiors want to be in sync with the source of money, which flows through the medical school structure, etc.

Of course, this is all made easy to swallow by massive propaganda blitzes from the pharmaceutical, surgical and medical supply industries and their representatives who come to the medical school, get to know the professors, the doctors and even the medical students (future customers) on a personal basis. They come armed with copies of studies showing the superiority of their products and with glossy brochures in hand, all free, of course, as are the samples of drugs and other medical products. These representatives of the branches of the medical industry also are equipped with obsequious attitudes, which are designed to please whoever they come into contact with and never to make any waves or create any upset or controversy. I remember them well.

It is very important that you understand this structure of mind control, for unless you understand it, you cannot grasp how an industry is able to hypnotize otherwise perfectly intelligent professors, doctors and medical students who are dedicated, in their hearts, to helping people.

So, while the answers to the pointed questions you ask your doctor about your cancer certainly come from what your doctor honestly believes is best for you, you must understand that, despite what your doctor believes, he may simply not know his subject in depth — and specifically he may not know much about the approaches to treating cancer which are "progressive,"except to say, as many doctors say about EDTA, "Well, I don't know much about that except that it is no good!" Or, "If that were any good, I would have learned about it in medical school." This type of statement from your doctor separates the thinking patients from the nonthinking patients.

Some people who think for themselves will survive their "incurable cancer," while almost all of those who blindly follow the blind will die from their cancer. One thing is for certain, if your doctor says your cancer is incurable — and you intend to be cured — then any statements from the doctor after that (such as "Why don't we use this or that treatment" or "Come to see me in two months") should absolutely be ignored. The diagnosis of "incurable" already has alerted you to the limitations of your doctor's knowledge.

As one reads case histories, one comes to realize that there is no type of cancer which has not, at one time or another, been cured! Your cancer may not be cured, but that does not mean your disease is "incurable." Do not let anyone sell you that point of view unless you want to die sooner, rather than later.

Theories About Cancer

What is cancer? As far as we know, there is no absolute cure for cancer. I may be wrong in saying that; however, it is not in my experience to report that there is an absolute cure for all cancers, although, as you will see, some cancer therapists claim that there is such a cure. However, as far as I know now, there is no absolute cure. That being the case, we should not accept anyone's theory about the cause of cancer as fact. Any explanation of what cancer is, which does not lead naturally to a cure for cancer, is necessarily simply a theory — and theory, regardless of how good it sounds, is not fact.

The only thing we know as certain about cancer is that it is an uncontrolled growth of cells. These cells have the ability to migrate to different parts of the body and grow out of control there as well. These cells may compress surrounding structures — especially in the skull and around the heart and lungs — and their waste products may be toxic to the rest of the body. By these means, they may usurp the function of organs such as the brain, liver, kidney, lungs and others and cause death by these means.

Why cells should be doing this is a mystery. Theories to explain what is happening abound.

The Internal Enemy Theory

The predominant theory of the medical establishment is that this wild overgrowth of cells is a kind of genetic rebellion within the body. According to this theory, one's own cells become the enemy and destroy the body which made them. It is a kind of biological decision for suicide.

If there is an enemy within, it only makes sense to form an army and go to battle with the enemy. The army may consist of surgeons who try to cut, slash and burn the cancer out of the body; it may consist of toxic medicines to poison these internal enemy cells, so that they die and go away; or it may be an army of electrons shot through the body during radiation therapy, killing both cancerous and normal cells.

In standardized medicine, these are the ways cancer is dealt with: cut, slash, burn, poison and shoot. This is the standard medical model, the paradigm or context in and from which doctors are required to think. People who think outside this paradigm are condemned by the cancer establishment. Their therapies are blacklisted, without investigation, by the National Cancer Institute (NCI) and the American Cancer Society (ACS) as "unproven, unaccepted" therapies.

How successful is surgery, chemotherapy and radiation? Because these are the dominant therapies, we can measure their success by the statistics on cancer over the last forty years. While it is true that cancer has increased in incidence by 44% since then, probably we cannot blame that on standardized treatment. For the answer to the increase in the incidence of cancer, we probably can look to the chemical industry and the flood of synthetic chemicals which are omnipresent in our daily lives. That subject is dealt with in the previous chapter.

Let us look at what happens after cancer is diagnosed. Did the prognosis for cancer improve between 1950 and 1990? Are a greater percentage of people with cancer being cured now compared to forty years ago? The answer is a resounding "No!" For whites, the five year survival rate is around 50% and for blacks, 38%. This is unchanged since 1950. This is hard to believe, but true. While surgery, chemotherapy and radiation may, in some cases, help people, with all the billions of dollars spent on research since 1950 and with the astronomical increase in the cost of treating cancer, nothing has been gained. If people have been helped or saved from cancer, an equal number have been fatally damaged by the treatment itself — statistics do not lie — nothing has changed overall since 1950!

Over one million people will be diagnosed with cancer in the U.S. this year. Two thirds of them will die of their cancer within five years. Chemotherapy will save two to three percent, primarily blood and lymph cancers, especially in children, which are diagnosed early. A combination of surgery, radiation and chemotherapy has achieved significant tumor eradication rates among certain rare tumors. Nevertheless, these people have eighteen times the probability of having a cancer later in life than other people. Is it possible that the treatment itself causes cancer? Epidemiologists think so.

Even though all of the FDA-approved, anticancer drugs are themselves toxic, immunosuppressive and carcinogenic and despite the fact that very few people can be helped with chemotherapy — despite all that, over fifty percent of patients with cancer will be given chemotherapy anyway. Why? It is a $750 million business from the medical/pharmaceutical side, and from the patient's side, well, people are desperate when their lives are at stake, so they are likely to follow doctor's advice.

With the average cost of treatment around $30,000 per person and the results so discouraging, it is little wonder that many people who are able and willing to think for themselves turn to progressive treatment when confronted with cancer. If you have cancer and accept chemotherapy, you may be saved, but statistically, the odds are better that you are going to die from complications of your treatment before you have time to die from your cancer. I guess you could say, ironically, that chemotherapy does prevent many people dying from cancer. They die from the chemotherapy instead.

President Nixon declared the "War on Cancer" in 1971 and initiated a major spending effort on the part of the federal government to develop a cure for cancer. The overall, age-adjusted cancer death rate has risen by five percent since 1971. Has the war on cancer succeeded? What do you think? Yet the NCI and ACS are likely to be calling you next week for another contribution.

The major thrust of the National Institute of Health, the American Cancer Society and the National Cancer Institute has been to promote the idea of surgery, radiation and chemotherapy to treat cancer (i.e., destroy the enemy within) and to degrade progressive means derived from alternative points of view. Do these branches of the cancer establishment have your best health interests in mind? What do you think?

Amazing, is it not? I know there are talented, intelligent, dedicated people in the medical establishment cancer research division. The fact that they are achieving no results, overall, indicates to me that there is something wrong with the entire paradigm within which they require themselves to think. Perhaps cancer is not simply "an enemy within." If the standard medical model is not the story, or at least not the whole story, perhaps this leaves an opening to consider other possible answers to the question, "What is cancer?"

Rather than abandon the standard medical model, I believe a rational thinking person would expand upon it. Let us look at other models, which are being quietly amalgamated into the traditional standard medical model.

The Environmental Toxin Theory

This theory holds that the runaway growth of cells is somehow stimulated by external toxins. The association made in many studies between toxins and cancer is so clear as to be irrefutable. Cancer prevention, and probably cancer treatment as well, has much to do with avoiding and eliminating exposure to these toxins.

The identification of these toxins is like pulling teeth. Most of us remember the pain and agony it was for our society to finally come to the conclusion that the use of tobacco and later alcohol, has something to do with cancer. Other industries which routinely use and build into their products chemicals which facilitate the development of cancer, consider tobacco a sacrificial lamb. "Tobacco and alcohol have been thrown to the wolves of medical epidemiologists. Why should we admit that our chemicals also are killing people?" There is only money to be lost and bother to be had in the changes which must happen to stem the tide of the cancer epidemic.

I believe the environmental toxin theory is very useful but, as with all paradigms, we must be careful not to accept it as the only approach to cancer, lest it limit our thinking. Probably, the many descriptions of what cancer really is, are the equivalent of men trying to describe the earth before space flight. There were many opinions of what the earth would look like, but they were no substitute for getting up there and looking at it. With regard to cancer, the day of clarity about the cause will come when the absolute cure arrives — if it hasn't already arrived and been suppressed.

The Invader Theory

The invader theory has it that cancer is caused, or at least triggered, by an organism or organisms from outside the body. This may happen by the production by the organism of a biochemical compound which causes cells to degenerate into a cancerous condition. These organisms may be viruses, bacteria, or parasites.

Finding an association between the presence of a virus and the development of cancer and proving viral causation are two different matters. While a virus may be present in, say, seventy percent of cases of a particular cancer, it may be that the virus did not cause the cancer but merely is allowed to exist in the body of a person due to damage to the immune system caused by the cancer or by the therapy designed to treat the cancer. In this sense, the virus is present as an opportunist rather than as a cause. Are flies the cause of the existence of rotten garbage? Certainly not; they are merely attracted to it. Are viruses the causes of cancer? Maybe, and on the other hand they may simply be attracted to it.

The Invader Theory also includes those explanations which blame bacteria and parasites. There seems little doubt that some viruses, bacteria and parasites have a statistical association with some cancers; however it is possible that they are merely attracted to the cancerous condition and are, therefore, present as opportunists. Their mere presence does not prove causation.

Many prominent, if somewhat maverick, researchers over the last seventy years have claimed to observe "pleomorphism" with the aid of dark field microscopes. A dark field microscope allows the experienced observer to see living tissue and living organisms within that tissue, whereas the standard light microscope and the electron microscope are designed to see only killed material. According to these researchers, it is necessary to see the living process to understand what really happens in the body which causes cancer. They say that subunits, which some have called "plastids," combine to form viruses and bacteria.

Pleomorphism is thus a paradigm which is based on the belief that plastids exist at all times in the body, that viruses and bacteria can evolve from them and from each other, and that these organisms represent different stages in the life cycle of microscopic life forms. Some of these researchers claim significant numbers of cures of "incurable" cancers using methods of killing these pleomorphic viruses/bacteria.

Pleomorphism is not accepted by mainstream medical microbiologists who also say that the human body is normally sterile, i.e., devoid of bacterial life forms. There is no convincing proof of this and a lot of evidence against it; it is medical dogma, and dogma does not die easily. Nevertheless, the routine presence of bacteria and/or viruses in the body does not mean they evolved from "plastids."

Pleomorphism also is a paradigm and, as you know about paradigms, they allow us to see what otherwise cannot be seen — and they restrict our vision for what is not included in the paradigm. The person who finally solves the cancer mystery will be, or was, a master of paradigms and not stuck to any particular paradigm.

Types of Cancer Therapies

With the above discussion behind us, we can now look at types of progressive cancer therapies. There are no reliable statistics on the results of cancer treatment by progressive therapies, because the "respected peer-reviewed" journals will not publish studies which threaten the profits of the cancer industry. Once again: how ethical is it to perform double blind placebo studies letting half the people in the study die to prove the effectiveness of a therapy? To me, it seems unethical in the extreme to carry out such studies if a cure for cancer seems at hand. The people who have some success in treating cancer in a progressive way are typically humanitarian healers, not researchers.

Many amazing reports have been recorded and continue to be recorded, in the lore of progressive cancer treatment. The medical establishment handles these in one of the following ways:

1. they are ignored;

2. they are explained as "anecdotal," implying that they are lies;

3. they are said to have undergone "spontaneous remission," i.e., unexplained recovery (that means the doctor has no idea what happened);

4. they are said to have recovered from the delayed effects of conventional therapy, which was administered weeks or months before the progressive therapy.

Let us examine the categories of progressive therapies one by one, with examples of each. I do not have room for complete discussions of these therapies. I write only to give you a taste of each therapy with resources listed for finding out more information.

Biologic Therapies for Cancer

The biologic therapies are those based on the idea that the body itself has methods of treating cancer, preventing cells from becoming cancerous and reverting them to normal once they do become cancerous. Therefore, from this point of view, the presence of cancer represents a breakdown of these defense systems. The task therefore is to restore, or replace, these defense systems.

Revici Therapy

Dr. Emmanuel Revici is a Romanian-born New York physician now in his nineties who has developed a unique way of dealing with cancer. Dr. Revici is considered by many of his colleagues as an innovative medical genius in the area of human biochemistry. His treatment is based on the restoration of what he believes to be an imbalance in the body's lipid chemistry and is designed to balance the anabolic and catabolic (build up and breakdown) processes of the body, which he believes are profoundly disturbed in cancer.

As usual with innovative medical genius, Dr. Revici has the distinction of having done battle with the representatives of standardized medicine who have tried, without success, to remove his medical license. When this struggle occurred in the 1980s, many of his former patients came to his aid and testified before the New York State legislature. Dr. Revici was allowed to keep his license and go on with his work.

For further information on Revici therapy:

Emmanuel Revici, M.D.
26 E. 36th St.
New York, NY 10016
(212) 685-0111

Hydrazine Sulfate

Hydrazine sulfate, a former unconventional therapy, has proven so useful as an adjunctive treatment in cancer therapy that it is now even approved by the FDA on a case by case basis. It restores lost appetite, one of the major problems in cancer, and reverses the wasting away which is a hallmark of cancer. In addition, it stops tumor growth, often causes tumors to shrink, and in some cases has made tumors disappear.

Hydrazine sulfate was first proposed as a cancer treatment by Dr. Joseph Gold, who waged a courageous battle over the last quarter century to gain acceptance from the medical establishment for this simple, off-the-shelf chemical.

For information:

Syracuse Cancer Research Institute
Presidential Plaza
600 E. Genesee St.
Syracuse, NY 13202
(315) 472-6616

Antineoplaston Therapy

Dr. Stanislaw Burzynski, who practices in Houston, Texas, has discovered that a group of peptides (short chains of amino acids) and amino acid derivatives normally are present in the body and serve to keep cells healthy and dividing normally. He also has discovered that people with cancer are critically short on these substances, which he has named "antineoplastons." He has particular success with non-Hodgkins lymphoma, as well as two brain cancers: glioblastoma multiforme and astrocytoma, both of which are incurable using conventional therapy. Most of his patients have been declared terminal and incurable by conventional doctors.

Dr. Burzynski is respected throughout the world for his work. Research into his ideas is progressing in many other developed countries and large numbers of patients say they have been cured with antineoplaston therapy. Despite all this, Dr. Burzynski is forced to engage in degrading wars with the FDA and the Texas Medical Society. He endures the snubs of the American Cancer Society and the National Cancer Institute and goes on with his work. As I write this, he is enduring harrassment by the FDA which, after going through numerous grand juries, finally found one which would charge Dr. Burzynski with a few false charges. For those who understand about the politics of medicine, his struggle is a kind of resumé which proves his worth.

You can contact the Burzynski Clinic:

Burzynski Clinic
6221 Corporate Dr.
Houston, TX 77036
(713) 531-6464 / 597-0111

Immune Therapies for Cancer

The human immune system is designed to defeat disease and restore order to the body. This includes the ability to combat cancer cells. It is now known that cells become cancerous routinely. We all have had cancer many times in our lives and were unaware of it because the immune system destroyed the cancer cells before they could grow and multiply out of control.

A combination of two methods exists for destroying cancer cells: antibodies and natural killer cells, specialized cells which track down and destroy cancer cells. NKCs (natural killer cells) are your first line of defense. If cancer cells escape the NKCs, T-lymphocytes detect the antigens given off by cancer cells and make antibodies to destroy these cells.

From this point of view, cancer is not an invasion of outside forces as much as it is a failure of internal forces to execute normal functions. Therapy therefore is designed to bolster the immune system so that it can do its job.

The orthodox medical establishment has a few biologic therapies. These are as follows.

1. BCG, which stands for bacillus Calmette-Guerin, is a tuberculin vaccine especially effective against malignant melanoma. This is used by both orthodox and progressive oncologists.

2. Interferon is a substance produced by white blood cells in response to viral infections. It is very expensive and has toxic side effects. At one time, it was hoped that interferon would be useful in a variety of cancers, but its use is limited now to the treatment of hairy cell leukemia and juvenile laryngeal papillomatosis.

3. Interleukin-2, a protein made by T-cells, is highly toxic, very expensive and not very effective. The original high hopes for this substance have vanished.

4. Tumor Necrosis Factor (TNF) destroys cancer cell membranes, but routinely has serious side effects.

5. Monoclonal antibodies are synthetic antibodies made by splicing the patient's cancer cell genes into the genes of his white cells. The resulting cells, when injected into the body, are supposed to manufacture antibodies specific to the cancer, to which chemotherapeutic agents can be attached. This all still is in the experimental stage, and the cancer establishment has high hopes for monoclonal antibodies as a method of treating cancer while making a shipload of money (because these little items are patentable).

All of the orthodox biological substances, except for BCG, are expensive in the extreme, and, except someday/maybe for monoclonal antibodies, very limited in treatment scope and loaded with side effects. Nevertheless, for some very specific conditions like hairy cell leukemia and juvenile laryngeal papillomatosis, they may be worth looking into.

The Coley Vaccine

Dr. William Coley (1862-1936) developed a vaccine made from bacterial toxins. These agents worked by stimulating immune response mechanisms in cancer patients and were said to have helped hundreds of people. After Dr. Coley's death in 1936, his daughter carried on with his work.

The Coley Mixed Toxin was available in the U.S. until the early 1960s. Park Davis (a large pharmaceutical company) manufactured their own weak version of the vaccine in the early 1960s, but theirs did not compare with the original.

The Coley Mixed Toxin was credited with a high percentage of tumor disappearances but was lost to history in the middle 1960s. Recently Donald Carrow, M.D., of the Florida Preventive Health Services, has recreated the Coley Mixed Toxin.

For more information contact:

Dr. Donald J. Carrow, M.D.
Florida Preventive Health Services
Henderson Center
3902 Henderson Blvd., Ste. 206
Tampa, FL 33629
(813) 832-3220
(813) 449-1050

The Camphor Therapy of Gaston Naessens

Gaston Naessens, a French biologist living in Canada, has developed an aqueous solution of nitrogen enriched camphor. This preparation is called "714-X." It is injected into the lymphatic system through the lymphatic channels of the groin. Its proposed mechanism of action is to strengthen the immune system, which then rids the body of cancer. Despite curing several hundred people who had been diagnosed as "terminal," his work has been blackballed by the medical establishment in Canada.

The Naessens remedies are available for export, including to the United States, with a doctor's prescription. They are widely available in Western Europe, as they are distributed by a Swiss pharmaceutical firm.

For information on 714-X, as well as a list of doctors in the U. S. who can provide additional information, contact:

C. O. S. E., Inc.
5270 Fontaine
Rock Forest, Quebec J1N 3B6
Canada   (819) 564-7883

or

Genesis West-Provida
P.O. Box 3460
Chula Vista, CA 91902
(619) 424-9552

Burton's Immuno-augmentative Therapy

In the 1960s, Dr. Lawrence Burton, then a senior oncologist at St. Vincent's Hospital in New York City, discovered four proteins which he found to be deficient in cancer patients. He found that replenishment of these proteins enables the immune system to fight the cancer on its own without side effects. He calls this Immuno-Augmentative Therapy or IAT.

Because Dr. Burton successfully treated patients with IAT before he put forth double blind placebo controlled studies, he alienated the cancer establishment, which then drove him out of the country. He now practices on Grand Bahama Island, where he has established an IAT Center. His clinic has treated over 4,000 patients and has established satellite clinics in Düsseldorf and Regensburg, Germany, with new clinics soon to open in Italy and Switzerland.

Since he left the U.S. in 1977, his blood proteins have been "discovered" by orthodox cancer research centers and are now, belatedly, being put to partial use with no credit, of course, to the originator. Dr. Burton's discoveries, on the other hand, have the distinction and honor of being put on the ACS and NCI blacklist of Unproven Methods — despite dramatic demonstrations of their effectiveness in two separate oncology seminars in 1966. Dr. Burton shares the common characteristic so often seen in people of genius — unwillingness to play the silly political games required to exist as a member in good standing within establishment medicine.

For more information:

Immuno-Augmentative Therapy Center
P.O. Box F-2689
Freeport, Grand Bahamas
(809) 352-7455

IAT Patients' Support Group
Mr. Frank Wiewel
P.O. Box 10
Otho, IA 50569
(515) 972-4444

Livingston Therapy

In 1947, Virginia Livingston, M.D., discovered a pleomorphic (i.e., form-changing) microbe (germ) which she named *"Progenitor cryptocides."* This name means, literally, "hidden, ancestral killer." Dr. Livingston was able to demonstrate the presence of this organism in all cancers, both human and animal. She also demonstrated that cancer would result in an animal when Progenitor was injected into that animal.

Dr. Livingston also found this organism to be universally present but ordinarily held in check by a healthy immune system. However, when the immune system fails due to stress, toxins, poor diet, or for other reasons, *Progenitor* divides and establishes itself at the levels found in cancer patients.

Once established, she found *Progenitor* able to produce a hormone almost identical to HCG (human chorionic gonadotropin), a hormone produced by the placenta which serves to protect placental cells from the antibodies of the mother. Dr. Livingston believed that HCG served to protect *Progenitor* and the resulting cancer cells from attack by the immune system.

Livingston Therapy is a shotgun approach designed to strengthen the immune system, so it can, hopefully, defeat Progenitor. Diet, antibodies and vaccines all are used for this purpose. Included under vaccines is, or at least was, an autogenous vaccine made from a culture of the patient's own bacteria.

In 1990, California health officials required Dr. Livingston to cease giving the autogenous vaccine. This action was taken in the absence of one single patient complaint and in the face of hundreds of patients who benefited from treatment with this unique preparation.

This represents the usual bureaucratic regulation of medicine, often spearheaded by doctors who no longer practice medicine (some never did). Their general attitude could be summed up like this: "If we don't agree with it, it must not work and if everybody is not doing it, it probably is dangerous."

According to this kind of thinking, a Big Mac, fries and a shake must be a very nutritious and healthy meal because everyone knows about it, and many people are eating this fare. On the other hand, an exclusively raw vegetable diet must be worthless and dangerous since few people have heard of it, and fewer still are eating it.

Dr. Livingston died of heart failure at the age of 84 three months after she testified before a congressional hearing regarding her therapy in March of 1990. Her work is being carried on by The Livingston Foundation Medical Center in San Diego, California and is managed by her daughter Julie Anne Wagner. I am happy to say, they still are treating patients.

For information:

Livingston Foundation Medical Center
3232 Duke St.
San Diego, CA 92110
(619) 224-3515

Issels' Whole Body Therapy

Agreeing with Virginia Livingston as to the cause of cancer and rendering a similar approach to treatment, Dr. Josef Issels, M.D., of Germany, achieved an independently verified complete remission rate of seventeen percent in people with terminal cancer who were given less than one year to live. This seventeen percent was free of any sign of cancer at five years. These remarkable results threatened the German and British cancer establishments so much that, through a series of prosecutions by the German government and an effective smear campaign by the British government, Issels was forced to close his clinic in the early 1970s.

Since 1984, his work has been carried on by Ahmed Elkadi, M.D., of Panama City, Florida. Dr. Elkadi calls this approach "multimodality immunotherapy." Another practitioner who carries on Dr. Issels' work is Wolfgang Woeppel, M.D., of Germany. Dr. Woeppel comes highly recommended by Dr. Issels.

For information:

Ahmed Elkadi, M.D.
Panama City Clinic
236 So. Tyndall Pkwy.
Panama City, FL 32404
(904) 763-7689

Wolfgang Woeppel, M.D.
Hufeland Klinik
Bismarkstrasse
D-97980 Bad Mergentheim
Germany
Phone No. from America: 011-49-7931-8185

Herbal Therapies for Cancer

Herbal therapies have been around for thousands of years and were widely prescribed by doctors until the late 1800s when the American Medical Association (AMA), a trade union of doctors committed to partnership with the budding pharmaceutical industry, used its economic and political muscle to suppress the use of natural substances. The use of herbs once was mainstream medicine but, because there is no great profit to be made from these unpatentable wonder drugs, they have become progressive therapies.

Nevertheless, although the AMA, NCI and ACS would prefer that you not know, several herbs produce patentable derivatives which are mainstays in the orthodox treatment of cancer. These herbs are "messed with," biochemically speaking, to produce unique, semi-synthetic compounds which retain some of the activity of the original herb and yet are patentable. Examples are vincristine, vinblastine and eteoposide. Taxol, a new experimental drug for cancer, is derived from the bark of the Pacific yew tree.

The fear of the cancer establishment is, of course, that people themselves would be able to treat their own cancer at least as well as the approved therapies for a tiny fraction of the cost, simply by finding the proper herb and preparing a tea or by eating the plant. For this reason millions of dollars are poured into the creation of synthetics and into the advertising necessary to convince people that laboratories can improve over nature.

We will focus on only a few herbal therapies, because it is not possible in the confines of this book to cover all the herbal treatments which may be effective in cancer. Besides that, only two percent of the herbs in nature have been tested as possible cancer therapies. It is certain that many effective herbs still lie undiscovered.

Essiac Tea

In 1922 Rene Caisse (pronounced as one would pronounce the words "Rin Case"), a nurse in Ontario, Canada, noticed an elderly hospital patient with a scarred and gnarled breast. When Rene Caisse asked about the scarring, she was told that twenty years earlier the woman had her breast cancer healed by an Indian medicine man using an herbal tea. This woman had been told by doctors that her breast must be removed. She refused this advice and decided to take her chances with the herbal tea. This woman handed over the information on this herbal remedy to Rene Caisse.

Rene Caisse put the formula aside, deciding that if she ever developed cancer she would use it. Two years later, one of her aunts developed stomach cancer and was told she had six months to live. Caisse remembered the herbal formula and, in partnership with her aunt's doctor, Dr. R. O. Fisher of Toronto, gave the herbal tea to her aunt. She recovered after two months and lived free from her stomach cancer for 21 years after that. Following this event, Caisse and Fisher began to treat terminal cases of cancer, curing many of them.

Not knowing what to call the stuff Rene Caisse spelled her own last name backward and came up with "Essiac." It seemed as good a name as any, so this is how it has come to be known. Rene Caisse, beginning in the 1920s until her death in 1978, offered this tea to thousands of people, many of whom were restored to health and many whose lives were prolonged and whose pain was lessened.

By 1937, the fame of Essiac had spread to the U.S. and Caisse was commuting to Chicago to treat patients at Northwestern Medical Center. After a two year evaluation the doctors at Northwestern concluded that Essiac tea eased the pain of cancer and prolonged life.

As with all such discoveries, Rene Caisse was forced to battle the medical establishment. This resulted in the formation, in 1938, of the Canadian "Royal Cancer Commission." Showing up to testify for Essiac were 387 of Caisse's patients. Of these, only 49 were allowed to testify. People who free of tumor after using Essiac after the failure of orthodox treatment were interpreted by the Royal Cancer Commission as "recoveries from orthodox therapies." In cases with no previous therapies, the interpretation was "misdiagnosis."

Rene Caisse, after years of harassment, and fearing imprisonment for her work, closed her clinic in 1942. Over the next thirty years she treated patients in great secrecy from her home, even while under surveillance by the Canadian Health Department, I suppose the "Royal" one.

As with most cancer treatments, orthodox, as well as progressive, some people respond and some do not. Undoubtedly, some people have been made free of tumor with Essiac, and others have died from their disease. As I read the literature on Essiac, it appears that its main use is to cause regression of tumor size and to reduce the pain induced by the tumor. It is thus an excellent adjunct to other therapies. If I had cancer I would choose several progressive therapies and not rely on just one. Essiac would be one of them.

Caisse sold the formula to the Resperin Corporation in late 1977 and died at age ninety just over one year later. It is still possible to obtain Essiac. You can buy Essiac Tea at well-stocked organic groceries. Essiac is, after all, a blend of herbal teas — not so easy for a government to regulate, although the government of Canada gives it a good try. They forbid the makers of Essiac to use the word "cure," so they simply distribute patient testimonials. If you have a condition for which Essiac might help, you can order it in quantity at a discount from:

Terrence Maloney
Essiac International
2211-1081 Ambleside Dr.
Ottawa, Ont. CANADA K2B 8C8
Phone (613) 820-9311
Fax: (613) 820-8455

The people at Essiac International also will work with you regarding a treatment protocol for your condition at no charge.

Hoxsey Therapy

Harry Hoxsey, who passed on in 1974 at the age of 73, was not a doctor but rather a self-taught healer who used a combination of herbs which he said was passed on to him by his father. Hoxsey's preparation helped many people with cancer, and his fame spread far and wide. In the 1950s, his clinic in Dallas and its seventeen satellite clinics represented the largest progressive cancer therapy approach in the world.

Naturally, his success drew the attention of the medical establishment and during the McCarthy era in the 1950s, Hoxsey was harassed by the AMA, FDA and NCI. They pronounced his therapy fraudulent without as much as a fact-finding mission to his clinic. (The FDA has not yet gotten the message that the McCarthy era is over.) Hoxsey closed his clinic in 1960 and three years later reopened in a freer country, at least from a medical point of view, Mexico. His clinic in Tijuana is known as the "Bio-Medical Center." It is run by Dr. Hoxsey's nurse, Mildred Nelson, R.N.

For further information:

Bio-Medical Center   Phone numbers from the U.S.
P.O. Box 727 01152-66-84-9011
Colonia Juarez   01152-66-84-9081
Tijuana 220000   01152-66-84-9082
Mexico   01152-66-84-9376

Iscador (Mistletoe)

Iscador is derived from the European mistletoe. Mistletoe is a parasitic plant often seen growing on trees. Mistletoe was used by the Celts hundreds of years ago. It was believed to be an aphrodisiac and was used as part of a month-long party when sexual license was given to everyone. Mistletoe was used to release inhibitions. What we have left of this is the custom of hanging mistletoe at Christmas time and kissing the lucky person who is found under it.

Although well-researched and available from doctors and hospitals throughout Europe, Iscador is still listed by the ACS as an "unproven therapy." Iscador both strengthens the immune system and directly inhibits tumor growth. In Europe it is used in conjunction with other treatments, especially before and after surgery and chemotherapy to prevent spread of the cancer from these procedures. Bladder, genital and digestive tract cancers are said to respond best to Iscador.

Doctors who use Iscador in the U.S. order it directly from its European manufacturers. The use of Iscador is associated with a philosophical movement called "anthroposophy."

For further information:

Physicians Association for Anthroposophical
Medicine
P.O. Box 269
Kimberton, PA 19442

Lukas Klinik
CH-4144 Arlesheim
Switzerland
011-41-61-701-3333

Chaparral

Chaparral is a hardy desert shrub native to the Southwestern U.S. and Mexico. This plant shows the ability to inhibit the germination of seeds from plants which may be in competition with it. This ability to inhibit plant germination may have something to do with its ability to inhibit tumor growth. Chaparral has been part of Indian folk medicine for centuries for treatment of a variety of illnesses, including cancer. Chaparral contains polysaccharides, which are thought to stimulate the immune system, and nor-dihydroguaiaretic acid (NDGA). NDGA inhibits glycolysis, the anaerobic breakdown of sugars on which tumors depend for their energy. So, like pau d'arco, chaparral both strengthens the immune system and directly inhibits tumor growth.

Chaparral is commonly available from health food stores in a variety of forms: tea, tincture, pill and capsule. As regards botanicals, the tea form is ordinarily the most effective. Binders and fillers, which are part of the preparation of pills and capsules, decrease and sometimes interfere with potency.

Pau D'Arco

Also, known as "Ipacho," "ipe rox o" and "taheebo tea," pau d'arco is derived from the inner bark of the Tabebuia tree of Brazil and Argentina. It is used in folk medicine in South America for the treatment of a wide variety of illnesses: colds, flu, malaria, gonorrhea and cancer.

In some cases, cancer remissions have been achieved; however, it is apparently necessary to keep drinking the tea for the rest of one's life to maintain the remission. Fortunately, this preparation is sold widely in health food stores.

The NCI sponsored a study of one of the ingredients of pau d'arco over twenty years ago. This ingredient is called "lapachol." It was found that a good blood level could not be achieved without producing severe side effects such as nausea, vomiting and spontaneous bleeding. The NCI concluded that pau d'arco is was not fit for treatment of cancer.

This narrow-minded approach is typical of the constraints of thinking imposed by the allopathic paradigm of one illness, one cure. The items in God's pharmacy (nature) come allied with each other, not separately. There is no vitamin B_6 tree, for example. There are twelve aromatic compounds in pau d'arco, which act synergistically. To isolate one item and test it in this manner therefore is absurd.

Pau d'arco is thought to act by inhibiting the formation of fibrin, which has the effect of preventing the formation of new blood vessels. New blood vessels are necessary for new tumors to form. Fibrin also is necessary for the formation of the protein coats, which surround and protect malignant cells.

When buying pau d'arco, let the buyer beware. There are many imitations on the market, which are ineffective. Read the label, and be sure you see the tree listed to be *Tabebuia impetiginosa* or *Tabebuia heptaphylla*. If you do not see one of these listed, do not waste your money. Ask the maker of the tea to supply names and phone numbers of satisfied customers. You also can have the product assayed for its level of lapachol.

When preparing the tea, use only a glass or stainless steel teapot. There should be no plastic in the packaging material. The pill form of pau d'arco is of no value.

Nutritional Therapies for Cancer

By 1984, after years of stonewalling, the American cancer establishment reversed itself and finally admitted that diet was a risk factor in the causation of cancer. Still, the ACS and NCI does not admit the usefulness of diet in the treatment of cancer. They dismiss the hundreds of cases of people who had cancer, went on a certain type of diet and then did not have cancer. "Anecdotal evidence," they say. In other words, "We don't know why, but these people must be making this up."

The fact is that your chances of cancer are less on a diet which is vegetarian, raw and free of hydrogenated fat and heated oil. It is no accident that your chances of becoming free of a cancer are increased by the same diet. Eventually, the cancer establishment will admit this also and, when they do, they will come on just as they did when they admitted that diet is a risk factor for the disease: like they discovered it themselves.

Let us talk about some of the more specific dietary treatments which have been shown to have a therapeutic effect on cancer. Research in this area is particularly humanitarian. There is no big profit to be made. It is a therapy which the individual can carry out for himself. It is simple and straightforward. When you learn about this approach to cancer therapy, and you do not adopt it to prevent or treat cancer, you are fresh out of excuses. Maybe Freud was right, there is a "death instinct."

When cancer is present, if one wants to survive, there is no room for half measures or rationalization. Pure food is healing; this has been demonstrated over and over, and impure food is cancer nurturing, this also is clear. When food is tampered with in the growing phase or later preserved or cooked, it is no longer pure. A large portion of plant nutrition is destroyed, and the food can rightfully be called "dead" — and it has a good chance of taking you with it.

In a society which has been duped by the illusory power of the synthetic drug lab, it is hard to hear this: food is your best therapy. All you have to do to enjoy this therapy is to stop eating dead animals and animal products and start eating a large variety of uncooked, organically grown vegetables, fruits and sprouted nuts and seeds.

Because our society is so addicted to dead foods, it is practically impossible for only one member of a family to make the transition to living foods. In the case of cancer, either the entire family wakes up to the problem and makes dietary changes as a family, or the person with cancer has no chance. It is just not possible for a person addicted to dead food to eat a healthy diet and see other members of the family gobbling down the food his addictions crave. The presence of cancer in one member of a family can be a great opportunity for the entire family to change to a style of eating which is vastly superior in its impact on health.

Macrobiotics

"Macrobiotics" include the dietary changes mentioned above with an emphasis on whole cereal grains and also lifestyle changes, which include exercise and spiritual clarity. The macrobiotic approach to cancer treatment, like all therapies, is not 100% effective 100% of the time. Nevertheless, thousands of people have handled their cancers while following this approach. Statistical estimates from practitioners of macrobiotics show that between fifteen and twenty percent of people are able to improve their condition through macrobiotics. This may not seem like so much, but when you realize that these are mostly people who have been pronounced terminal by orthodox oncologists, it is not bad at all. It probably is true that the earlier one begins to use this approach and the sooner one rejects the immune-depressing therapies of standard medical treatment, the better are one's chances. Usually people turn to macrobiotics when there is nothing else left.

To successfully utilize the macrobiotic approach, the average person needs a lot of support and a lot of relearning regarding nutrition. When one is in this position, it is important to realize that the typical family doctor has had no formal training in nutrition beyond the brainwash we all got in grade school, and his or her advice in the area of nutrition should be valued accordingly. Many people who have done well on the macrobiotic approach have suffered relapse back into cancer upon taking doctor's advice to add meat and/or dairy to their macrobiotic diet in the name of getting in enough protein. Even the NCS and the NIH recognize the nutritional sufficiency of the macrobiotic diet.

Please understand that I am not referring here to the Zen Macrobiotic Diet popularized by George Ohsawa. That may be a sufficient diet for a Zen master but not for ordinary people. A modern macrobiotic diet is rich in all nutrients and includes an astounding array of tasty foods.

For information:

Kushi Institute of the Berkshires
P.O. Box 7
Becket, MA 01223
(413) 623-5742

Wheatgrass Therapy

Many nutritionists believe that wheatgrass is especially nutritious and recommend wheatgrass combined with the diet described above. Here is a list of places where you can ask for information or seek treatment including wheatgrass.

Ann Wigmore Foundation
196 Commonwealth Ave.
Boston, MA 02116
(617) 267-9424

Hippocrates Health Institute
1443 Palmdale Ct.
West Palm Beach, FL 33411
(407) 471-8876

New Hippocrates Health Institute
1 Shipyard Way
Medford Square, MA 02155
(617) 395-1608

Health Institute of San Diego
6970 Central Ave.
Lemon Grove, CA 91945
(619) 464-3346

Creative Health Institute
918 Union City Rd.
Union City, MI 49094
(517) 278-6260

Moerman's Anti-Cancer Diet

After fifty years of struggle with the medical authorities of the Netherlands, Dutch physician Cornelius Moerman lived to see his methods approved as effective in the treatment of cancer. The following year he died at the age of 95, a vigorous man to the end, a beneficiary of his own treatment methods.

The Moerman Association has a membership of 10,000 people, including many former cancer patients. The Dutch Ministry of Health issued a report in 1989 concerning 350 recovered cancer patients. Thirty-five percent were certified by the Ministry of Health to be in complete remission with the Moerman Diet as their only treatment. Ten of these people had been sent home to die by orthodox doctors.

The Moerman Diet emphasizes vegetables and also allows some dairy and believes strongly in the nutritional value of egg yolks. It also emphasizes the value of nutritional supplements particularly citric acid, iodine, sulfur, vitamins A, B complex, C and E.

For more information:

Mrs. G. G. Strating-Ijben
Moerman Vereniging
Postbus 14
6674-ZG Herveld
Netherlands
Phone number: 011-31-8880-51221

Metabolic Therapies for Cancer

The metabolic therapies are based on the belief that cancer is a complex breakdown in normal body chemistry which requires intervention at many levels to interrupt the cancer growth. Detoxification procedures such as colonic irrigation, and liver and gallbladder flushes are used. Dietary changes, similar to the ones listed under "Dietary Therapies" above, are used.

Metabolic agents such as vitamins, minerals, glandulars, enzymes, EDTA, DMSO, ozone, hydrazine sulfate, bovine and shark cartilage and the often maligned (by the cancer establishment) laetrile (vitamin B_{17}) are used to attack the tumor at the biochemical level. The vaccine approach is used, as is live cell therapy and psychological counseling.

When reading about metabolic therapy for cancer, one gets the image of pointing fifty shotguns at a rabbit, so that even though many pellets go astray, some also will hit the target. Politically speaking, it is so difficult to practice metabolic therapy in the United States, many dedicated doctors have moved their practices just across the border to Mexico, most of them being located in Tijuana. If you want to know more about these clinics, you can contact:

The Cancer Control Society
P.O. Box 4651
Modesto, CA 95352
(209) 529-4697

Hans Nieper, M.D.

Dr. med. (as they call it in Germany) Hans Nieper is an oncologist now practicing in Hannover, Germany. He applies various metabolic therapies in his own unique way, using many of the approaches already mentioned. He terms his approach "eumetabolic therapy." He employs the usual vegetarian/fruitarian approach along with, among other things, vitamins, minerals, BCG, laetrile, squalene for chromosome repair and bromelain (600 to 1200 mg. per day) to dissolve the membrane around cancer cells allowing T-lymphocytes (which he builds up with thymus extract and zinc orotate) to attack them.

Dr. Nieper's therapies are unique for each individual and are based on the type of tumor and the results of extensive lab tests. As with all these therapies, there is much more to know about Dr. Nieper than we have room to cover here.

Dr. med. Hans A. Nieper
Sedanstrasse 21
D-30161 Hannover
Germany
011-49-511-348-0808

Gerson Therapy

Max Gerson, M.D., was a refugee from Nazi Germany who immigrated to the U.S. in 1936 where he practiced the dietary and detoxification therapies he had developed during his distinguished medical career in Germany. He came under severe persecution for his methods by the New York State Medical Society. His methods still are listed under the "Unproven Therapies" blacklist of the ACS, even though his diet for cancer has an uncanny resemblance to the ACS diet, adopted in 1984, which is recommended to prevent cancer — 48 years after Gerson first applied these principles to the treatment of cancer in the U.S.

Gerson Therapy emphasizes fresh, organically grown, raw vegetables and fresh juices made from same. The primary detoxification method is the coffee enema, which allows the liver to relax its drainage system and discharge accumulated toxins. All types of cancers are said to respond and, during his lifetime, Gerson reported a thirty-percent, five-year survival rate for the "incurable" cancers in advanced stages. Gerson Therapy is most effective in lymphoma and melanoma and least effective with leukemia.

Dr. Gerson died in 1959 and his work is carried on by the Gerson Institute in Bonita, California.

For more information:

Gerson Institute
P.O. Box 430
Bonita, CA 91908
(619) 472-7450

Centro Hospitalario Inernationale del Pacifico, S. A.
Playas, Tijuana
Mexico

Kelley's Nutritional Metabolic Therapy

A Kansas dentist, Dr. William Donald Kelley, developed a program for dealing with a variety of degenerative diseases, including cancer, based on the idea that the primary deficiency in cancer is the inability to digest proteins. Dr. Kelley believed that the primary deficiency was located in the pancreas, which does not produce enough enzymes to digest protein completely. He said that even if a tumor is surgically removed it probably would return if this metabolic deficiency were not corrected.

Every biology student knows the pancreas releases enzymes into the small intestine to digest food. What usually is not taught is that the well-functioning pancreas also releases enzymes directly into the blood stream where they reach all tissues and destroy cancer cells by digesting them.

Kelley's therapy, therefore, focuses on diet, detoxification, enzyme and vitamin replacement and glandulars. Psychological and spiritual exploration and a prayerful relationship with God also are encouraged.

After a five-year, case- by-case analysis of Kelley's patients, Dr. Nicholas Gonzalez of New York was inspired to carry on with Dr. Kelley's work.

For more information:

Nicholas Gonzales, M.D.
737 Park Ave.
New York, NY 10021
(212) 535-3993

Adjunctive Therapies for Cancer

There is a short list of treatments that are usually used in combination with other therapies, which have powerful healing properties of their own. Each one is occasionally used exclusively in the treatment of cancer, with life-saving results. These therapies are: chelation, ozone, hydrogen peroxide, hyperthermia, DMSO and live cell therapy.

Chelation Therapy

This subject is well covered in the first chapter of this book. Its role as an adjunct to cancer treatment lies in the fact that it is a powerful antioxidant and in its ability to clear toxic heavy metals from the body. No one proposes that EDTA cures cancer; however, as an adjunctive treatment, it is believed to potentiate other approaches to cancer therapy. Informal studies indicate that very few people who are fully chelated go on to develop cancer after chelation. Its power to prevent cancer is estimated to be about ninety percent: a full course of chelation serves to prevent ninety percent of cancers which otherwise would happen.

Cancer is a complex disease, and its successful treatment is a complex process. When the final story is written, and all the politics are finally processed out of the chelation debate, I predict that EDTA will assume its rightful position as a powerful adjunct to the treatment of cancer. This process, however, may take a century.

Hyperthermia

As a treatment for cancer, raising the body's temperature — called "hyperthermia" — is designed to make life hard on cancer cells which cannot stand prolonged temperatures over 107° Fahrenheit. High temperatures collapse their vascular systems.

This procedure is carried out using ultrasound, microwaves and radio frequency waves for local treatment. For systemic treatment, either heated blood is reinfused or whole body wraps in rubber blankets with circulating hot water are applied. The objective is to raise body temperature to 108° and hold it there for two hours. General anaesthesia is used.

There are proponents for and against using hyperthermia alone. Those who are against this idea believe that it works best if combined with radiation and/or chemotherapy. And guess what? The FDA approves, probably because it does not interfere too much with the surgery/radiation/chemotherapy industry.

Despite FDA approval, I still consider hyperthermia a progressive treatment for cancer because it had the honor of being disapproved by the ACS and the FDA for so long (until 1977 and 1984 respectively) and because few people have heard of it. University medical centers are about the only places where it is available at present.

For information:

Valley Cancer Institute
12099 W. Washington Blvd., Ste. 304
Los Angeles, CA 90066
(310) 398-0013
(800) 488-1379

DMSO Therapy

The subject of DMSO therapy has been covered elsewhere in this book. I want to focus here on its use in cancer therapy. DMSO has many characteristics which make it a good adjunctive treatment for cancer. Recall from our previous discussion that DMSO is a super-solvent. It binds to water (which makes up around 65% of the body) better than water does. This gives DMSO the ability to penetrate every single cell of the body, so whatever its other effects may be, they will be spread systemically through the entire body. Whatever is administered with DMSO tends to bind with the DMSO and is carried to the inside of cells along with DMSO.

Animal studies show that DMSO, by itself, inhibits the growth of breast, colon and bladder cancer, as well as leukemia, in animals. The fact that this list is not longer probably reflects the fact that DMSO has not been studied in other cancers.

If cytotoxic drugs are given to fight a cancer, they are more effective when given with DMSO to escort them to the inside of cancer cells. DMSO also relieves the pain of cancer and, by being a free radical scavenger, reduces the side effects of radiation therapy.

But, it's the old story! As with most effective and affordable cancer therapies, it is not approved for that use by the FDA. This, despite the presence of more than 6,000 articles attesting to its safety and effectiveness and despite the fact that almost every civilized country approves of DMSO treatment for cancer except, you guessed it, the USA.

Nevertheless, some doctors do offer DMSO in the US. Because DMSO is approved for one rare bladder condition called "interstitial cystitis," it is possible for doctors to use it for any other purpose. The FDA's authority extends to the determination of whether or not an item is safe, and it is up to the doctor to determine its correct use. While the FDA specifies approval only for treatment of interstitial cystitis this specification has no teeth.

Ozone

One of the many sad facts of standardized American medicine is the great difficulty encountered by doctors who use ozone to treat anything. Despite the fact that ozone is an accepted, safe and effective treatment for a variety of conditions in almost all other countries, the FDA clings to the position that it is potentially dangerous to human health! They have that wrong. Ozone is safe. The FDA, on the other hand, is dangerous to human health — at least in the USA.

Other than safety, the other feature about ozone is that it is relatively inexpensive and cannot be patented because it is abundant in nature. This is the real problem for the medical cancer establishment. Some doctors offer ozone in the US despite the restrictions. Some states do not choose to harass doctors who offer ozone therapy. Others choose to take their licenses.

There is a lot of confusion about ozone. We hear about it in two places: the ozone layer in the atmosphere and as part of industrial pollution. The ozone layer in the upper reaches of the atmosphere absorbs UV light and protects us from skin cancers and cataracts. Thus, it prevents death and blindness. Not bad. Even the FDA does not object to the presence of ozone in the ozone layer.

Ozone also is part of the mix of industrial pollution. It is created when petroleum ignites inside an internal combustion engine, like the one which turns the wheels on your car to take you to work. Because it comes in this form and is easy to measure, it is used to gauge the degree of pollution — so people in Los Angeles will know what they are dying from just before the moment of asphyxiation.

However, while petrochemical pollutants are dangerous to human health, ozone is not a petrochemical. It is merely oxygen in a *menage à trois*. Oxygen, like human beings, usually prefers to come in pairs, or diads: O_2. However, also like human beings and in about the same proportion, oxygen occasionally gets kinky and comes as a triad: O_3.

Ozone, or O_3, is much less stable than O_2. Probably, three-way love affairs are as explosive at a molecular level as they are at human level. O_3 is looking for an opportunity to become O_2 plus singlet oxygen (O^-). When this happens, singlet oxygen, O^-, combines with another singlet oxygen and forms O_2 again. If no singlet oxygen is available, O^- combines with other surrounding molecules. This is called "oxidation," and it is particularly hard on cancer cells, killing some outright and stunting the growth of others.

The route of administration of ozone is rectal, intravenous and aural (infusion into the ear canal allowing the ozone to absorb through the ear drum).

If you want ozone therapy you must find one of those courageous doctors living in one of those states which do not harass these sorts of docs, or you must travel abroad: Mexico, Europe, the Bahamas, notably.

For further information and a physician's referral list:

International Bio-oxidative Medicine Foundation
P.O. Box 610767
Dallas, TX 75261
(817) 481-9772

Hydrogen Peroxide

The subject of hydrogen peroxide (H_2O_2) has been covered elsewhere in this book. It is more acceptable to, although not exactly smiled on by, medical orthodoxy. In most states, you can find doctors who offer this therapy. The mechanism of action is the same as ozone, and the route of administration is intravenous.

The question comes up as to which is more efficacious: ozone or hydrogen peroxide. Theoretically, they should be the same, because the mechanism of action — boosting oxidative metabolism and damaging and killing cancer cells, bacteria and viruses, as well as boosting the immune system — is the same. I know of no studies which compare the two, so this question will have to remain unanswered for the moment.

For further information and a physician's referral list:

International Bio-oxidative Medicine Foundation
P.O. Box 610767
Dallas, TX 75261
(817) 481-9772

Live Cell Therapy

The injection of fetal or embryonic cells, usually of calf origin, was developed by Paul Niehans in Switzerland in the early 1930s. Unapproved by the FDA, it is offered by a number of clinics in Tijuana, Mexico as part of a nutritional/metabolic approach to cancer therapy. It also is used to treat a wide variety of other diseases.

In cancer treatment with live cell therapy, the thymus gland is targeted, because it plays an important role in immune function. Shark fetal cells are favored, because it is believed they contain a substance which accounts for the fact that sharks almost never get cancer.

Even live cell therapists admit that by itself live cell therapy is not a cure for terminal cancer. They also believe it is very useful as part of an overall nutritional/metabolic approach. The earlier the cancer is diagnosed and the earlier treatment is instituted, the more effective it is.

For further information:

American Biologics - Mexico Hospital and Medical Center
1180 Walnut Ave.
Chula Vista, CA 92011
(619) 429-8200
(800) 227-4458

Energy Medicine in the Treatment of Cancer

Something animates the body. What exactly it is which gives life to otherwise dead meat may not be knowable in scientific terms. However, there are many manifestations of this force. When one considers a living being, one must consider what can be seen and what cannot be seen. When you walk by a telephone line you do not see something which would indicate to you the thousands of conversations whizzing back and forth over that line. Nevertheless, those conversations are happening. Likewise, when you look at the body, you cannot necessarily see the communications happening between the billions of cells. Nevertheless, those communications are happening. If they were not happening, life would not be happening.

The physical energy of the body is expressed as electromagnetic fields. These fields are not visible, and yet they can be measured. The results obtained through acupuncture and homeopathy, for example, are based upon the ability of these therapies to alter these fields. This is the paradigm which gives meaning to these therapies.

Within this paradigm, it should be possible to treat all illness, and cancer should be no exception. In the profound disturbance which is cancer, there should be an electromagnetic component, which, if correctly altered, should give a solid push toward recovery.

Bioelectric Therapy

The term "bioelectric therapy," in relationship to cancer, refers to the work of Raymond Rife (1888-1971). This Nebraska-born, scientist/inventor, who lived out his professional life in San Diego, California, developed a light microscope capable of magnification to 60,000X with a resolution of 31,000. This was remarkably superior to ordinary light microscopes and even superior to the electron microscope, in that it made possible the study of living cells under fantastic magnification. (With an electron microscope, whatever is being studied must first be killed. Therefore, what one is actually studying is a corpse.)

To his amazement, Rife was able to observe bacteria in the living state transform into viruses. He found that these same viruses were present in the blood of ninety percent of people with cancer, and that injection of these viruses into experimental animals produced cancer. Rife concluded that bacteria, at least the bacteria he was observing, could change form — demonstrating, similar to the manner of parasites, different forms in different stages of life. Concurrent to these observations, Rife developed a frequency generator and was able to kill the organisms he saw under the microscope with specific frequencies.

In 1934, Rife was invited by the University of Southern California Medical Clinic to undertake the treatment of sixteen terminal cancer patients. After treatment, fourteen of the sixteen are said to have been cured by a panel of supervising doctors. The treatment consisted of three-minute sessions, three times each week on the Rife Machine.

The AMA and the California State Board of Public Health undertook a systematic campaign of suppression of Rife's work through harassment of physicians who were working with him. Doctors were threatened, one associate was shot at, another had his lab, which was working to independently duplicate Rife's results, burned to the ground — proving once again that capitalism and humanitarian medical genius cannot live together in the same country without one becoming a predator of the other. A cheap, simple approach to cancer treatment could not be allowed to put the cancer industry out of business.

There now are many "Rife-like" machines out there — it is said about twenty varieties — and many people who treat cancer with these machines who are not doctors. There is no way to verify quality control of these machines, however, and if the technology is wrong, there is the possibility that more harm than good can come from it. If I were in the situation of wanting to have my cancer treated in this way, I would go to American Biologics in Mexico or Dr. Bjoern Nordenstroem in Sweden.

Another bioelectric therapy has to do with the use of magnets to treat cancer. The resource to find out more about this technology is Bio Health Enterprises listed below.

For further information:

Bjoern Nordenstroem, M.D.
Solnav 1
S104-01 Stockholm
Sweden
011-46-834-0560

American Biologics - Mexico Hospital and Medical Center
1180 Walnut Ave.
Chula Vista, CA 92011
(619) 429-8200
(800) 227-4458

Bio Health Enterprises, Inc.
P.O. Box 628
Murray Hills, KY 42071
(502) 753-2613
(800) 626-3386

Homeopathy

Homeopathy rests upon three fundamental paradigms. These paradigms are as follows:

1. Each substance has a unique energy.

2. This energy not only remains in a solution of the substance but increases (paradoxically) as the concentration of the substance in the solution decreases.

3. Illness can be cured by administering the energy in the form of a dilute solution of a substance which produces symptoms (in a healthy person) of the illness one wants to cure.

In successful homeopathy, when the correct substance and the correct concentration are chosen and administered, the patient goes through a "healing crisis," in which he first becomes more symptomatically ill and then recovers from the illness.

There is disagreement among homeopaths as to the value of homeopathy in the treatment of cancer. Some feel it has little value. Others, presumably those with experience in treating cancer in this way, report results any oncologist would envy. If you choose to have homeopathic treatment of your cancer, I suggest you screen the homeopath by phone before making an appointment. How long have you practiced homeopathy? Do you treat cancer homeopathically? If so, what are the results you have observed? Can you put me in contact with satisfied cancer patients you have treated? These questions will lead naturally into other related questions.

For further information and referral information:

Homeopathic Educational Services
2124 Kittredge St.
Berkeley, CA 94704
(510) 649-0294

National Center for Homeopathy
801 No. Fairfax, Ste. 306
Alexandria, VA 22314
(703) 548-7790

Chinese Medicine

Acupuncture, herbal preparations, meditation and also breathing, movement and relaxation disciplines constitute the heart of traditional Chinese medicine. The body is believed to conduct vital energy, or "chi," through channels called "meridians," making a complete cycle every 24 hours. Proper energy flow is deemed vital to health, and restoration of this flow is considered essential in treating disease.

Many of these principles of Chinese medicine are combined in a discipline called "chi gong," which combines the slow movements of tai chi with breathing and meditation. There are numerous reports of people helped through chi gong.

Cancer is the leading cause of death in China, probably due to their high level of industrial pollution. To cope with this situation, the Chinese have tried to integrate allopathic techniques into their treatment approach — surgery, radiation, chemotherapy.

Here are some resources for further information:

Amer. College of Traditional Chinese Med.
455 Arkansas St.
San Francisco, CA 94107
(415) 282-7600

Amer. Academy of Med. Acupuncture
2520 Milvia St.
Berkeley, CA 94704
(415) 841-7600

Ayurvedic Medicine

The world's oldest existing medical system, Ayurveda has been practiced for over 6,000 years. It has developed, in some way, in a parallel manner to Western allopathic medicine, although it is millennia older. There are hundreds of medical schools which offer basic medical training, as well as training in specialties bearing some of the same names they are given in allopathic medicine: obstetrics, pediatrics, ophthalmology, etc. Therapeutic diet, herbs, detoxification, breathing exercises and massage constitute the main avenues of approach to treatment.

The basic difference between Western medicine and Ayurvedic medicine is this: in the Ayurvedic paradigm, consciousness is conceived of as primary; in Western medicine, material is considered primary. The Ayurveda holds that we are thoughts which created bodies. In Western medicine we are material (body) which creates thoughts.

From the point of view of an Ayurvedic physician, the allopathic method of treating illness is at best crude, at worst dangerous, in that it treats only part of the patient: the part which is conceived of as being ill — the material part. In every aspect, Ayurvedic medicine treats the whole person in the belief that one cannot safely split a person into parts. For example, the Ayurvedic doctor may work extensively with the way the patient thinks, believing that thoughts manifest themselves in the biochemistry of the body.

The pharmacopeia of Ayurvedic medicine is massive, with hundreds of herbs used. The active ingredients of many of these herbs have long been utilized by Western medicine. Of course, as usual, our pharmaceutical companies have tried to isolate a few active ingredients, then alter, synthesize, patent and market the altered form. Reserpine, for the treatment of hypertension, is but one example.

Although Ayurvedic (which literally means "the science of life") medicine is the most ancient on earth, it is by no means resting on its laurels. Research is carried on with vigor, and many new herbal compounds are available, some of which, like MAK-4 and MAK-5 are suitable for treatment of cancer.

Some doctors in the U.S. have incorporated the principles of Ayurvedic medicine into their practices. For a referral to one of these doctors, or for more information on Ayurvedic medicine:

Maharishi Ayur-Veda Medical Center
P.O. Box 282
Fairfield, IA 52556
(515) 472-5866

The Cancer Hospitals of Mexico

Special mention of the cancer hospitals in Mexico is in order. Unlike the US government, the government of Mexico is not dominated by the financial interests of a mammoth pharmaceutical industry, and therefore has not outlawed therapies for cancer which are both effective and inexpensive. It is there many people go when the toxic, destructive therapies offered by the US medical establishment have failed. Many of them come home free of tumor. Following is a short list of reputable hospitals in Mexico. This is not an exhaustive list. If you want to check out such hospitals, there is a bus tour offered in Tijuana which takes you through twenty hospitals. Your travel agent should be able to make arrangements for you.

Bio-Medical Center		American Biologics	Oasis Hospital
P.O. Box 727	01152 -66-84-9011	Mexico Hospital and Medical Center	2247 San Diego Av. #235
Colonia Juarez	-66-84-9081	1180 Walnut Ave. (619) 429-8200	San Diego, CA 92110
Tijuana, Mexico 220000\ -66-84-9082		Chula Vista, CA 92011 (800) 227-4458	011-52-668-01850

The Anti-parasite Approach to the Treatment of Cancer

Hulda Regehr Clark, Ph.D., N.D., is in a class by herself, although what class that is we are not yet sure. She alone states categorically that she has discovered the cure for all cancers. That is the title of her book: *The Cure For All Cancers*.

Dr. Clark writes that all cancers are caused by a parasite, *Fasciolopsis buskii*, the human intestinal fluke. She seems to have discovered this not by massive research but by simply noticing it. She noticed that all cancer patients have two things in common: the presence of the human intestinal fluke and exposure to isopropyl alcohol (ordinary "rubbing alcohol"). Normally, the human intestinal fluke is unable to live in organs other than the intestine. They are able to gain access to the blood stream though microscopic tears we all have in our intestinal wall from time to time. When the eggs hatch, producing a stage of the fluke called "miracidia," the liver normally destroys them.

However, a person with isopropyl alcohol in his body cannot destroy the miracidia. Dr. Clark states that the miracidia are able to set up shop and produce the next stage called "redia." Each fluke produces millions of eggs, each egg produces 25-30 miracidia, each miracidia produces forty redia and each redia can produce forty more redia! Let's see, 25 x 40 x 40 = 40,000, and one million eggs going through this cycle would produce 40,000 x 1,000,000 = 40,000,000,000 (40 billion) redia! These redia, says Dr. Clark, migrate to weakened tissues such as smoker's lungs, enlarged prostate, benign breast tumors, etc. The redia reproduce for several generations and then change into a new stage with a tail called "cercaria." The cercaria then find a place in your body to glue themselves; they shed their tails and become metacercaria surrounded by a tough shell.

There it should end with metacercaria in hibernation. But, for some reason (perhaps the isopropyl alcohol?), the tough shell dissolves, allowing the metacercaria to develop into adult flukes in your tissues. When this happens in the liver, a growth factor, ortho-phospho-tyrosine, is released and this causes cancer by provoking the host's cells to divide out of control. Ortho-phospho-tyrosine is designed to provoke growth of the fluke itself but has the secondary, unintended result of causing cancer formation in humans, according to Dr. Clarke.

Dr. Clark says: purge the parasite and cure the cancer. She gives a rigorous recipe of herbs to accomplish this. She also recommends eliminating all contact with isopropyl (rubbing) alcohol. If you have no further contact with isopropyl alcohol, it will leave your system by evaporation. These two steps together, according to Dr. Clark, constitute a definitive cure for cancer. I do not know if Dr. Clark is right. If she is even only partially right, it is a monumental breakthrough. However, I promise you that if she is right, it will not be easily embraced by the cancer industry. If you find this approach intriguing I suggest you find a copy of *The Cure For All Cancers* and read up.

With the exception of the last-mentioned approach, if you want to read deeper and have more details, I suggest a book called *Options, The Alternative Cancer Therapy Book* by Richard Walters.

Burzynski Clinic
6221 Corporate Dr
Houston, TX 77036

Emanuel Revici, M.D.
26 E. 36th St.
New York, NY 10016

Syracuse Can. Res. Inst.
Presidential Plaza
600 E. Genesee St.
Syracuse, NY 13202

C. O. S. E., Inc.
5270 Fontaine
RockForest
Quebec, Canada J1N 3B6

Genesis West-Provida
P.O. Box 3460
Chula Vista, CA 91902

Florida Prev. Hlth. Ser.
Henderson Center
Tampa, FL 33629

Immnno-Aug. Ther.Ctr.
P.O. Box F-2689
Freeport, Grand Bahamas

IAT Patient's Supp. Gr.
Mr. Frank Wiewel
P.O. Box 10
Otho, IA 50569

Livingston Med. Ctr.
3232 Duke St.
San Diego, CA 92110

Ahmed Elkadi, M.D.
Panama City Clinic
236 So. Tyndall Pkwy.
Panama City, FL 32404

Hufeland Klinik
Bismarkstrasse
D-97980
Bad Mergentheim
Germany

Bio-Medical Center
P.O. Box 727
Colonia Juarez
Tijuana 220000
Mexico

Elaine Alexander
6690 Oak St.
Vancouver,B.C. V6P 3Z2
Canada

Physicians Association
 Anthroposophical Med.
P.O. Box 269
Kimberton, PA 19442

Lukas Klinik
CH-4144 Arlesheim
Switzerland

Ann Wigmore Found.
196 Commonwealth Ave.
Boston, MA 02116

Kushi Inst. the Berkshres
P.O. Box 7
Becket, MA 10223

Mrs. G. G. Strating-ljben
Moerman Vereniging
Postbus 14
6674-ZG Herveld
Netherlands

Hippocrates Health Inst.
1443 Palmdale Ct.
W. Palm Bch., FL 33411

Cancer Control Society
P.O. Box 4651
Modesto, CA 95352

Gerson Institute
P.O. Box 430
Bonita, CA 91908

New Hippocrat.Hlth. Ins.
One Shipyard Way
Medford Sq., MA 02155

Nicholas Gonzales, M.D.
737 Park Ave.
New York, NY 10021

Dr. med. Hans A. Nieper
Sedanstrasse 21
D-30161 Hannover
Germany

Health Inst. of San Diego
6970 Central Ave.
Lemon Gr., CA 91945

International Bio-oxidat.
 Medicine Foundation
P.O. Box 610767
Dallas, TX 75261

Valley Cancer Institute
12099 W. Washington
          Blvd. #304
Los Angeles, CA 90066

Creative Health Institute
918 Union City Rd.
Union City, MI 49094

American Biologics
Mexico Center
1180 Walnut Ave.
Chula Vista, CA 92011

B. Nordenstroem, M.D.
Solnav 1
S104-01 Stockholm
Sweden

Bio Health Enterprises
P.O. Box 628
Murray Hills, KY 42071

Homeopathic Educ. Ser.
2124 Kittredge St.
Berkeley, CA 94704

Natl.Ctr. for Homeopathy
801 No. Fairfax, Ste. 306
Alexandria, VA 22314

Ayur-Veda Medical Ctr.
P.O. Box 282
Fairfield, IA 52556

Coll. of Trad. Chin. Med.
455 Arkansas St.
San Fran., CA 94107

Acad. Med. Acupuncture
2520 Milvia St.
Berkeley, CA 94704

Oasis Hospital/Contreras
 Med. Ctr.., Mexico c/o
2247 San Diego Av. 235
San Diego, CA 92110

AIDS

AIDS

Between November 1980 and April 1981, Michael Gottlieb, a researcher at the UCLA Medical Center in Los Angeles, reported on five young, actively homosexual men with a curious wasting syndrome — loss of vitality and weight — involving immune deficiency with low helper lymphocyte (T-cell) counts. These five men contracted infective diseases — systemic yeast infection and *Pneumocystis* pneumonia — usually associated with people whose immune systems have been damaged by cancer chemotherapeutic agents, diseases to which healthy people have immunity.

Turned down by a "respected peer-reviewed" medical journal for quick publication, Gottlieb took his findings to the Center for Disease Control (the CDC). The CDC was happy to announce this new disease to the world and thus create activity for itself. At that time the CDC was smarting from congressional chastisement over its media oriented handling of "Legionnaire's Disease," which turned out not to be the epidemic advertised by the CDC. As Gottlieb was making his report, the CDC was receiving other reports of similar illnesses, which also involved Kaposi's Sarcoma, a previously rare blood vessel cancer. Within one year, these cases were demonstrated to have occurred in clusters; i.e., the cases were coming from specific geographic locations, notably San Francisco, Los Angeles and New York.

When the investigators at CDC looked at what these people had in common, they found them all to be active male homosexuals who used the drug amyl nitrate in the gaseous form. Known as "poppers," because they come in small capsules which are broken apart (popped) releasing the gas which is then immediately inhaled.

The medical use for amyl nitrate is in childbirth. When the time for delivery comes, the woman is offered this gas which puts her into a state of temporary anaesthesia and, not incidentally to the gay community, also a state of temporary euphoria. For the homosexual, this temporary euphoria facilitates anal intercourse through temporarily clouding consciousness, inducing euphoria and lowering inhibitions.

The CDC had a problem: did this new syndrome have something to do with amyl nitrate, or was it related somehow to the promiscuous, homosexual, drug-oriented lifestyle? And here the first error was made. Reasoning that if amyl nitrate could cause immune deficiency, that fact would have long ago been uncovered, the CDC decided that either all of these people were inhaling poppers from one contaminated batch or the amyl nitrate hypothesis was incorrect. They quickly determined that these people could not have been inhaling poppers from the same batch, and therefore the amyl nitrate popper hypothesis met a premature death.

The CDC overlooked, or more probably chose to ignore, the possibility that repeated long term use of amyl nitrate might indeed cause immune deficiency. Overlooking this possibility, the CDC declared the arrival of a new infectious epidemic disease transmitted somehow through sexual contact in homosexuals.

The toxicological — amyl nitrate — explanation for this new syndrome was swept under the carpet, and many people can no longer remember ever having heard of it. The priority agenda at CDC became the tracing of sexual contacts in a population of highly promiscuous homosexual men immersed in a culture of avid pursuit of sexual pleasure as the number one purpose in life. Most of these people had an enormous number of contacts through the bath house scene which was popular in that culture in the late seventies and early eighties. This exposure was in the range of several hundred contacts each year.

The "latency period" of a disease is the time from infection to onset of disease symptoms. The latency period of this new disease was postulated, at that time, to be one year. Therefore, the possible numbers of contact links in a population of people with hundreds of contacts per year became truly staggering.

Not surprisingly, a sexual contact trail leading from one disease victim to another was readily discernable. However, a sexual contact link in the gay bath house scene could be made between almost any two individuals. It all seemed to make sense, never mind the political bias of the CDC for an infectious cause of what would be named, in July of 1982, "AIDS": the autoimmune deficiency syndrome.

History and Personalities

To comprehend what happened next, it is necessary to understand that the field of virology was given a tremendous boost in the 1950s through the conquest of the poliomyelitis virus by Jonas Salk and Albert Sabin. Prior to that event, virology languished as a curiosity in science. After that event, uncountable millions of dollars flowed into virology, inflating the number of people going into that field and the budgets of research departments in university medical schools throughout the country.

Despite the expenditure of such vast amounts of resources, virology produced very little of use to human health through the 1960s and '70s. When the 80s' rolled around, virologists were desperate for an epidemic, any epidemic, to which a viral cause could be assigned. Without such an event, virology was headed to the status of a museum piece in science, and many virologists were going to learn how to pay the bills some other way. Thus, when the new epidemic was announced in 1981 and named "AIDS" in 1982, there was a loud rumble of activity in the virology laboratories throughout the nations.

Now, enter one Robert Gallo, an individual working at NIH (the National Institutes of Health), who had embarrassed himself on a couple of previous occasions by announcing discoveries which turned out not to be accurate. Searching frantically for a cause of AIDS, he settled on the idea that a convincing case for some type of human retrovirus might be made.

Through 1983, he fought a loosing battle to convince his peers that a retrovirus named "HTLV-I," which he himself had discovered, was the culprit. This virus, and possibly a variant named "HTLV-II," was already thought to cause T-cell leukemia in humans, and this presented a serious problem. How could the same virus cause leukemia, which makes T-cells grow out of control, and also cause AIDS, a disease in which the virus is supposed to kill T-cells?

Meanwhile, Luc Montagnier, of the Pasteur Institute in Paris, had isolated another human retrovirus and named it "LAV." He asked Gallo to assist him in presenting LAV to the scientific community as a possible cause of AIDS. Montagnier sent Gallo a sample of his LAV virus for study.

Soon after that, Gallo claimed to have isolated an almost identical virus, which he named "HTLV-III." Gallo probably renamed the LAV virus discovered by Montagnier claiming the "new" virus as his own. When later confronted with this, Gallo was to claim that Montagnier's virus somehow "contaminated" his test tubes. Although fraud was suspected by a few well-trained virologists in 1984, it was not investigated by NIH until 1989, and Gallo was not convicted of scientific fraud until 1992. (Somehow, despite this, Gallo is hailed by the popular media as one of the great scientific minds of our times!)

All of that was in the future. Back in 1984, Gallo was busy plotting to pin AIDS on HTLV-III. Finally he felt he could make his move. He called a press conference on April 23, 1984 and announced that he had isolated the virus which causes AIDS.

A press conference is against all scientific protocol which requires that evidence be published in peer-reviewed journals and then checked by independent research. Since Gallo was the big gun in virology at NIH, he had the weight of a large portion of the medical research establishment behind him, as well as the authority of the federal government, when he made his surprise announcement to the press.

Very few people at that time even knew enough to challenge Gallo, and the few who did realized that the *coup d'etat* had been successful, and that they had better jump on the bandwagon or loose all research funding. When the HTLV-III virus was renamed "HIV," the "human immunodeficiency virus," the dogma was set in concrete.

All research into other possible causes of AIDS ceased and almost the entire scientific herd thundered off in the direction of a viral cause of AIDS. Those scientists willing to think for themselves and speak the truth of their findings were left in the dust of a money/prestige-hungry research establishment herd. Meanwhile, Gallo quietly sent in his application for a patent of his test to detect "HIV antibodies" and from this patent a veritable fortune has been made.

Koch's Postulates

To begin to think for yourself about AIDS, it is necessary to review the basic assumptions regarding infectious disease. A German medical doctor, one Robert Koch, published a landmark paper in 1876 announcing that he had proven the cause of anthrax, a disease of cattle, to be caused by a microorganism with a tubular shape, a "bacillus." This was the first convincing evidence to show that some diseases are caused by animals so tiny that they cannot be seen with the naked eye.

Koch demonstrated his proofs along a line of logic which became known as "Koch's postulates," even though the first part of the hypothesis was created by another German doctor, Jakob Henle, in 1840. Henle stated that if a microorganism was to be shown to cause a disease, that microorganism would have to be isolated from diseased tissue and grown outside the human body.

Yet another German doctor postulated, in the 1870s, that such a microbe also must be shown to cause the same disease when introduced into another animal. Thus, did the germ theory stand when Robert Koch published his finding. Koch's postulates set the gold standard for identifying infectious diseases.

Therefore, the basis for a new biological science was laid down in eloquently logical terms in 1876. Some diseases were definitely caused by microbes; however, to avoid a gross abuse of the new theory, these logical postulates were required to be fulfilled before any disease could be said to be infectious, i.e., caused by a microbe.

It became generally accepted that in order for a microbe to cause a disease it must have the following characeristics:

1. It must be found in sufficient quantity and in proper distribution to fully explain the symptoms of that disease;

2. It must be isolated from the infected tissue;

3. It must be cultured (grown) in pure culture outside the human body;

4. It must, without fail, cause the same disease when introduced from this culture into a second animal, human or otherwise.

Any exception to any of these requirements, even one single exception, would be enough to debunk the entire hypothesis of a particular microbe causing a particular disease.

Koch's postulates were laid out in this manner to prevent the temptation to blame microbes for disease states in which they have no causative relationship. After all, microbes are everywhere, and usually they have nothing to do with disease states. Koch's postulates were defined for just such a scientist as Robert Gallo.

When we apply Koch's postulates to the theory that "HIV" causes the disease known as "autoimmune deficiency syndrome," we are immediately in very hot water. Let us see why.

Koch's First Postulate

The virus must be found in sufficient quantity and in proper distribution to fully explain the symptoms of AIDS, in all cases.

First, according to Koch's postulates, the virus must be found in everyone with AIDS. Is it? Certainly not. Autoimmune deficiency has been present in the world since there have been lab studies to measure its parameters. I graduated from medical school in 1969. The syndrome was well-known at that time. There still are many people with AIDS who do not have HIV. Therefore, HIV fails Koch's first postulate.

Koch's Second Postulate

The "HIV" virus must be isolated from the infected tissue, in all cases.

Since the virus is not even present in everyone with AIDS, it cannot be isolated from the tissue of those people. Koch's second postuate: *geht kaput.*

Koch's Third Postulate

The virus must be grown in pure culture, outside the human body.

This postulate is not fulfilled, as it requires the presence of T-cells to grow the virus in a test tube or on an agar plate. You can argue that these T-cells are outside the body, and even if you grant that Koch's third postulate is fulfilled, the other three postulates must be fulfilled also to make the case for HIV as the cause of AIDS.

Koch's Fourth Postulate

The virus must, without fail, cause the same disease when introduced from this culture into a second animal or human.

Koch's fourth second postulate is that the virus must cause the same disease when introduced into another animal. Does it? Well, granting species specificity for a virus, the jury is still out on that one.

The experimental animals for a species-specific organism can only be other members of that species, in this case humans. We cannot ethically inoculate humans with HIV, so we must study the disease in its natural state. If we find someone who has turned "HIV positive," we presumably have a case to study.

But, what happens if such a person does not become ill? In that case, we must postulate a "latency period," a period of time between the presence of the virus and the onset of illness. No one knows what a virus is doing during a latency period — perhaps drawing up battle plans for the war ahead?

In 1983, the latency period was said to be one year between infection and onset of AIDS. When many people with HIV antibodies did not develop AIDS, the latency period was pushed back year by year. The latency period is now up to thirteen years. This self-serving latency period is designed to get around the question of why these people are not developing AIDS.

To fulfill Koch's fourth postulate, the HIV virus must cause AIDS in every person who has the virus. This appears not to be the case.

And what about people who are exposed to the virus but do not develop antibodies? It is said that about 1000 sexual exposures are necessary, in the average case, to result in a presence of HIV antibodies in the recipient.

What happens the other 999 times? Could it be that the healthy person, who does not already have a deficiency in immune functions, simply kills the virus on contact? Perhaps having the antibodies to AIDS is evidence of former infection successfully erdicated. This is what such anitobodies mean in all other cases in which the person is healthy.

Therefore, Koch's postulates are failed at every turn. The only way to believe that HIV causes AIDS is to either have insufficient knowledge to think for oneself or to have a vested, financial and/or ego interest in the theory being true. That includes over 99% of the population, so the HIV theory of AIDS is the banner of a thundering herd of virological and public opinion.

Inflated Statistics

So if AIDS is not caused by HIV — or at least some infective agent — how do we explain the "explosion" of AIDS in the population? The fact is, there has not been an explosion of AIDS. The predicted explosion of AIDS never happened.

The only way the CDC has been able to create the appearance of an increase in the rate of AIDS is by almost yearly adding one more disease to the list of diseases which are said to result from AIDS. Now, diseases which have been around forever are said to be a manifestation of the AIDS virus: candidiasis, cervical cancer, dementia, Kaposi's sarcoma, lymphoma, *Pneumocystis carinii* pneumonia, thrombocytopenia and toxoplasmosis. All one needs to have AIDS, by CDC definition is the HIV virus and one of these diseases. Just about any disease is fair game to be added to this list, as long as the person also has the HIV virus.

Meanwhile, in Africa, people who are HIV positive are not manifesting AIDS with the same complex of diseases, but rather are showing up with signs and symptoms of wasting: weight loss, loss of appetite, diarrhea — in other words the signs of calorie deficiency malnutrition. Of course, malnutrition is endemic to most of Africa. It seems that the World Health Organization is willing to do the same job overseas that the CDC is willing to do in the U.S., namely take whatever endemic (meaning always present) diseases are present and call them AIDS when seen in combination with an HIV positive blood test.

Let us therefore rethink AIDS. Although it is not of epidemic proportions as previously advertised by the CDC, there certainly is more autoimmune deficiency around than there was in 1969. It also is true that a large percentage of those people who are ill are carrying antibodies to the HIV virus. Is there an alternative way of looking at this situation, perhaps one which would make a bit more sense than the HIV hypothesis of AIDS?

Another Possible Cause of AIDS

Let us remember that an ever-increasing amount of petrochemicals are produced each year: 500 billion pounds at the present time. Probably, this stands behind the cancer epidemic. During the average day, the average American is exposed to 500 xenochemicals (chemicals foreign to human biochemistry), molecules which have not existed in nature during the evolution of the human immune system. These xenochemicals are added to the soil which grows our food. They are added to animal feed fed to livestock, and they are added to food to prevent the growth of bacteria.

Some of these xenochemicals are xenobiotics, chemicals which the FDA actually approves of introducing directly into the human body for therapeutic purposes, for example, antibiotics. The word antibiotics means, literally "anti-life," and you better believe it. Antibiotics severely suppress the immune system, and no other category of medication has been so commonly used, overused and abused in this century — so much so that bacteria have gained enough experience with them to develop wide-spectrum resistance. This is another problem of epidemic proportions, as is cancer. The cancer epidemic may be nothing more than another manifestation of immune suppression rendering the immune system incapable of performing its usual function of killing off cancer cells before they can multiply out of control.

While it is very difficult to prove that minute amounts of any single petrochemical produces cancer or immune deficiency, it stands to reason that when there is exposure not to one or even a few petrochemicals each day, but rather something on the order of 500 different chemicals, it becomes obvious that they may work synergistically to cause cancer and AIDS. While it may be true that you are safe from being eaten by any one of the small animals of the forest, it also is true that if they all attack you together, you are dead meat.

It also may be that most street drugs, as well as drugs which are sold through the pharmacy and over the counter, are immunosuppressive. Probably, the immune system cannot distinguish those drugs of which the FDA has approved and those of which is has not approved, both being equally dangerous to immune function.

What About HIV?

So what about the presence of the HIV virus in many people with AIDS? It seems far more likely to me that this virus is a so-called "passenger virus," in other words just going along for the ride.

No other retrovirus has been thought to produce illness in human beings, so why this one? It is well-acknowledged that the HIV virus is cleared quickly out of the body. The mechanism by which it is cleared is through the production of an antibody, which is specific for the virus. What can be found in an "HIV positive" individual is this antibody, not the virus itself. The virus itself is undetectable, and this is explained away by the AIDS establishment as a "latency" period. How does a virus which is not present do progressive damage to an immune system?

If an immune system is already weakened and on its way to a decompensated state, it is well-known that all kinds of weak viruses can exist in the body which would not be allowed in by a competent immune system. This does not mean that these viruses cause illness, it only means that they are along for the ride, they are passenger viruses. HIV probably is one of these viruses.

While it may be true that the retroviruses have the ability to cause the cell to produce more viruses, if those viruses are causing no problem, it is just not relevant. It may even be that, at the end-stage of AIDS, there is a sudden increase in HIV virus particles. However, this does not mean that HIV is causing the final collapse of the immune system, but vice-versa: the final collapse of the immune system allows large numbers of HIV particles to exist.

No one yet has proposed a reasonable mechanism by which the HIV virus might actually damage cells, and in all likelihood it is as harmless as the other retroviruses. Nevertheless, if the immune system eventually decompensates from multiple toxic exposures, it is easy to blame a virus which is going along for the ride. It also fits the allopathic paradigm of one disease, one cause.

Multiple contributory factors causing one disease is too complex and unpredictable for the allopathic paradigm to accommodate. Likewise, multiple contributory treatments for a disease process are thought not to be "scientific," even if they work.

If the allopathic paradigm were applied to criminology, all criminal acts would be committed by individuals and never by groups and there would be only one cop for each criminal. Therefore, in Tombstone there could not have been a "Clanton gang" and there would have been only one cure for one Clanton, i.e., one Wyatt Earp, not his brothers and not Doc Holliday. The shootout at the OK Corral never happened. Ah, well, I digress.

The Psychological Impact of the HIV Hypothesis

It is probable that the HIV causation hypothesis of AIDS and all the scare tactics which go with it are a hoax — of which some sharp scientists are well aware but who are not yet talking.

It is estimated that there are one to two million HIV positive individuals in the U.S. That figure has not changed, because AIDS is not an epidemic. Nevertheless, many people who are HIV positive have become aware of it through Robert Gallo's patented HIV antibody test. Except for the HIV dogma, those people would be going about their lives blissfully unaware of anything to be worried about regarding their health. Now these people live with a death sentence hanging over their heads.

The Psychosocial Impact of the Aids Hypothesis

This has changed lives. It has caused depression and lethargy. Many productive citizens have given up and are waiting to die. Some have committed suicide in despair and anticipation of a future of suffering and certain death from AIDS. Many relationships have been smashed asunder by the knowledge that someone is "HIV positive." The toll in psychological suffering is impossible to calculate, but it must be staggering.

All this would be excusable, if the CDC knew, as a fact, that HIV always leads to AIDS and death. This is just not the case. The idea of the inevitability of an AIDS-related death for people with an HIV-positive blood test is a wild guess for which there is no proof. It is a thundering herd of paradigm-dominated, research grant-motivated opinion.

The Interpretation of an HIV Positive Blood Test

In my opinion — the best guess of a person who has examined the evidence — a positive HIV test means one of two things: your immune system is in serious trouble from exposure to immunotoxic chemicals (which can include amyl nitrate), probably on a life-long basis, or there is a curious "hole" in your immune system, which allows the virus to exist in your body long enough for your immune system to make a special antibody to get rid of it.

An almost decompensated immune system probably is much more common than a singular defect which allows the virus to exist. I cannot tell you how to distinguish between these two conditions. If you become "HIV positive," it would be prudent on your part to assume that your immune system is in trouble and to clean up your life style to support a healing process. A thorough reading and application of the principles and knowledge contained in this book would be an excellent beginning.

The Checkered History and Deadly Presence of AZT

In 1964, Jerome Horwitz of the Detroit Cancer Foundation, synthesized the drug azidothymidine in an effort to find a treatment for cancer. The action of azidothymidine is to block the replication of DNA in the dividing cell. Horwitz's hope was that azidothymidine would kill cancer cells without serious toxic effects in the patient.

However, when he conducted experiments on mice with cancer, it must have failed miserably, because he did not bother to publish his results — nor did he apply for a patent. Probably, he found that his mice died before their cancer was affected, an outcome similar to that in most patients treated with chemotherapy to this day. Thus, azidothymidine joined a host of other failed chemotherapeutic agents on the shelf destined to gather dust in the annals of what might have been.

Then came AIDS. In an environment with people dying by the score everyday from AIDS, with doctors and patients alike feeling impotent, the drug companies knew there was a fortune to be made in the chemotherapeutic treatment of AIDS. The trick was to get FDA approval, and the stampede would be on.

Burroughs-Wellcome, the British pharmaceutical giant with an American division, looked into a handful of off-the-shelf, out-of-the-past chemicals and found azidothymidine, also known as "AZT," a powerful blocker of replication of the HIV virus.

Full of enthusiasm, with dollar signs in their eyes and loaded with influence at the FDA, three individuals, Barry, Broder and Bolognesi of Burroughs-Wellcome, published the results of their studies. In an environment of intense political pressure, particularly from the gay community, to find an effective treatment for AIDS, Burroughs-Wellcome struck a deal with the FDA to shortcut the process of approval of AZT and rushed it to market after studies which were, in retrospect, clearly flawed in design and execution. In 1987, with FDA approval in the bag, AZT became the standard of treatment for AIDS.

If one takes the time to read the label of possible side effects of AZT, one realizes a paradox. Here is a drug for treating autoimmune deficiency which causes autoimmune deficiency. When one sees the result of treatment with AZT, the list of possible side effects becomes the list of probable, almost certain, side effects. When AZT hits the scene, T cells are killed by the millions. Loss of appetite, nausea and vomiting (of blood), muscle wasting, severe fatigue, bloody diarrhea and slowed growth in children are the results which the doctor can count on seeing in the person taking AZT.

And yet, paradoxically, these all are signs of AIDS. It only becomes a question of what really causes AIDS: HIV or AZT.

Now, take this information and add it to the fact that, in 1990, AZT was approved by the FDA for the preventative treatment of AIDS, and you can guess what happens. In comes a patient, probably with an infection, to see the doctor. Doc says "OK and let's get an HIV test just to be on the safe side." The test comes back positive, doctor explains the death sentence and says, "Well, we don't have a cure, but if you take AZT perhaps we can prolong your life until a cure is found." Doctor wants to help, patient wants to live, Burroughs-Wellcome and the local pharmacy want the business, FDA approves and — *voila!* — another AZT prescription.

Patient, who was perfectly healthy, by the way, begins to take AZT. On the next visit to the doctor, weight loss is noted and patient is not feeling so well. T-cells are down. Doctor says, "Well, too bad to say, but it appears that you are in the early stages of AIDS. We had better increase the dose of AZT." You can see what happens next. It happened, for example, to Arthur Ashe, who was informed, but not convinced, of this information, so he continued taking AZT. "Besides," he said, "what will I tell my doctors?"

Now, there are a few other drugs — ddA, ddC and ddI — which are approved by the FDA for the treatment of AIDS. They have the same mechanism of action as AZT and also the same result. AIDS, like cancer and vascular disease, is a disease which selects out those people able to think for themselves and willing to inform themselves. Those who blindly follow the blind will, well, both fall into a ditch. Darwin lives!

An Alternative Treatment of AIDS

If HIV does not cause AIDS — and I am persuaded that it does not — its presence is an indication of probable impending compromise of the immune system. The last thing a thinking person would do in that case, if he wishes to live a long life, is further damage his immune system by taking immunosuppressant drugs like AZT and its buddies. If you think about it, there is no way to damage an immune system other than by allowing substances into your body which have that effect.

You can empower yourself to be healthy in two ways: educate yourself and find out what is in your food. Read labels. At least partial truth and partial completeness is required to be printed on the labels of all packaged foods. Knowing what is on the labels and what it means, is a good beginning.

Beyond that, do all things which are in the interest of your health. What that is, you must decide based upon your efforts to educate yourself. I can give you my thoughts, which is what this book is all about; however, only the knowledge you put into your mind ultimately will make a difference in how you treat your body. Educate yourself. Think for yourself. Do not blindly follow others, not me and not other doctors. Remember, the thundering herd of public opinion may just be headed for a cliff. This is the same public opinion which once was certain that the earth was flat. Anyone who thought otherwise was an idiot.

Obviously, stay away from all drugs toxic to your immune system. Obviously, find a source of organically grown foods, or grow your own. Obviously, drink pure water, not that stuff out of the tap. Obviously, lay completely off tobacco, alcohol and all prescription and over-the-counter drugs not required to save your life. Antibiotics are just what the name says: against life agents. Obviously, lay off the street drugs.

Take the opportunity for a spiritual transformation. The presence of HIV in your body can be a wonderful opportunity for spiritual awakening. Nothing brings home the preciousness of life like the possibility of losing it. And nothing brings God closer than loving life. Do not fear death, and yet love life.

A Prediction

I predict that, over the next few years, even virologists will back down to the position that HIV is at most a "risk factor," or perhaps only a "marker," and not the cause of AIDS. Probably, they will all pat themselves on the back for "discovering" this through their multi-billion-dollar research programs. Already the process has begun through media events with titles like "Why Some People Have a Natural Immunity to AIDS."

One should always keep an open mind. I keep an open mind for the HIV hypothesis and yet, as it appears now, it would be the strangest thing in science if it should turn out to be true.

Further Reading

You can read the whole sordid story about the HIV hypothesis of AIDS in a book entitled *Why We Will Never Win The War On AIDS* by Peter Duesberg and Brian Ellison, imminent virologists who lived through the whole thing and have become champions of the "HIV ain't it" community of scientists. This community grows by several hundred people each year, and it will not be long until its voice must be heard. Duesberg and Ellison's book can be ordered through Inside Story Communications in El Cerrito, California.

A Final Word

Please understand what I write here is an inquiry into medical science. This is not to be construed as a green light to abandon the concept of safe sex. Nor is it advice to have no concern for the potential risk to others in case you are HIV positive. On the outside chance that HIV really does, after all, have a direct causal role in AIDS, I suggest you follow all precautions which are commonly recommended to prevent spread of this virus. I know a doctor who is so certain that HIV does not cause AIDS that he intentionally infected himself in front of an audience of hundreds of people. I would not have done that. Nor should you, in my opinion.

> **See page 358 for instructions on contacting my office for a referral to a doctor experienced in the treatment of AIDS by progressive, nontoxic methods.**

ADDICTIONS

WHAT THEY ARE,

WHAT THEY COST YOU

ADDICTIONS

The purpose of this section is to help you illuminate all your addictions, so that you can be able to choose to have them or to discard them. The conditions which make addiction possible are summarized in the following statements.

1. Who you *are*, really, after all that you *have* is stripped away, so that who you are is revealed, is an enlightened soul.

2. This soul you are is at perfect peace and constantly in the experience of bliss and ecstasy.

3. Your soul is bound into your body, and the presence of your body obscures awareness of peace, bliss and ecstasy.

4. The body is always in a state of hunger: for food, excitement, affection, recognition, safety and security.

5. This state of hunger constitutes a pain, which could be said to be the pain of separation from the soul.

6. As life goes on, you become more and more identified with your hungers; that is to say, your consciousness exists in the pain of hunger and not in the awareness of peace, bliss and ecstasy.

7. Anything which lowers your consciousness serves to make you less aware of both the hunger and the ecstasy.

With these seven conditions, the stage is set for addiction. When you experience something which lowers consciousness, you want more of it because it provides relief from the pain of life. When you get more of it, you want even more, and soon you can hardly get enough. This, then, is a state of addiction.

Addictions are rationalized, so that you do not recognize them as addiction. People are not engaged in looking for their addictions, rather in looking for ways to conceal those addictions — not only from others, but from themselves. I can suggest that you are addicted, and you will listen only because you have made a commitment to better health through self-examination. I presume that if you have addictions, you want to know about them. That usually is not true for people.

For example, in alcoholism, the alcoholic usually is the last to notice the addiction and will lie to himself to conceal it from himself. Alcoholism is merely an obvious example. The mechanism concealing all addictions is the same.

Therefore, you cannot rely on your own evaluation of your addictions except to simply suspect them. The task is to identify some possible areas of addiction, to raise them to the level of suspicion. I will outline some common addictions to bring your attention to the possibility of these addictions in your life. Your job is to make a list of possible addictions. For now, do nothing about them, simply identify possibilities.

Handling Addictions

Any addiction you may have makes you less conscious than you are supposed to be. In a state of less-than-perfect consciousness, you will miss what your life is all about. Nothing clouds your consciousness like an addiction.

It is important that you understand what you are up against. A true addiction will fight you to the bitter end until you have gone back to feeding the addiction, or until one of you is dead. Many people resolve to give up an addiction only to soon go back to feeding the monster. Success with killing an addiction lies in the realization of who is senior and who is junior, who created and who was created.

What I can promise you as a result of kicking all addictions is (initially) great discomfort and (after that) increased awareness of life and of being alive. Let us talk about the initial discomfort, specifically about what you can expect, at least for the first few weeks.

Here are the common experiences you can expect followed by the addictions, the giving up of which will bring up these experiences. Primal pain is the pain derived from abandonment of the soul. It comes disguised as boredom, depression, vulnerability and physical symptoms.

Boredom is the result of giving up these addictions:

> listening to music
> talking on the telephone
> working
> studying
> reading
> writing
> watching television
> excitement
> drama in your personal life
> entertainment
> exercise
> gambling
> shopping
> accidents
> sleeping more than needed
> staying up too late every night

Sadness, depression, loss of a false sense of self and loss of self-esteem are the results of giving up these addictions:

meditation
compulsively telling your story
gossiping (about self and/or about others)
sex
relationship
a particular person

The uncomfortable position of being responsible for success and failure is the result of giving up this addiction:

setting yourself up to lose

Vulnerability, helplessness and a sense of being used are the results of giving up these addictions:

acting tough (intimidating others)
being right (winning arguments, having the last word, etc.)

Various physical symptoms such as fatigue, headache, insomnia and irritability are the results of giving up these addictions:

alcohol
nicotine (cigarettes, chewing tobacco, cigars, etc.)
caffeine (coffee, tea, chocolate, etc.)
sugar (candy, soft drinks, added to tea, coffee, etc.)
calories
fat
chewing and/or swallowing
milk and/or milk products (cheese, yogurt, etc.)
meat
salt (highly salted food or adding salt to your food)
tranquilizers
hallucinogens (LSD, marijuana, peyote, hash, etc.)
designer drugs (ecstasy, MDA, 2-CB, etc.)
nitrous oxide
narcotics (heroin, demerol, morphine, etc.)
cocaine, crack, crank, etc.
speed, amphetamines, etc.

Addiction To Sugar

"Sugar" is a term applied loosely to any of a number of chemical compounds. They all are simple carbohydrates, soluble in water, colorless, odorless and form crystals at room temperature. Sugars come in molecules with as few as three carbon atoms per molecule, to as many as nine carbon atoms per molecule. These are known by the family names trios, tetrose, pentose, hexose, heptose, octose and nonose. In each case, the carbons are formed in the shape of a ring with the "last" carbon atom being attached to the "first." Sugars come as single-ring, double-ring and triple-ring molecules called "monosaccharides," "disaccharides" and "trisaccharides," respectively.

Although all these forms are found in nature, by far the most common are the hexoses: six carbon structures with the empirical formula $C_6 H_{12} O_6$, which simply indicates the presence of six carbon atoms, twelve hydrogen atoms and six oxygen atoms.

The most important of the hexose sugars in human metabolism are glucose and galactose. One other "-ose" is important: the five carbon molecule (pentose) called "fructose" (also known as "fruit sugar").

The human body manufactures these simple sugars in the so-called "Kreb's cycle" (also known as the "citric acid cycle"), which is designed to release the energy which is the driving force of life. Glucose is the major source of energy for the muscles and nervous tissue of the body. The body knows very well how to maintain a perfect balance of glucose unless it is presented with unnatural amounts.

Sugar is not ordinarily ingested into the body in the form of these simple monosaccharides, but rather as the disaccharide sugars maltose, lactose and sucrose. The body treats these disaccharides with enzymes and acid and quickly breaks them down to their component parts: two molecules of glucose in the case of maltose, one glucose and one galactose in the case of lactose and one glucose and one fructose in the case of sucrose. Sucrose is ordinary table sugar. The major source of lactose is milk and milk products and the major source of maltose is barley grain.

In human nutrition, the major source of concern for a person who wants to live a healthy life is sucrose and, to a lesser degree, lactose and maltose as all three frequently are used as food additives in processed foods.

As a basic foodstuff, sucrose supplies approximately thirteen percent of the energy derived from food. This is an average figure, of course, with some foods having more sucrose than others.

Food in natural form presents no metabolic problems when consumed in variety. Consuming a variety of fruits and vegetables, for example, presents no metabolic problems a normal body cannot readily deal with.

Sucrose is present in limited quantity in many plants including various palms and the sugar maple. However, sugar beet and sugarcane are the only commercially important sources with sugarcane being the more important of the two. Sugar is extracted in similar manner from sugar beets and sugarcane, and this extraction technique is less than 200 years old. In both cases, the plant is crushed to produce juice in a process called "grinding." During grinding, hot water is sprayed over the crushed material to dissolve out additional sucrose. Lime is added, and the mixture is heated to boiling.

During this heating, organic acids form insoluble compounds with the lime, and this is then filtered off along with other solid impurities. The juice is then treated with gaseous sulfur dioxide to bleach it and passed through further filtration. The resulting clear juice is heated to evaporate off the water content. All of this is done in a partial vacuum. The sugar becomes sufficiently concentrated to crystallize. The part which does not crystallize is called "molasses," and it is forced out through rapidly spinning the entire mixture in a large centrifuge, leaving what is called "first sugar." This first sugar is sprayed with water to remove any molasses still present, then redissolved, decolorized and recrystallized.

The final product is table sugar. Not only is this product at a concentration unknown in nature, even in the sugar beet or the sugar cane, it also is stripped of any redeeming nutritional value that may have been present in the original plant.

The purpose of outlining this process for you is to allow you to see for yourself just how unnatural commercial sucrose — table sugar — really is. It would be a miracle if the body were prepared to deal with this stuff, given that nothing like it exists in nature.

The unfortunate fact of life is that this stuff also adds good taste to whatever it is added to and, to make matters even worse, it is strongly addicting. It can be no surprise that sucrose is used as an almost universal constituent of processed foods, all with government approval as long as the package is clearly marked to indicate the presence of sucrose. This is a classic example of the government's hands-off attitude toward the food industry: *caveat emptor* - let the buyer beware.

When this process of purification of sucrose was first invented, it was carried out by hand and only small quantities of table sugar could be made. It was so expensive, only royalty and other very rich people could afford to consume it as regular fare. Degenerative diseases were once the privilege of the rich. Now everyone can afford them.

To make matters worse, all food manufacturers know of the taste and addiction qualities of sucrose, and almost all of them are willing to use sucrose, or its breakdown product glucose, as a food additive without discrimination to increase their sales of processed foods. Glucose is used as a cheap filler and tastes less sweet than sucrose, disguising from your taste buds the large amount of simple sugar you are introducing into your body. On the label, all this masquerades as "syrup," usually "corn syrup." Thus your mind is deceived, along with your sense of taste.

The Effect of Simple Sugars on the Human Body

The key to health is the moderate consumption of complex carbohydrates — from natural food sources, such as fresh vegetables and, to a lesser extent, cooked vegetables — balanced with intake of protein from a clean source, such as organically grown soy products. Anything less than this is a compromise and will eventually affect your health and/or longevity. While it is true that this stuff breaks down to simple sugars in a few hours, if you take your carbs in this fashion, the quantity will be tolerable, and it will come with other nutrients.

It is very likely that you are addicted to sugar. A sugar addict can find ways to rationalize the addiction. Sugar addiction is so common in industrialized Western nations as to be unrecognizable. If you grew up in a culture where everyone — every single person from the time a cigarette could be held in the hand — smoked and where practically nothing was said about it, you would come to accept it as a natural fact of life. (Europe is almost such a place.) You would not think of yourself as addicted to tobacco, as there would be no one in your environment with whom to compare yourself. They would all be busy smoking, just like you. Thus, it is with sugar. Fish in the ocean ask no questions about dry land.

Probably, you are saying to yourself, "Yea, I eat a little sugar but not too much." This is what I call "addict's logic": "I can smoke a cigarette here and there without becoming a smoker again"; "I can have just one drink without becoming an alcoholic again"; "I will just have a little cake, or a candy bar here and there." Certainly, and then revert to sucking down large quantities of hidden sugar in processed foods. Just because it's in the grocery store does not mean it is good to eat. *Caveat emptor*! Let the buyer beware!

Degenerative diseases caused by regular sugar consumption include the following.

hypoglycemia	diabetes
chronic constipation	chronic stomach upset
intestinal gas	arthritis
asthma	headaches
osteoporosis	heart disease
obesity	chronic Candida infection
tooth decay	inflammatory bowel disease

This is not a complete list of the diseases believed to be caused by chronic long-term sucrose consumption, but these are the diseases in which it is easiest to see a relationship. Other diseases in which the consumption of sugar is implicated are:

psoriasis	cancer
multiple sclerosis	canker sores
gall stones	cystic fibrosis

You can have any of these degenerative diseases and be unaware of it for years.

Your point of view may be "Okay, Dr. K., but I do not have any of these diseases." Right, you may not, and if not, it is only because you are young and have not yet done sufficient damage to the systems of your body. The diseases people ordinarily die from are degenerative diseases, and it requires at least several years to create a clinically symptomatic degenerative disease. Degenerative diseases exist long before they become obvious. If you are a sugarholic, you are somewhere to be found in the degenerative disease process.

Here is a list of the minerals required to digest sugar: calcium, phosphorus, chromium, magnesium, cobalt, copper, zinc and manganese. These minerals are the so-called "co-factors" necessary for the proper functioning of the enzyme systems, including the enzyme systems required to metabolize sugar. These minerals have been stripped away in the refining process which produces sugar. Also, the mechanisms which produce glucose from complex carbohydrates, proteins and fats simply shut down from disuse when you continue a steady diet of simple sugars. If you don't use it you lose it.

Thus, you become dependent on an outside source of glucose, i.e., addicted. This source usually is sucrose. Also, you lose the ability to metabolize sugar and keep it in a healthy range within the cells. You may have a normal blood sugar and a normal glucose tolerance test. Under these conditions, your doctor will tell you "no problemo." Don't believe it! A normal blood glucose and/or glucose tolerance test only proves that your pancreas is still healthy enough to shunt a large load of sugar to inside the cells. It is within the cells themselves where sugar does its damage.

The evolution of our enzyme systems required millions of years, and throughout those millions of years purified sugar was not available. Therefore, your body simply is not programmed to handle anything more than the quantity of simple sugars present in, for example, a couple of peaches or a couple of apples. Those peaches or apples, by the way, come with their mineral supply — and loads of other nutrients — intact. You can even overdose on natural foods and take a large hit of sugar from fruit, for example, especially dried fruit. It also is easy to juice six apples or six oranges and gulp your juice down in ten minutes whilst thinking what a wonderful thing you are doing for your body.

The first enzyme systems of your body which are upset by refined sugar are your digestive enzymes, because these are the first encountered by the sugar you put in your mouth. Because these enzymes are disabled by abnormal concentrations of sugar, food passes through your digestive tract in an undigested or a partially digested state.

Some of these large molecules enter your body through the walls of your small intestines in this undigested or partially digested state. Your body recognizes these large molecules as foreign tissue and makes antibodies to them. Thus, do food allergies develop.

Most people get twenty percent of their calories from refined sugar, an average of 130 pounds (59 kilos) per year. This is a massive and continuing upset for the body.

The usual calcium/phosphorus ratio in the serum is 10:2, a ratio of ten mg. calcium for every two mg. phosphorous per liter of serum. The ingestion of sugar alters this ratio by decreasing the phosphorus and increasing the calcium. Because calcium and phosphorus work together in the enzymatic systems of the body, a phosphorus deficiency is sensed by the body as a calcium deficiency as well as a phosphorus deficiency. The body has no readily available source of phosphorus; however, it certainly does have a ready source of calcium. Therefore, your bones and teeth are robbed of calcium to deal with this imbalance, and the result is osteoporosis of bones throughout the body and weakened tooth structure.

This extra calcium, without a complement of phosphorus to balance it, is toxic. Calcium can be in deficient supply, even though the concentration may be above normal, because insufficient phosphorus is present to enable the body to use it. Therefore, the odd situation arises of toxicity from calcium, which also is in deficient supply as far as availability to the enzyme systems is concerned.

This is called "nonfunctioning calcium," and it leads to kidney stones, arthritis, hardening of the arteries, cataracts and plaque on the teeth. In extreme imbalance, massive calcium tumors may form in the body.

Calcium caseinate, along with oxidized cholesterol, is a major component of atherosclerotic plaques found on blood vessel walls in people with hardened arteries. This is the major cause of heart attack, and this situation can develop at a very young age thanks to degenerative illness driven by habitual simple sugar ingestion.

Addiction To Salt

The particular salt we refer to in human nutrition, unless otherwise specified, is sodium chloride. It is plentiful and cheap, but it wasn't always so conveniently available. Sodium chloride once was considered a great delicacy to be used sparingly because it was difficult to obtain and expensive. Roman soldiers of antiquity were often paid in salt, and this was called their "*salarium*," from which our word "salary" is derived. It was said a soldier was "worth his salt," a term still used for a worthy person. Once paid with salt, it could be used as money in exchange for other goods.

Sodium and potassium individually combine with bicarbonate, phosphorus or chlorine, to make the six major salts in the human body. Potassium and sodium are metals forming positive ions (cations, i.e., missing an electron) each with an electrical charge of +1. Phosphate, bicarbonate and chloride are negative ions (anions) with a negative charge of -1, having an extra electron. All these ions are found in the human body. In health, they all work together along with the kidneys to maintain the acid/base balance of the body within a very narrow, slightly alkaline range. Each cation is balanced by an anion, existing in an almost 1:1 ratio, with a slight excess of anions. Bicarbonate is a buffer, able to absorb and neutralize both acid and base, thus holding the acid/base balance within the narrow range necessary for life.

The concentration of these salts is very close to the concentration of the same salts found in ocean water, out of which our distant ancestors walked a few hundred million years ago to begin animal life on land. Our cells have maintained the memory of sea water from which our ancestors came.

Of all the salts present in the sea and in our bodies, the ones made from sodium are by far the most abundant. Therefore, sodium serves to maintain the concentration of salts in the body necessary for life. It exists in dynamic relationship with potassium — excessive amounts of one will result in depletion of the other — in order to maintain the proper concentration of salts in the body.

The kidneys work by filtration through glomeruli, millions of tiny filtering devices, and then reabsorption through the renal tubules, the passageways from the glomeruli to the bladder. In the distal (second) part of the renal tubules, there is a mechanism called the "Sodium Pump." Each renal tubule has such a pump, and there are millions of renal tubules. The Sodium Pump mechanism is a cellular/chemical way of recovering sodium from the urine before it is sent to the bladder for excretion. The amount of sodium recovered is related to the degree of need the body has for sodium. If the body is overloaded with sodium, most of the sodium filtered through the glomeruli is allowed to leave the body. If the body is sodium depleted, a large percentage of sodium is recovered and put back into circulation in the body.

There is no pump for potassium in the kidneys comparable to the Sodium Pump — so, we must have continuous replacement of potassium because the kidneys cannot conserve it. Plant foods are rich in potassium but low in sodium, in line with the needs of the body. Animal-derived foods and processed foods usually are the opposite.

Sodium is the pivotal actor among the important cations in the mechanism maintaining the all important acid/base balance of the body. As sodium goes, so goes the acid/base balance of the body. The problem with sodium, as with phosphorus, is not one of deficiency, rather of excess. Salt is plentiful in the soil, and all plants grown in such soil are sufficient in sodium. No supplementation is necessary. Nevertheless, almost all processed food manufacturers *add* sodium chloride to food for taste, promoting an addictive state in order to sell more of their product!

Sodium chloride (common table salt) is the usual form of sodium added to food, so common that the word "salt," in layman's language, refers to sodium chloride, although in the language of chemistry there are hundreds of different salts. To make matters worse, the social convention is to keep a salt shaker at the ready to add even further salt to food.

At age forty, the kidneys begin to lose their ability to rid the body of excess sodium, and, as you grow older, sodium sickness becomes more and more likely, especially if you salt your food and/or eat processed foods.

The body can deal with excess sodium by storing it in the spaces between cells (collectively called the "interstitial" space) to protect the acid/base balance of the blood. This condition is called "edema." It appears first around the ankles as puffy tissue, which, upon pressing with moderate force, will hold the impression of your finger for several minutes after pressure is removed. This is called "pitting edema."

When sodium is shunted to the interstitial space, anions are attracted there to balance the electrical charge of the sodium. To maintain the proper concentration, water also is drawn in with this soup. This all has serious consequences for the cells, which must keep out this excess of sodium using their own version of the Sodium Pump. If this mechanism fails in a cell, that cell dies. This pumping action burns a lot of calories, which should be used for other cellular processes. The cells become overworked keeping out the excess sodium.

When this line of defense has reached its limit, sodium appears in the blood in excessive quantities. The same phenomenon then happens, causing increased circulatory volume, elevated blood pressure, stress on the heart and depletion of potassium. If this process continues unchecked, the result is congestive heart failure and death. In affluent societies, elevated blood pressure is found in 25% of adults and 12% of children!

Recent research suggests that the chloride content of table salt is more important in the elevation of blood pressure than is sodium. Nevertheless, the solution is the same, since the two come together: restrict sodium chloride intake.

Sodium *is* necessary for proper transmission of impulses along the axon of every nerve in your body, and necessary for muscle contraction as well. Deficiency of sodium is difficult to achieve, because sodium salts are everywhere in nature.

Do not worry about deficiency of sodium. Be concerned instead about excess. While the daily requirement for sodium chloride is 50 mg., the average adult consumes 5,000 mg., 100 times more than is needed! Even a young person whose kidneys can handle sodium will feel much better restricting salt: more energy (the Sodium Pump drains a lot of energy), fewer headaches, and better sleep.

Love of the salty taste of salt is an addiction similar in quality to the addictions to alcohol, tobacco, sugar, caffeine and a host of others. The same principles apply to kicking the salt habit as apply to kicking any addiction.

Unless you have one of the conditions causing lowered sodium such as adrenal insufficiency, salt-losing renal disease, colostomy, or chronic postural hypotension, I strongly recommend that you get out of the habit of salting your food. Do not drink beer (25 mg. of sodium per 12 oz.), avoid baking soda (sodium bicarbonate), monosodium glutamate (MSG, a popular preservative), baking powder, sodium-laden laxatives (most are), and home water softener (adds sodium to the water). Do not eat meat. Do not drink diet soda. Look for the words "salt," "sodium," or the symbol "Na" when reading food labels.

Consume the following salt-laden items sparingly: dill pickles, soy sauce and canned vegetable juices. Stay far away from **all** prepackaged foods and processed foods until you have carefully read the label and discovered no added salt, sugar, or preservatives (practically impossible). Do not eat salted popcorn or peanuts, and do eat only fresh foods, organically grown. Also, avoid salt substitutes, because they employ potassium, and an accidental overdose of potassium can be fatal.

That is what not to do. Here is what to do. Learn to enjoy the natural flavors of food. Your taste buds have been overstimulated for years with salt, among other items, to the extent that they cannot detect and enjoy subtle tastes. You may use spices in making the transition to the enjoyment of natural flavors. I suggest thyme, tarragon, paprika, sage, basil, dill and oregano. After the transition, you will discover that spices are unnecessary in most cases and the natural food tastes irreplaceable.

Remember, the preference for salt is learned, not natural, and it can be unlearned. If you use salt, use only sea salt, which contains all the other minerals your body needs in a balanced mixture, and use it sparingly.

If you kick the sodium chloride addiction, all things being equal, you will add vitality and a number of wonderful years to your life.

See page 358 for instructions on contacting my office for a referral to a doctor experienced in the treatment of addictive states.

EXERCISE:

AEROBIC HEALTH

AND

MUSCULAR CONDITIONING

AEROBICS

The name of the cardiovascular-respiratory system game is **delivery of oxygen to the cells of the body**. Oxygen is the source of the consciousness of the cells of your body. Without it they die within minutes.

The purpose of this section is the development of aerobic habits in your life for the purpose of expanding your health and vitality to a higher level. To develop and maintain aerobic habits, it is necessary to develop a body of knowledge of aerobics and a body of aerobic attitudes.

With the exception of plants, blue-green algae and some primitive bacteria, all of which burn carbon dioxide for fuel, life as we know it depends on oxygen to fuel its activities. Oxygen is one of the basic elements found on the periodic chart of elements. It has an atomic weight of sixteen — reflecting the presence of eight protons and eight neutrons in its nucleus.

The source of oxygen in the universe is atomic fusion in stars. All elemental oxygen is created by fusion in stars with lighter elements fused together to form heavier elements. In the fusion process, a small percentage of matter is converted to energy, which is given off as heat, light, radio waves, x-rays, etc.

Eventually, a star of mass at least ten times the mass of our sun reaches a certain stage of its development, collapses, then explodes to become what we call a super-nova. Super-novas release massive amounts of heavy elements into the surrounding space, some of which eventually are attracted into the gravitational field of new stars forming from swirling clouds of hydrogen and helium left over from the Big Bang. Among these heavy elements contributed to new solar systems is oxygen.

Your body contains heavy elements derived from exploded stars, elements such as carbon, sodium, chlorine, silicone, magnesium, iron, to name only a few and, of course, oxygen. You are, quite literally, a star, or at least you are made of 100% star stuff.

When life first evolved on the earth, the first organisms, blue-green algae, used the gaseous form of carbon dioxide for fuel. The source of this CO_2 was the earth itself which spewed forth massive amounts of carbon dioxide from volcanoes. This CO_2 was the result of the fusion of carbon and oxygen contained in molten lava rocks.

Carbon dioxide is a molecule of one carbon and two oxygen atoms. Organisms which we call "anaerobic" use carbon from carbon dioxide to construct their cells and liberate oxygen as O_2, a gas which is, from their point of view, a toxic waste product. To these early organisms oxygen was poison, and this became a problem over the next billion years as this toxic waste product built up in the atmosphere of the earth.

These blue-green algae, and other evolved anaerobic organisms, banished themselves to the cracks and crevasses of the world where they could escape the heavy concentrations of oxygen with which they themselves had poisoned the atmosphere. There they remain to this day.

Meanwhile, aerobic bacteria had evolved. The first bacteria were anaerobic, burning CO_2 for fuel. They were poisoned by the advent of large quantities of O_2. To survive, some bacteria figured out how to use oxygen as a primary fuel, and these revolutionary organism, called "aerobes," released carbon dioxide as a byproduct of their metabolism. To the aerobes, carbon dioxide is poison to the extent that it replaces necessary oxygen.

This happy development was a case of symbiosis: living in a condition of mutual benefit. The anaerobes breathe in CO_2 and breathe out O_2. The aerobes breathe in O_2 and breathe out CO_2. Each makes continued life possible for the other.

You, of course, are an aerobe. You are busy breathing in O_2 and breathing out CO_2. You eat carbon atoms in the form of plants, animals — and animal products, if you are not a vegetarian. You combine this carbon you eat with the oxygen you breathe to make CO_2.

The plants, anaerobic bacteria and blue-green algae of the world are glad you are here. They use your CO_2 as fuel. You should also be glad they are here. They supply not only the carbon necessary to construct your body but also the oxygen which is the necessary fuel to carry out that construction.

This is one reason there is so much concern about the destruction of the rain forests. Without the green things of the earth, we lose most of our source of oxygen, and most of the earth's capacity to recycle carbon dioxide, the buildup of which traps heat from the sun. This buildup favors global warming through the greenhouse effect, leading to melting of the polar ice-caps, flooding of coastal areas and destruction of cities, farm land, etc. As an aerobe you have a big stake in this matter. It is important for you to be conscious of, and understand thoroughly, the role of oxygen in the creation of your consciousness. For you, oxygen is the breath of life.

The air you breath is twenty percent oxygen. The other eighty percent is nitrogen, carbon dioxide, a few trace gases like argon, and a few other greenhouse gases derived from industrial processes. Ideally, only oxygen is absorbed into your body from the air you breathe, although some toxic gases also are absorbed (e.g. carbon monoxide and methane). Hemoglobin in your red blood cells is specifically designed to extract oxygen from the air. Only the oxygen in air is necessary for life. The other gases are breathed out in the same concentrations in which they are breathed in, except for carbon monoxide, which also is bound by hemoglobin.

If you take a trip to the countryside or to a forest, you can experience the "freshness" of the air. That freshness is a concentration of newly liberated O_2 from the plants in the area, relatively free of other gases. There you can experience the sensual pleasure of breathing oxygen.

Your Relationship With Your Heart

Your heart is a muscle located in your chest between the right and left lungs. Consult the encyclopedia for a diagram of the human heart. The heart, in the state of contraction, is about the size and shape of your hand when made into a fist. Your heart is held in place by the pericardium — a sac of fibrous tissue — and by its attachment to the great vessels, which carry blood to and from the lungs and the body. The most amazing fact about the heart is that it never ceases to contract and relax as long as you live.

All the blood in your body passes through your heart every sixty seconds. The heart is divided into four chambers, two light-weight chambers above and two heavily-muscled chambers below. The function of the light-weight chambers, called "atria," is to pump blood into the heavy chambers and the function of the heavy chambers, called "ventricles," is to pump blood on to the lungs and to the body.

Imagine yourself to be a red blood cell. You are loaded with hemoglobin, a complex protein carrying an atom of iron in such a way that each hemoglobin molecule can bind oxygen with iron and release the oxygen to the cells of your body, all of which run on oxygen.

As a red blood cell, you contain one million hemoglobin molecules. You have just completed discharging your oxygen to some cells in need and this oxygen has made its way through the capillary wall. You have done your job, and you are pooped. You need a vacation.

The pressure from the heart, now far upstream, as well as the movement of your body pushes you through tiny vessels called "capillaries," which are thinner than you are wide. To pass through, you have to fold backward into the shape of a parachute.

Once through the capillaries, you enter the slow moving venous system. In this system you have nothing to do, so you take a little rest. This rest lasts about thirty seconds and then you find yourself in the first chamber of the heart, the light-weight right atrium. The right atrium heaves you into the right ventricle, and from there, on the next beat of the heart, you are blasted into the lungs. In the lungs, you encounter a massive amount of fresh oxygen. Your hemoglobin eats an enormous amount of oxygen, and suddenly you feel great — all fatigue has disappeared.

Now you find yourself in the left atrium, which quickly shoves you into the massive, powerful left ventricle. From here, you are rocketed out the aorta, a hose-sized artery looping behind the heart and feeding both the upper and lower parts of the body with fresh blood.

And that is what you are now — fresh blood — brimming with oxygen. Soon you find yourself surrounded by cells which need oxygen. You discharge your payload and take a rest in the venous system for a leisurely ride back to the heart.

This is hard work, but you are a sturdy red blood cell built to last, and you are able to last four months before you burst with fatigue. During that four months, you will have traveled much further than the best made automobile can travel before it falls apart. When you finally die, you release all the nutrients contained in your little body, and some of these are recycled; others are processed and then excreted. Some of these nutrients find their way to your bone marrow where they are used to build a replacement for you.

During your four-month lifetime, you had a powerful relationship with the heart, which is designed to give a lift to you and your buddies for over 100 years, providing it is treated right. You are glad to have served such a powerful organ. You lived out your life in great respect for this powerhouse, the heart.

The heart is the source of vitality for the body and the mind. When it is treated well, it is much stronger than required for ordinary needs and able to respond to emergency situations with ease. When not responding to an emergency, your well-treated, vital heart is a source of inner peace and well-being in times of rest, and the source of great courage under stress. The condition of your heart has everything to do with your ability to express yourself and to fulfill your destiny. It also generates a powerful field of energy affecting your ability to think clearly and relate powerfully with others. The heart is more than a physical organ. The effectiveness with which it can do its job, physical, as well as spiritual, is clearly connected to its physical condition.

The heart is made strong through use, like any other muscle. If you place it under stress, it responds by enlarging and becoming more powerful. This is reflected by a lowering of the resting heart rate. The unconditioned heart requires 70-100 beats per minute at rest to do its job. The conditioned heart runs between thirty and sixty beats (depending on age and condition) per minute at rest, pumping the same amount of blood as the unconditioned heart does at 70-100 beats per minute. Needless to say, the conditioned heart undergoes much less wear and tear to do its job than does the unconditioned heart.

Your Relationship With Your Lungs

Working on cardiovascular health is incomplete until the place of the lungs is considered. In evolutionary development, the lungs evolved from a bag of air a certain lazy fish invented a billion years ago to control his depth in the water without all the effort of swimming toward the top or swimming toward the bottom. By compressing this little bag of air he could sink, and by releasing the compression he would rise in the water — very convenient for dropping in on smaller fish for dinner.

Some of these fish developed the ability to breath with this bag and evolved into creatures similar to today's lungfish, who, as adults, use only air for respiration: the exchange of O_2 and CO_2. It was these primitive lungfish who evolved into amphibians and who are our ancestors. As an embryo you had gill slits, just like fish embyros. However, they all disappeared except for one, which became your ear canals.

To bring your lungs into your consciousness, it is very important to have an accurate visual image of them. Consult your encyclopedia for the appropriate diagram. We will now take up a discussion to begin to build that image. If you can arrange to see some color photographs of the lungs, or anatomical specimens of lung tissue, all the better. I suggest a library — even better a medical library or the pathology lab of your nearest medical school. Such labs have permanent displays of dissection specimens and usually are open to the public like a museum.

Your lungs are made of several million tiny sacs called "alveoli." The tubes leading from them are called "bronchioles." They lead to the larger bronchi, which lead in turn to the trachea: the pipe in the middle of your throat through which you breathe. Each tiny bronchiole serves 8-10 alveoli.

There is a thin, one-cell-thick layer of tissue holding all the lung structures together called the "pulmonary pleurae." The alveoli present a total surface area of several hundred square meters from which to absorb oxygen and expel carbon dioxide. In the unsmoked, living condition, this tissue is a beautiful pink color. In appearance, the lungs are more alive than any other tissue. To gaze upon the living, healthy, breathing lung is an almost mystical experience — its beauty and vitality unspeakable.

The adult lungs can inhale from 3.3 to 4.9 liters of air in one breath. This is called the "vital capacity." A healthy person's vital capacity is twenty times what is needed for life in the resting state. That is to say you can destroy 95% of your vital capacity and still, conceivably, continue surviving on the remaining five percent. Realistically, however, you could not, in this condition, take a walk. That would call for more vital capacity than you would have.

Many people lead normal lives after the removal of one lung. The lungs are very elastic and the remaining lung simply expands to fill the chest cavity maintaining almost normal vital capacity.

Because the lungs, like the heart, are out of sight, we are tempted to abuse them. The lungs present such a large surface area that whatever you inhale into them has a good chance to enter the body through the pulmonary capillaries.

Smoking tobacco is, of course, the most common insult to the lungs. The reason nicotine can enter the body so easily through the lungs, despite the fact that it is a relatively large molecule, is that there are only two cell layers between the air you breathe and your blood. These are the cells of the alveoli and the cells of the pulmonary capillary next to them. Between these two layers of cells there is a potential space. Ordinarily, this space is not present because there is nothing to go into it; it is like one bag fitting snugly into another, slightly larger, bag.

When you smoke, while the nicotine disappears into the body, the carbon molecules from the cigarette simply are too large to enter the body. Carbon in smoke is arrange into dodecahedrons, also known as Bucky Balls, after Buckminster Fuller who first described the utility of the dodecahedron, a perfectly symmetrical 32-sided geometric shape. These carbon-constructed dodecahedrons have a very large molecular weight. They pass through the alveoli and become stuck between the two cell layers and there they remain for years. The body tries to remove these little dodecahedrons by sending in macrophages — white blood cells that ordinarily scavenge for dead tissue. However, the carbon (also called "tar") is heavy and difficult to move, and many years are required to cleanse the lungs completely of all the carbon from even one cigarette.

To gaze directly upon a smoker's lungs is the same experience as seeing a large bag of rotten garbage dumped on the altar of a beautiful cathedral. The accumulated tar gives the appearance of coal transplanted into the lungs. One cannot help but think "If only they knew..." This is the dilemma. The lungs and heart are out of sight and too often out of mind. If smokers had to wear the tar from their cigarettes on their faces for years after smoking, there would be considerably fewer smokers in the world.

The leading cause of death in Western countries is lung cancer. This is true for men and for women. The cause/effect relationship between smoking and lung cancer is no longer debated. It is. It exists. Even breathing the smoke from other people's cigarettes (secondary smoke) is known to be carcinogenic: eight hours of second-hand smoke is equivalent to smoking twenty cigarettes. The relationship of smoking to the development of emphysema also is unquestionable.

Emphysema is the breakdown of the walls between individual alveoli, forming sacs of bubble-like tissue, which, at best, is useless for respiration and, at worst, will burst and cause air to enter directly into the chest cavity (pneumothorax) and threaten life.

Smokers who exercise, thinking they are protecting their lungs from smoke, delude themselves. There is no evidence that aerobic exercise benefits the lung tissue itself. The lung is a passive organ designed to serve the rest of the body on an as-needed basis. It does not become stronger with use. There are no muscle fibers in the lung to become stronger. The diaphragm, the muscle which drives the lungs, does become stronger with use; but more about that later.

Care of the lungs before they become diseased is primarily a matter of do nots rather than of dos. Do not smoke. Anything. Ever. If you smoke, stop, now. Avoid smoke from other people's cigarettes. When you drive, drive with your windows up and without ventilation to the outside traffic. If you live close to a factory which belches smoke, move, now. Arrange to live in, or close to, the country or in a smaller town away from industrial areas, close to the ocean is ideal.

Doing It

The importance of the aerobic habit cannot be over-stated. It is the one instance of over-consumption which is absolutely good for you. The more oxygen you move through your body, the greater will be your awareness of life and, ultimately, your consciousness of who you are.

Your relationship with your heart is your relationship with life. If you are fully committed to life, you are fully committed to your heart. There is no difference between these commitments; one is an important part of the other. The aerobic habit is created by **doing** aerobics. Each aerobic session you do further strengthens the aerobic habit.

Thinking about it does not get the job done. Like anything else which is a priority, it must be written into your schedule and then done when scheduled. Beginning is the most difficult step. After a certain number of aerobic sessions it will become as natural as eating, something you will hunger for if you do not do it. Believe it or not, it becomes fantastic fun. What the body actually needs is rather simple: a twenty minute aerobic workout every other day. This amount every day, or much more, is no problem for the body, but the actual need, based on my experience, is twenty minutes every other day. I have such fun doing my workouts, I have a hard time holding it down to only that much.

The benefits of having a strong aerobic habit? Here are a few: the ability to think clearly and creatively, a strong sex life, courage under stress or in emergency situations, the experience of well-being, a body that tends to find its ideal weight without effort, rejuvenating sleep, and healthy appetite for food and for life itself. There are many more. I invite you to discover all of them by developing a strong aerobic habit. **You don't have enough time not to develop such a habit**.

The form of the exercise is up to you and should be what you enjoy most. Swimming, bicycling and walking are possibilities. I recommend against regular running because of the cumulative damage done to the delicate tissues of the spine, particularly the lower back.

Before you begin an aerobic program, you should get a cardiovascular physical exam from a good doctor specializing in this area. When you have your doc's okay, you are ready to begin. Do not overdo it. You should be able to hold a conversation while exercising and, if you cannot, you are going at it too hard. You can achieve just as much at a more sensible pace.

While conventional wisdom is not to exercise to the max, the benefits of exercise go up exponentially with degree of exertion, particularly the release of growth hormone from the pituitary, in response to anaerobic exercise, and the creation of new insulin receptor sites which accompanies increased lean muscle mass. Growth hormone and insulin receptor sites work long-lasting beneficial changes in the body.

On the other hand, you must stay in a safe zone, particularly if you have some degree of cardiovascular disease. Your doctor should be able to give you an answer to this question. The best choice would then be to work with an exercise physiologist to design the best possible workout for you, given your limitations if you have any.

You should be shooting to maintain a sustained heart rate in a certain range for twenty minutes every other day. You can determine this range with the following formula: 220 minus your age in years multiplied times 0.6 and 0.8. This first figure represents the rate you want to achieve or exceed. The second figure represents the rate you want not to exceed. For example, if you are forty years old, 220 minus 40 is 180. 180 x 0.6 = 108. 180 x 0.8 = 144. Therefore, if you are forty years old, you want to equal or exceed 108 heartbeats per minute during exercise but not exceed 144 heartbeats per minute.

See page 358 for instructions on contacting my office for a referral to a doctor experienced in advising you in the area of aerobic exercise.

THE VALUE OF PUMPING IRON AT ANY AGE

So far, in this section of the book, we have been engaged in creating a relationship with the environment and with the body itself in order to sustain, experience and enjoy life. It is this relationship which is important.

To live your life appropriate to who you are, it is also critically important that you have a living relationship with the earth, its history, with the atmosphere and its history and with life and its history. When all that is in place, you are ready to begin to create your place in this incredible world.

The first step in creating your place in the world is to learn about your body. We have begun the process of gathering the information you need to appreciate the miracle that is your body. We have considered the heart and the blood which it pumps and the system of vessels through which it is pumped. We also have considered the organ responsible for gathering O_2 from the atmosphere and the common insults to that organ: tobacco smoke and air pollution. There is only one thing left: skeletal muscle.

Skeletal muscle is a unique kind of tissue, which has the ability to contract and relax at your command, thus the ability to do work. Biologists are just beginning to fully understand how muscle contracts and that discussion is too long and technical for this discussion. However, consider how miraculous it is to have a living tissue that can make itself longer or shorter on command and do work.

The skeletal muscle of your body makes up fifty to seventy percent of the tissue through which blood is pumped. For your heart to have a chance to do the best job possible, it is important that skeletal muscle be conditioned.

Skeletal muscle does not condition itself naturally. It must be exercised to be properly conditioned. Only when conditioned are the channels clear through which blood must pass. In a muscle which is disproportionately fatty, as the unconditioned muscle is, regardless if you are "fat" or "skinny," the capillary beds through which blood must pass are compressed. The overall effect is to raise blood pressure, so that the heart must pump harder and do more work to get the job done. Only when your muscles are conditioned can your body find its natural blood pressure. Also, when your muscles are conditioned, you feel better and are more able to concentrate on your activities.

There are hundreds of separate skeletal muscles in the body, and each of them has an attachment to two bones (an "origin" and an "insertion"). It is in the movement of the skeleton that work is done — therefore, these two attachments are absolutely necessary.

Skeletal muscle runs on the same energy source as does the nervous system: oxygen. A muscle can do its job only when supplied with sufficient oxygen. Oxygen arrives in the muscle via arteries, which branch over and over until capillaries are formed. Five factors determine the amount of oxygen delivered: (1) the condition of the arteries, (2) the condition of the muscle, (3) the strength of the heartbeat, (4) the oxygen exchange capacity of the lung and (5) the oxygen-carrying capacity of the blood.

One of the muscles of the body is the *diaphragm*. For life to be happening, the diaphragm must contract. It is the only compulsory skeletal muscle. It must continuously contract and relax; this activity is compulsory for life to continue.

All other skeletal muscles are noncompulsory. For them to contract requires the activity of the command center located in the cerebral cortex coordinated through reflex circuits in the spinal cord and the cerebellum.

Consult your encyclopedia for a diagram of the skeletal muscles of the body. Look under "muscles."

The diaphragm is run by the respiratory center located in the brain stem. Superior conditioning of the diaphragm is achieved through aerobic exercise. Superior conditioning of the rest of the skeletal muscles, likewise, requires special attention. This is called a "weight training program." When you think of a "weight training program" you probably will think of lots of time spent pumping iron, expense, Arnold Schwarzenmuscle, etc. That is not it. I am not recommending that you become muscle-bound; however, I do want to introduce you to your muscles. We will take them by groups, rather than as individuals, and find out how easy they are to condition.

The body can be thought of as a collection of sticks connected by joints. The sticks are the following: feet, legs, thighs, thorax-abdomen, upper arm, lower arm and neck. That is a total of twelve sticks. Each stick has two basic movements — flexion and extension — except for the neck, upper arm and thigh, which have five basic movements: flexion, extension, abduction, adduction and rotation. For exercise purposes, we can forget about rotation and adduction. Arnold and his friends must worry about those movements, but we do not have to.

Let us begin with your foot. In a sitting position, flex your foot back and then extend it forward. To flex your foot back, you used your anterior tibial muscles. Place your hand just over your shin-bone, and feel this flexion. To extend your foot, you have used your *gastrocnemius*. Place your hand on the back of your leg, and feel the action of that muscle. Now, do the same for the front and back of the thigh, the *quadriceps* and the *hamstrings* respectively. You need to stand up and flex your knee backwards to feel your hamstrings in action. These two muscle groups are responsible for extension and flexion of the leg (foot to knee), respectively.

Now, consider the movement of your thighs. These are moved by muscles attached to your pelvis. Stand up and, keeping your right thigh and leg straight, kick as if you were kicking a ball. Now, the left. This movement is accomplished with a muscle buried deep in your abdomen called the *psoas*. You will be unable to feel the action of the psoas with your hand. Now, kick in the same way, except backward. As you do this, put your hand on your buttocks. The muscles which do this action are called the *gluteal group*. Let us hope yours is cute! Now, kick to the side and, as you do, find with your hand the muscle that does this action. It is called the *tensor fascia lata*.

Now, on to the thorax-abdomen. Those muscles that form little waves on your belly (if and when you become skinny) are called the *rectus abdomini*. These muscles flex the thorax-abdomen in relationship to the thighs. Do a sit-up, keeping your hands on your belly to feel the action of these muscles. Now, get in a crawling position and raise the upper part of your body to the position of standing on your knees. As you do this, arch your back. The muscles that do this are located on both sides of your vertebral column and are known as "extensors" of the spine.

Now, consider your upper extremities (arms, forearms and hands). First, let us look at the shoulder joint. Stand with your arms outstretched as if to fly like a bird. Now, bring your hands together back-to-back over your head. The muscle doing this action is the *deltoid* and is what you refer to as your "shoulder." Now, resume the flying position; imagine yourself upside down, and bring your arms from that position to your sides. These muscles are the *latissimus dorsi*. They originate from your rib cage about where your elbows are when you are typing or playing piano, and they attach ("insert") to the inner aspect of the upper arm just below the shoulder. Find them with your hands.

Now, lie on your back with an object of two to ten pounds in each hand with your arms spread-eagled straight out from your sides. Keeping your arms straight, bring the two objects together in front of you. The chest muscles which have done this action are called the *pectorales* (*pectoralis* is the singular form). Find them, and inspect their action.

Now, stand next to an armless chair with your right knee on the seat of the chair. Bend forward until your trunk is horizontal with the floor, and support yourself with your right hand on the chair. With a moderately heavy object in your left hand, and that hand at floor level, pull that object upwards until your elbow is at the level of your back. Keep your elbow flared out and away from your body. One of the muscles in this action is the *trapezius*, and it spreads out over your back like a sheet, attaching to your shoulder blade and stabilizing your shoulder blade, while other muscles (*teres major* and *minor*), attached to your shoulder blade and arm, elevate your arm. The *trapezius* also attaches to the neck and the spine from the upper neck to the mid-back.

Now, take a moderately heavy object in each of your hands, stand up and, with your hands facing forward and your arms hanging at your side, lift the object to your chin with the palms of your hands turned toward your face. These muscles are the *biceps*.

Now, take the object, and hold it directly over your head. Let your elbow bend and your hand come down behind you with the shaft of your upper arm pointing to the ceiling. With your other hand, resting on your biceps and holding in place your upper arm, raise the object again over your head keeping your elbow in the same place. The muscles which have done this action are the *triceps*.

Now, find the *flexors* and *extensors* of the *wrists*. These muscles are located on the front and back of your forearm respectively, and they bend the hand back and forth.

That leaves the neck. Disregarding rotation, the neck has four movements: flexion, extension, abduction and adduction. These muscles groups are named for what they do: *neck extensors, flexors, abductors* and *adductors*. Flex and extend your neck and find those muscles. Point your head to the right and the left, and find the muscles which do that.

There are hundreds of muscles in the human body, but if you pay attention to them in the manner I have outlined and work them regularly, all muscles will be well-conditioned. I distinguish between becoming muscled up and being conditioned. It is not necessary to be muscled up to be conditioned.

However, it is necessary to exercise each muscle group twice each week. To achieve our purposes, each muscle group needs to be matched to an appropriate weight and worked to exhaustion two times each week. This represents about thirty minutes of your time, less than one-half of one percent of one week.

Worked to exhaustion means that the last repetition is the last one you can possibly do. The number of repetitions should be between eight and twelve. The weight is adjusted up or down until exhaustion occurs after eight, nine, ten, eleven, or at most twelve repetitions.

This is called "anaerobic" exercise because you are using stored energy rather than straight oxygen. Believe it or not, anaerobic exercise is an important part of aerobics. **It creates muscle tissue through which your heart can pump blood with minimum effort**. It also creates more insulin receptor sites and changes the insulin/glucagon/eicosanoid hormone balance in a very positive way. A usual effect is to lower blood pressure, even if your blood pressure is only in the high normal range. See pages 114-122 for a full discussion of insulin, glucagon, and the eicosanoids.

Getting Started

How to get started? This is a process of education. If you are not already accustomed to this, you need a teacher. If you are accustomed to weight training, and you are not actually doing it, you need to further educate yourself about the benefits. When you know enough, and if you love life, you will do your program. It will be a high priority. If you join a fitness club, they will provide someone to set up a program for you. When you become very practiced at it, you will be able to take this activity into your own home and make it a part of your regular routine. You brush your teeth, you wash the dishes, and you lift your weights.

The proper diet to follow for maximum benefit from exercise is covered on pages 110-113 under "Human Growth Hormone."

See page 358 for instructions on contacting my office for a referral to a doctor experienced in anaerobic exercise.

PSYCHOLOGICAL

HEALTH

THE EMOTIONS

This chapter is designed to allow you to become more familiar with, and clear about, your emotions. Nothing could be more important for your health than the unimpeded expression of emotion. Unfortunately, this is not something our culture promotes. The result is that unexpressed emotions express their energy in the living systems of the body, frequently disrupting those systems.

Every doctor is familiar with the "cancer personality," that person down in room 204 of General Hospital with a new diagnosis of some sort of cancer. "The nicest person in the world," say his friends and relatives. "This should not have happened to him!"

It is only now being recognized that most arthritis is caused by, at least in part, repressed emotions, and that the changes which happen with joints and discs are accelerated by, and perhaps initiated by, repressed emotions.

The mind acts on the body in whatever way is necessary to divert your attention from the emotions it considers unacceptable. These emotions are repressed out of consciousness. The result is pain and dysfunction in any of the organ systems of the body. Any repression of emotion presents a health hazard to the body.

Emotions are expressions of thoughts manifested in the body. Obviously, crying and laughing are emotions, as are depression and elation, sadness and ecstasy, anxiety and bliss. Some emotions, you think of as good — those that provide release of tension, pleasure, or escape from pain. Other emotions, you consider bad — those that hold tension in place and create pain.

Good emotions derive from adding to your reality something or someone which you believe will bring pleasure, or by letting go of something or someone you believe has brought you pain. This is called "happiness" and "relief" respectively.

Bad emotions are related to adding to your reality something or someone you believe will bring you pain or discomfort or by letting go of something or someone you believe has brought pleasure or comfort to your life. This is called "dread" and "grief" respectively.

Happiness, relief, dread and grief are the only true emotions. Anger, which is commonly thought of as an emotion, is actually a projection of responsibility. True emotions, when experienced, lead to a state of peace. Anger, when experienced, leads to a state of agitation. It is important to consider the situations in your life in order to make contact with your emotions **because** — and this is important — by living in the modern world, you have lost track of how you feel — you have lost track of your emotional life. The only variable here is how much you have lost track of your emotional life, not whether or not you have — because you have. No one has escaped this fate. Men, generally, are further away from their emotions than women. However, considering how lost everyone is, the difference between the predicaments of men and women is almost insignificant.

I am not recommending that you learn to wear your emotions on your shirt sleeve, and put it on other people like some kind of holy water. Your emotions are your own, and sharing them should be done only with people with whom it is appropriate to share them. Like an exclusive party, this sharing is by invitation only.

You have no one to thank or to blame for your emotions. They all are yours, caused and owned by you and by no one else. Nevertheless, they are related to the way you handle the comings and goings in your life. When good things come happiness is natural. If you do not feel it, you are blocking an essential part of who you are. When good things go from your life, sadness is natural. If you suppress the experience of this sadness, it will show up in other ways — pain in your body, loss of sleep, altered behavior, or impaired judgment, for example. When bad things come to your life, dread is natural. If you do not experience this dread, you cannot be appropriate and handle your life in the best way. When bad things go from your life, relief is natural. If you do not experience that relief, you are left with the tension related to the item which is now gone.

Therefore, there is a certain value to experiencing the emotion appropriate to any situation, as that situation appears. However, there is a big problem here. That problem is unconsciousness. Your emotions have become, partially at least, unconscious. The appropriate question relates to how to make unconscious emotions conscious.

Any experience which exists in your reality has some degree of permission from you to exist. Otherwise, it could not exist in your reality, for you created that reality, and all things come and go only with your permission. On the other hand, some experiences come with such great strength that they require very small permission from you to exist. If I send you a new Porsche Carrera, even though you may be a person not given to laughing and dancing in the street, you may have some difficulty suppressing just such a celebration. If the one you love most in the world dies, even though you may have an image of yourself as a very tough person, you will weep for this loss.

So, for an emotion to be expressed requires some degree of strength of experience combined with some degree of permission from you. You have an emotion, experienced or unexperienced, to every event of life, regardless of how seemingly trivial.

Happiness

Happiness is the emotional response to the coming of things or people into your life from which or from whom you expect pleasure. This is so plain and obvious as to need no further discussion.

Grief

Grief is the emotion associated with letting go of someone or something which you believe has brought pleasure to your life. For our purposes in this book, we will consider the letting go of people, even though the same principles apply to things like a wrecked car or a burned-down home.

Grief is natural to the loss of someone you believe has brought pleasure to your life. Grief is healthy and leads to new beginnings. New beginnings full of joy and expectation are possible only when you have made peace with the past.

Making peace with the past constitutes letting go of someone who once was in your life. However, letting go of someone is made impossible by the failure to have acknowledged. Prolonged grief is certain evidence of the failure to have acknowledged. When someone passes from your life and is no longer around you, that person exists in the past, even if that person is still alive and living on the other side of town. When someone is in the past, it is necessary to let go of that person in order to get on with your life. Letting go in the absence of acknowledgment is not possible.

The purpose of this section of the book is to review the last ten years of your life in a search for prolonged grief. This is not as simple as it seems. A common chain of events goes like this:

1. someone disappears from your life (death, breakup of a relationship),

2. you experience an acute grief reaction,

3. you complete the relationship with a **negative** acknowledgment,

4. you renew your life with your grief in a state of unconsciousness.

Grief exists in a state of unconsciousness when you have not acknowledged the perfection of a relationship. Perfection in relationship includes the fact that it ended. If, in your experience, it "should have" gone on, you are not in touch with the perfection of the relationship, and your grief exists in a prolonged and perhaps unconsciousness condition.

Prolonged unconscious grief has the effect of limiting the possibilities of your life. Reality must show up consistent with the stand you have taken about the nature of people, the victim-stance, which in that system explains circum-stance, the "condition around." Prolonged unconscious grief also binds the amount of vital life energy necessary to maintain the grief in a state of unconsciousness.

Relief

Relief is the emotion appropriately experienced when letting go of something or someone you believe has brought you pain. Like all emotions, it is acceptable to have it, and it has its appropriate time and place for expression. Relief often comes in combination with grief. For example, if someone you love dearly, with whom you also have struggle and conflict, dies or otherwise disappears from your life, the appropriate emotions are grief and relief. Many a married person is, at this moment, daydreaming of the sudden and unexpected death of his or her spouse, wishing for the relief that death would bring without the price tag of responsibility for ending the relationship. If it were to happen, there would be grief, relief, and a psuedo-emotion: guilt.

Relationships without some degree of struggle and conflict are very unusual, almost nonexistent. Therefore, some degree of relief is expected with the end of almost any relationship. Now comes the problem: rarely is that relief experienced and what takes its place is guilt and shame. Where relief should exist, guilt and shame actually do exist. This guilt and shame blend in with the grief which is appropriate to the loss which has happened and prolongs that grief in an unnatural way. The experience of relief at the death of a person or the dissolution of a relationship is inadmissible to consciousness — it makes you look bad to yourself, because you wished for that death in your daydreams.

There is a deeper, more pervasive lie going on here: that relationship with people you love is supposed to be free of struggle and conflict. To admit relief to yourself at the end of a relationship would be to admit that the relationship was not free of struggle and conflict. Struggle and conflict are uncomfortable experiences, and you do your best to eliminate uncomfortable experiences from your awareness. The result: relationship becomes a pretense. You pretend that you have no struggle or conflict with a person, and you do your best not to give away the presence of that struggle and conflict in your behavior or the things you say.

So the advantage of admitting and experiencing relief at the end of a relationship is that authenticity is reintroduced into the relationship, even if the relationship is over forever in terms of interacting with each other. Authenticity is one of the qualities which allows for completion in relationship: the experience that nothing is left over which should be dealt with.

The alternative to admitting the presence of struggle and conflict and resolving issues openly is deadening to relationship. You may look good for a while, but when the relationship is absolutely dead, it looks as good in your life as a dead horse would look in your living room. Here is the natural flow of experiential transformation: the experience of relief is made conscious and more fully owned → greater authenticity in current relationships → awareness of the presence of struggle and conflict in present relationships follows naturally → open and fair conflict resolution begins to have a chance → the experience of love and intimacy becomes more possible.

Dread

Dread is that emotional experience appropriate to the situation of adding something or someone to your reality which you believe brings you, or will bring you, pain or discomfort. The definition of the word dread is: anticipation of pain and/or discomfort.

Dread is a normal and useful emotion as long as it remains fixed on the potential danger for which it is designed. Dread moves you toward taking precautions against danger. If, while driving, you see a large truck approaching through your rear-view mirror and that truck is swerving from right to left without regard for other vehicles, dread is the normal emotion to that situation. It moves you to take action — to remove your vehicle and thus your body as well, from the possibility of pain and discomfort. Dread in such a situation may even save your life.

If you are considering working with a person in a job situation and experience dread when you interview with that person, you had best heed this emotion. If you are thinking of marriage to a person and dread keeps coming up, you should pay attention to that experience. The kind of toughness we have developed, to allow us to continue functioning in a world in which people killing people is an accepted form of conflict resolution, makes us unable to acknowledge the presence of dread. When dread is unacknowledged, it presses itself forward for recognition and in such a situation can grow out of proportion to the situation and become paralyzing.

Franklin Roosevelt said at the beginning of World War II, "We have nothing to fear but fear itself." That was not the truth, but it called forth toughness and repressed for some the experience of dread. Since you are not going to war in day to day life, it is not to your advantage to repress dread. Rather, acknowledge its presence, and take it into account. It means something. It can be very useful in living your life successfully, but only when it is recognized and acknowledged. Properly integrated into your life, dread can save you from disaster.

THE PSYCHE

The Psyche I: The Result of Repression

Knowledge of the psyche is of critical importance in the maintenance of perfect health and vitality. The influence of the psyche over the health of the body is not just important, it is complete, absolute and total.

A thorough review of psychoanalytic theory would not only be inordinately long, it also would be confusing and not very useful. Your ideas about the psyche, in order to be effective, need to be incisive, direct, powerful and applicable.

All ideas about the psyche are paradigms; they cannot be proven or disproven, but are looking glasses with which to interpret the events in life. Please read the following comments with this understanding: this is not "The Truth," there is no "The Truth." Nevertheless, these comments reflect my direct experience. Take them for what worth they can be to you.

The Essential Identity

The first and possibly most difficult notion to accept without some direct experience is that there is more to you than just your body. You are an eternal spirit, once unified with God and in possession of all knowledge. With your conception, your consciousness was severed from God, and you came to this physical reality as a lonely individual, unified with matter: incarnated in a body. In that event you lost all memory of your relationship with God and all knowledge disappeared from your awareness. You came into the world to strengthen yourself: to master the ability to love and the ability to experience being loved. You are one spirit. You are not made of parts. You are made of peace, bliss and ecstasy.

When your body ceases to live, you still will be present, probably to your great amazement. This fact is born out in the reported experience of tens of thousands of people who have faced physical death, yet have been revived and lived again. I am one of those people.

The Apparent Identity

Although you are one spirit, you appear to yourself as many parts. This is the inevitable result of occupying a body and identifying with that body. Physical reality presents itself as parts. The central experience which makes this fragmentation possible is fear. The drives of the body inevitably bring you into conflict with the world, for you inhabit an animal among animals. This animal you inhabit demands satisfaction of its needs. It wants to reproduce itself, and it wants to destroy all threats to its survival.

While your essential identity is in harmony with the world, this animal identity is inherently destructive to all that appears to threaten it and, therefore, destructive to itself as well. When this animal appears dangerous to the animals of other people, it places itself in jeopardy.

Therefore, you are obligated to control this animal, and to do this, you develop a mechanism commonly called the "ego." It is this ego, this control mechanism, which you think of as yourself. You give this mechanism control over everyday functions, thought processes and the voluntary muscles of your body. The ego is your Apparent Identity, it seems to be who you are.

The Emergency Identity

Despite the size and power of the ego, the animal in you threatens to break through to consciousness from time to time. On the less serious side, the animal would have you eat without utensils, never bathe and never brush your teeth. This is mild fare compared to wild and crazy thoughts about sex and violence which you think only criminals should have. You have them also, and admitting them into consciousness is painful.

As Freud discovered through dream analysis — almost one hundred years ago — to protect yourself from the painful awareness of these aggressive instincts, you give great power to a branch of the ego to judge and condemn these criminal thoughts as wrong in yourself and in others.

To protect yourself from awareness of your own animal, you repress awareness of the animal in you and project it onto others. You become very concerned about controlling the behavior of other people. In the extreme, you become cynical about human nature and the world at large, and you may align yourself with rigid religious systems to allay your fear and make yourself right. This empowered branch of the ego is called the "superego."

When the animal raises its ugly head, this is considered a grave emergency by the ego and superego. The ego and the superego together repress the thoughts and desires of the animal, or "id," as Freud called it.

The memory of very traumatic events also may be repressed because of the violent, sadistic nature of the thoughts the animal has in response to these events. The purpose of repression is to maintain your identity as a socialized human being in your own eyes. The superego is a right/wrong machine designed to push the animal into unconsciousness in emergency situations. The superego is your Emergency Identity. It functions in the emergence of repressed animal experience into awareness.

These structures of the mind: animal, ego and superego, are created by you, the essential identity or who you are. However, you never think of yourself as that eternal spirit, but rather as the structures it creates. Your unwillingness to include this animal you are into your consciousness causes illness in the body. The animal is never absent, only repressed. Repression does not mean disappearance, it means transmutation into another realm. Repressed experience can go into the interpersonal sphere and make your relationships with others difficult, or it can go into the sphere of the body and alter the normal functioning of the body. When this happens in the realm of the voluntary muscle system, it is experienced as involuntary movements: tics, false seizures, etc.

When repressed experience reappears in the sensory systems of the body, the result is "hysteria": unexplained sensations, loss of sensation, or paralysis in parts of the body. These phenomena have no physical explanation. When repressed experience reappears in the involuntary systems of the body, the results can be conditions such as asthma, ulcers, colitis, arthritis, skin disease and cancer.

The avoidance of these kinds of conditions is achieved by allowing into consciousness all of one's experience. In your animal self, you have all the base thoughts which criminals have. There is no difference between you and a criminal except that you have created mind structures which successfully repress out of awareness all thoughts of wanton sexuality and violence.

You have gone a step too far. You only need to prevent these thoughts from transforming themselves into action, but you have gone further than that: you have repressed them out of your consciousness. You do not accept these thoughts of the animal within your consciousness and because you do not accept them, you project them into your perception of the thoughts of others, into the vital systems of your body, or both. This damages your relationships and your health. Damaged relationships will, in turn, cause damage to your health in the form of increased stress.

The Psyche II: Personality Types

The personality is the ego's way of relating to other people. It is a massive collection of behavioral traits, stimulus/response pairs, the sum total of which is your presentation to the world.

While you think you are your ego, the personality is who other people think you are, and the success of your personality determines the degree to which other people will allow you to succeed. Clearly your success in life is, in large measure, derived from how much other people will allow you to succeed.

How well you succeed has a large impact on your health through stress or the lack of it. A person who is succeeding is, all other factors being equal, under less stress than a person who is failing. The purpose of studying the personality is to create the space for more success in your life, thus less stress and greater health and vitality.

Like it or not, your success depends on your relationships with other people. You will be allowed by others to succeed in proportion to how much you are "liked," and whether or not you are liked depends on the *flexibility* of your personality. Herein lies the problem. To some degree you are *inflexible* in your response to people and situations. Let us see what that means.

When you were born, you did not have a personality. Newborns are pretty much alike from one to the other. Some are more irritable than others, but that is the only difference one can see. This remains the case for several months, and during this time, as a developing child, you were unconcerned about your future survival, simply because you had not figured yourself out to exist in a body. When your body finally became real to you, and when you identified with and made it your essential identity, it became possible for you to conceive of not surviving. In that moment, you began to devise strategies for survival.

This occurred in relationship to the person who cared for you, who you would later identify as "mother." However, before she was mother, she was simply your only lifeline to survival. You took it as your job to make sure she continued to show up with the food. You thought you had something to do with her decision to feed you. You were unaware that she had made a life decision to take care of your needs.

There were three ways you could change yourself, and you selected one of these three to (you thought) cause your mother to continue returning with food. These changes were first described by neo-Freudian psychoanalyst Karen Horney.

Going Along to Get Along: The Pleaser

You may have decided to become a pleasing baby, to make very little trouble for your mother, and in this way, you thought, persuade her to continue to show up with food. If you made this decision, you became the talk of the Mother's Club — you were the "good" baby, the baby every mother wished her baby would be like.

When you entered school, you made good grades, not because you wanted to but to please your parents. Behaviorally, you either blended in with the wall, so that teacher did not know you were there, or you became teacher's pet. After your school years, you did not continue to develop your intellect.

When adolescence came, you did not rebel but rather identified with your elders, trying to be more like them, and you distanced yourself from rebellious peers. During adolescence, your pleasing ways became compulsive and rigid, your automatic first reaction to stress, and in this condition you entered adult life.

As an adult, you enter relationships meekly, and as long as you feel insecure in relationship, you are super nice. When you begin to feel secure, however, you turn very mean and destructive, much to your partner's surprise. As a compulsive pleaser tremendous pressure builds up inside you, and you take it out on the person closest to you.

Opposition for the Sake of Opposition: The Rebel

If, on the other hand, you made a different decision in the crib on that fateful day, things turned out very differently. You may have been one of those babies who decided that if you raised enough hell, made enough noise and caused enough trouble, mother would stay and take care of you. However, when she disappeared around the corner one day, you concluded that she was gone forever, and you let out a mighty scream. She came running back into the room, and you decided that she must somehow like your screaming. After that, you did a lot of screaming, making sure, so you thought, that mother would stay for all that entertainment provided by your mighty lungs and your big mouth.

When you entered school, you were a model of misbehavior. On many occasions, you had to bring a note home for your parents to sign, detailing your misbehavior. You did not make good grades, but at least you had a chance later in life to develop your intellect, not to please anyone but based on your own interests.

In adolescence, you rebelled like a volcano, and you spent your time with other kids who were rebellious like you. You thought adults were stupid, and you did your best to dissociate yourself from them, beginning with your parents.

As an adult, you enter intimate relationship with your rebel banner flying proudly. You are unlikely to pass up any opportunity to argue or debate a point. You don't let anything slide by. However, when the argument is over, it is done, and you recover quickly. As a compulsive rebel, you release pressure as soon as it builds up.

Withdrawal: The Hermit

There is a third possible choice: withdrawal. On that day when you thought about how to keep your mother coming back to take care of you, you may have come to the conclusion that if you did not respond to stimuli she would become concerned about you and try to persuade you to come out and play. This persuasion was just the attention you liked, so you worked your withdrawal act to an art form.

When you went to school, you made excellent marks, not to please anyone, but simply because you had so few friends, books filled the void where relationship could have been. In your isolation, you desperately hoped someone would come and try to persuade you to come out to play. A few people did, but not many. In a condition of loneliness, you may have decided to yourself that you were better than others.

In adolescence, you participated in withdrawal, not rebellion. You probably went for a higher education and may have become a professional. Many distinguished scientists and scholars are this sort of personality type. In intimate relationship, you are primarily the entertainee, not the entertainer. You hate arguments, although you will participate in them. You consider yourself a better person than the kind of person who would engage in an argument, and when you do argue it damages your self esteem. You are a hermit from participation.

I have described here the three basic personality types in pure culture. In this description, you can probably find yourself described but only approximately, needing additions and deletions. Being a personality type is not a problem. Everyone has one of these personalities at the core, and there are only three. The problem comes when one never outgrows the **rigidity** of one's personality, so that one reacts in a stereotypical way to each stressful situation. This plainly does not work for other people and, as a result, you will not be likable, and people will not allow you to succeed. This will cause stress and damage your health.

When you find your personality type, the job is to begin to develop other ways of acting and reacting, so you have a choice under stress. A flexible person is a happy person and a person others like to be around and empower to succeed in life. Most important, flexible people are under less stress and therefore live longer, more vital lives.

The Psyche III: Intimacy and Health

"Honor your father and your mother, as the Lord God has commanded you, *that your days upon the earth may be prolonged*, and that it may go well with you..." The fifth of the Ten Commandments, Deuteronomy 5:16 (emphasis mine).

A clean clear relationship with your mother is vital to your health. It is well-known that stress in interpersonal relationships has a detrimental effect on one's health. Until your relationship with your mother is clean, clear and full of love and the experience of being loved — until that time, your health is at risk. The relationship between health and relationship is not as obvious as the relationship between health and diet, only because it is not in our culture to consider such a possibility. Nevertheless, it is very real.

"Mother" is that person who nurtured you in the earliest years of your life. That may or may not have been your biological mother. It could have been an aunt, a sister, even an uncle or a brother. Around your experience of this person, you created your personality and your relationship with intimacy.

This is the usual, almost inevitable sequence of events:

1. perfect harmony with Mother, from birth to age two years, six months;

2. testing Mother to learn about people — particularly people who love you — begins at age two years, six months;

3. playing the game that Mother failed — for the purpose of learning her reaction (withdrawing your acknowledgment of her love, as a game) - begins at three years of age;

4. making real the game that Mother failed — happens in early adolescence; at this time, you repress the memory of her loving you right, and the past is transformed into a story proving that she never loved you right;

5. living in the reality that Mother failed and creating the struggle to change her — early adolescence to the time you leave home, or Mother dies;

6. parting from Mother with the point of view that she failed, did not love you right and refused to change.

After that, you go into the world with the reality that the person with whom you are closest cannot love you right. This point of view becomes a piece of your identity. Then you search for a cure: someone who will love you and love you right.

You then find such a person, but there is a problem. Your reality dictates that the person with whom you are closest cannot love you right. In contradiction of that paradigm, here is a person loving you and loving you right. Something must change, one of these items must win out over the other.

The reality you stand for is always stronger than the reality in which you live, and it will chisel on that reality until it is resculpted into something you can interpret as consistent with the reality for which you stand. In other words, the pattern you played out with your mother from early childhood will repeat itself. Here is how it looks:

1. perfect harmony with the partner: romantic love;

2. testing the partner to make sure he/she loves you;

3. playing the game that the partner does not love you right and thus has failed you;

4. making real the game that the partner failed — the honeymoon is now over;

5. living in the reality that the partner failed, and struggling to change her/him;

6. leaving the partner with the point of view that the partner failed, did not love you right and refused to change.

"Leaving" the partner can take one of two forms: (1) responsible leaving and (2) irresponsible leaving. In responsible leaving, one packs one's bags and hits the road or drives the other person out. In irresponsible leaving, you become so obnoxious the other person leaves you. Irresponsible leaving is also, usually, unconscious leaving.

The experience you are left with is that you have been unfairly abandoned. Then you practice your abandonment story and sell it as reality to your friends and to yourself. After that, you repeat the process, which by now has become a pattern.

Unless your relationship with your mother is perfect, and by that I mean that your experience of your mother's love for you was and is perfect, you can find your life somewhere within steps one to six above. You are trying to move to the next step while consciously resisting. You probably have noticed that movement backward from the direction of six toward the direction of one is almost impossible.

So how to get out? Focusing on your partner is not the answer, because that is not where the pattern gets its power. The pattern receives its power from your incomplete relationship with your mother. Your relationship with your mother is the origin of the paradigm that the person closest to you cannot love you right.

Of course, about now you are saying, "Okay, Dr. K., all this will change for me when my mother changes." That gives you a life sentence in your prison without possibility of parole, because your mother is not going to change. You may already have figured that out.

What needs to change is your **experience** of your mother, not your mother! Your experience of her will change back to the stage of perfect harmony when you return yourself to the condition of being a **living** acknowledgment of her love and not before.

How to do that? This is not some easy process that you just go do and then you are done. For most people, this will be a project requiring years of work. It involves a promise you give about the relationship between your experience and life events. Here is the promise:

I PROMISE TO FUSE MY IDENTITY WITH THE IDEA THAT ALL EXPRESSIONS ARE EXPRESSIONS OF LOVE.

That sounds simple, doesn't it? However, you live in the opposite reality: that some expressions (comfortable ones) might be expressions of love and other expressions (uncomfortable ones) definitely are not expressions of love.

Therefore, this involves the intentional recreation of reality. For this to be possible requires that you know reality to be created by you, not to exist as some kind of Truth. This is the one that gives people problems, because one becomes convinced that one's reality is The Truth, and what fool would dare to argue with The Truth?

Because you can have it any way you want it, and because how you really want it is to be loved and be loved right, you can have it that way. Here is what you must give up: trying to change other people. Here is what you can have: all expressions as expressions of love. To the degree that you have this experience, you will live a longer, more vital, healthy, satisfying life.

The most useful place to begin to create this reality is with your mother, because exactly there did you give up your grace and divinity.

The Psyche IV: Authority and Health

Your relationship with authority is critically important to your health. Few events in life can stress your body as much as conflict with authority. People in authority are most appropriately experienced as partners in your life who have seniority over you in certain areas of living.

Your relationship with authority was derived in relationship to your father. Maturation in relationship to authority cannot happen until you can fully experience your father's love for you.

"Father" is that person who first presented the ground rules of life to you along with consequences for breaking those ground rules. The nature of these consequences was that you could not tolerate them. Father could conceivably have been an uncle, a brother, or even a female person in your life. Around your experience of this person, you created your relationship with authority, and from this person you derived your ability to discipline yourself and get the job done. Your relationship with this person is your relationship with all authority in the world.

There are three possible ways to deal with this person, and each has profound consequences for your relationship with the world. You can become agreeable to this person, you can rebel against this person, or you can withdraw from this person.

The problem is: confrontation, early in life, with someone much bigger than you, who is willing to say, or do, whatever it takes for you to pay attention to the ground rules.

The solution to this problem is: a stand you take about who you are, in relationship to authority. It is very likely that you chose a favorite method of dealing with this person. This becomes the method you use for dealing with authority in general, all through life. You become an expert on this method and, under any degree of stress, you revert to this method on which you are an expert.

If you become agreeable with this person, you lose the ability to generate initiative and creativity, and you go through life being a follower looking for a leader. If you rebel against this person, you set yourself up in life to have conflict with people who have real or imagined authority in your life. If you withdraw from this person, you acquire the lone ranger complex and become detached from the world and from your place in it.

Determine now which solution you chose in relationship to father:

1. agreeableness;

2. rebellion;

3. withdrawal.

Regardless of which one you chose, you have painted yourself into a corner. You become an expert on how to survive in relationship to authority, and the price you pay is self-determination and creativity. Your solution to this situation in life becomes a part of your personality, just as it did in relationship to your mother.

The way out is to become a living acknowledgment of your father's love for you. That means that every single time your father sees you or hears from you, he feels acknowledged. This, for many, becomes a life-long project. If you achieve it, you are a new person in relationship to authority, and you are at a new level of effectiveness and ability to contribute in your chosen work.

I have devised a one year correspondence/telephone course for the transformation of relationship from its core: the relationships with mother and with father, extending that transformation to all relationships. Its name is *The Man Woman Course*. If you are interested in taking this course and would like to receive a prospectus to help you with your decision, send your request to:

Ron Kennedy, M.D.
P.O. Box 2909
Rohnert Park, CA 94927

WEIGHT

CONTROL

WEIGHT CONTROL

Studies demonstrate that each pound you carry on your body, over and above your ideal weight, costs you one year of your life, on avergage. So a man at his ideal weight for the first half of his life, and twenty pounds overweight for the second half of his life, all other factors being equal, on average will live ten years less than he otherwise would live. Since your years can be full of vitality, these ten years are a high price to pay for being overweight.

However, the pure number of pounds you weigh is not the whole story. The habits that number reflects mean much more than the number itself. If you starve yourself to your ideal weight, you will induce a state of malnutrition and decrease your vitality and longevity. A healthy ideal weight is achieved through healthy living, not through starvation diets.

Following is a list of factors which cause your weight to be what it is. If you want to achieve your ideal weight in a healthy way, become a warrior in these areas and I promise you, your weight will be at its ideal level within one year.

Selection of Food

Nothing is more important than your selection of food. The body is made for a balanced intake of protein and complex carbohydrate. Let the fat content be determined by whatever amount of fat comes with your other food sources.

A proper balance of protein to complex carbohydrate regulates your insulin/glucagon, and thus your eicosanoid hormone system. You can do so with no fat or some fat.

Our culture is, mistakenly, fat phobic. Read carefully. Organically grown food. Ten parts carbohydrate to seven parts protein. Organically grown food. Ten parts carbohydrate to seven parts protein. Organically grown food. Ten parts carbohydrate to seven parts protein. Organically grown food. Got it?

Balance of Emotions

Eating to suppress experience is ever so common. Stay in communication with your emotions. Experience the way you feel, and tell the truth about it. This is not advice to stay calm or stay happy. Simply be honest with yourself, and you will not have to put a mountain of food on your experience to suppress it.

Regular Aerobics

"Regular" means at least, *at least*, <u>at least</u> twenty minutes of vigorous aerobics three times each week. Regular aerobic exercise keeps your metabolic rate at the perfect level, and this burns calories which otherwise would show up on your thighs and waist.

Colon Health

Keep your colon clean. See a colon therapist at least twice a year. As you grow older, you may need an herbal stimulant (aloe vera, for example) to maintain a transit time of no more than 24 hours. A transit time of more than 24 hours results in putrefaction of food in the colon with resulting toxic overload of the liver. This calls for more nutrients through the mechanism of increased hunger.

No Addictions Allowed

In the modern world, constant vigilance is required to guard against addictions. Any addiction you allow into your habits calls up its friends, including food addiction. Most food addictions involve sugar and fat with storage of these extra calories around the body. It is possible to be an overweight vegetarian. If you eat enough vegetables, you will be overweight. It is possible to be addicted to quantity of food and to stay overweight on "healthy" food. Addiction has an emotional basis, so the complete discussion of this topic includes the earlier information on balance of emotions.

Juice Fasting One Day Every Two Weeks

Juice fasting resets the body's entire biochemical makeup toward a normal condition. After a lifetime on a typical affluent western diet, fasting is an extremely valuable tool. If you fast one day out of every two weeks, you should not need longer fasts, although you may choose to have them for the clarity and euphoria you can achieve that way.

No Simple Sugars

Simple sugars are so common in the typical diet that the best approach to handle the problem is simply to allow no simple sugars into your diet. Fortunately, you have a set of simple sugar detectors on your tongue. If it tastes sweet (with the exception of some chemicals you also should avoid), it contains simple sugars.

Defensive Food Shopping

Smart people drive defensively, because everyone knows the location of the second most dangerous place in the world: the road. Few people know the location of *the* most dangerous place in the world: the food store. If you buy it, you probably will eat it. If it does not fit with what you know to be healthy food, do not buy it or allow it into your house. Do not use the excuse that you are buying it for your guests. Have enough respect for your guests not to offer them food items which damage their health. They can do that on their own time, if they must. Spend a minimum of time in restaurants and, when you do go there, order salads and vegetable dishes.

Plenty of Water

Water is the medium of biochemical exchange in the body; it is the river which the body uses to cleanse itself. Drink plenty of water. Eight ten-ounce glasses per day of steam distilled or carbon/reverse osmosis filtered water provides wonderful cleansing of the body. Thirst comes partially disguised as hunger, which makes some sense because the water content of food partially satisfies thirst. Consider yourself hungry only when your thirst is satisfied.

Pancreatic Health

Partially digested food causes hunger to return before it should, resulting in bloating of the abdomen, putrefied food in the colon and excess food in the upper digestive tract. Pancreatic enzymes are an important component of digestion. Supplementation of your diet with digestive enzymes, in the form of raw food or the powder form of pancreatic extract, frees up enzymatic energy throughout the body which, among other things, burns fat.

Completion with Parents

It is important to be on good terms with your parents. If you are not on good terms with your parents, this condition unbalances all the other relationships in your life and, in turn, unbalances your emotions — resulting in anxiety and depression with compensatory overeating. Do your body a favor by honoring your mother and your father.

Nutritional Supplements

Although this is slightly controversial, I believe the use of high-quality nutritional supplements balances the nutritional needs of the body and quiets the fires of hunger for calories. However, do not waste your money on cheap supplements. There are several grades of supplements, and only the best will do in terms of bioavailability and bioactivity. The best costs more. What's new?

Zero Intake of Extra Salt

Plain food contains abundant salt, and your body has the ability to retain the salt which it needs. The only reason to add salt to your food is for taste, and this is, in itself, an addiction. Salt retains extra water in the body, increasing weight, slowing down the cleansing process and elevating blood pressure. Throw your salt shaker away along with that container of salt in your kitchen cabinet. The exception to this is the person who has weak adrenal function and secondary low blood pressure. This person should add salt to his or her food, and the best salt to add is sea salt.

A Good Sex Life

See pages 344-347 for a discussion of this subject. Suffice it to say, a good sex life decreases the craving for comfort foods.

Do Not Try to Restrict Calories

Calorie restriction diets do not work. You may loose weight, but when you go off the diet you will gain it back plus more. Then it will be even more difficult to loose that weight than before.

Controling Your Appetite: Ephedra Tea

If you find difficulty in controling your appetite, I suggest ephedra tea, also know as *Ma Huang* and *Ephedra sinica*. Make a strong brew of several cups, in the morning, add honey and drink a cup every few hours. You will find that you do not think about food so much, and you will be able to eat appropriate to your nutritional needs. It also has a mind stimulating effect, less dramatic and more subtle than caffeine, but longer lasting. The active ingredient is ephedrine, which promotes burning of fat in the liver and formation of muscle tissue, in addition to suppressing appetite. It is far less expensive, and more effective, than the various diet pills containing ephredrine. However, if you have an enlarged prostate, hypertension, thyroid disease, diabetes, take a MAO inhibitor or any other prescription drug, are pregnant or nursing, you should first consult with your doctor before using ephedra.

Be Patient

If you are overweight, just remember that Rome was not built, or torn down, in a day. Follow the principles outlined above, and watch your weight fall gradually over the period of six months to a year to the ideal level. Slow weight loss is likely to be permanent weight loss, because it is based in good habits, not in crash programs.

See page 358 for instructions on contacting my office for a referral to a doctor experienced in the treatment of the problem of overweight.

THE ROLE

OF SEX

IN HEALTH

SEX AND HEALTH

Your health and vitality are profoundly affected by the flow of sexual energy in your life. If this energy flows freely, all other things being equal, you will live longer and have far greater vitality. If sexual energy is blocked, it will adversely affect your health and predispose you to a host of illnesses which you otherwise would avoid. These assertions have been proven over and over in scientific studies and surveys.

Unfortunately, there is a myth that sexual energy must wane with age. This simply is not true. There are many documented cases of people who are very sexually active well into their eighties and some into their nineties. This, of course, cannot be if you allow your health to deteriorate through poor dietary habits, lack of exercise and general ignorance about maintenance of the human body. This, however, need not apply to you if you apply yourself to the content of this book.

If you follow the ideas presented in this book you will have a strong sex drive, regardless of your age. Nevertheless, it will still be possible to suppress your sexual energy due to fixed negative ideas about sex and thus reap all the negative rewards of this kind of thinking. If this barrier is lifted, you should have the sex drive commonly associated with being eighteen years old — okay, 21 at least.

Your ability to enjoy yourself in sex must begin with your relationship with your own body. You must love your own body to accept and experience the love another person may have for your body. You must be able to be sensual with yourself to be sensual with another person. Otherwise, you look to the other person for the source of pleasure, and this is a misidentification of the source of pleasure. It will not work for long.

Only a few weeks after birth, you began to explore your own body. This exploration began after you identified your hands (using your eyes to do so) and associated them with your identity. Your hands soon found your feet, and, for a while, who you were to yourself was a pair of hands and a pair of feet with a consciousness observing them. Then your hands went to work exploring your body and slowly, bit by bit, your body was incorporated into your identity. This exploration was a very pleasurable experience.

Finally, all the body parts were identified, except for the back, through manual exploration — not only identified but identified **with**. What was identified with, however, were the sensations — not a visual image of the body but the sensations of the body itself. (While the growing infant is identified with the sensations of the body, pleasure exists in abundance.) Sensations were sharp and clear, and pleasure was at a level which is almost unreachable as an adult.

Then came the fateful day when you were placed in front of a mirror, and once again, as on many previous occasions, your parent pointed to your mirror image and said something like, "That's you!" On this fateful day, it all fell into place for you, and you saw that image in the mirror as a reflection of your essential identity. This was the beginning of your flight away from the direct experience of sensations. Your identity was no longer what you felt but what you saw. From then on, what you felt had to agree with what you saw, or worse, what you thought you should be seeing.

You exist in a culture which does not value feelings but values, rather, appearance. The sensations you experience in your own body, therefore, become secondary in importance to what you see in the mirror. If you watch TV or read magazines, you are presented with standard images. Unless you look like those images, you come to resent your body.

You also live in a society which suppresses normal sexuality in favor of an image of sexuality as it rationally and ideally should look. This combination — worship of image and suppression of normal sensuality/sexuality — shows up in your life as alienation from your own body. As a consequence, people are busy disregarding their bodies (and their health) in the pursuit of ego pleasures, image, or "looking good."

The recovery of physical intimacy, and the ability to experience and share physical pleasure, begins with the recovery of your relationship with your body, so you can experience pleasure in the way you did before you identified yourself as an image. Sensuality/sexuality is a continuum. If you cannot have deep physical pleasure massaging your own foot or your arm, for example, it is not possible to have full pleasure in direct pursuit of sexuality. Deep pleasure exists in the absence of judgment about image — whether it is good or bad, right or wrong, or looks the way it "should."

Alienation from the body, and the natural pleasures of the body, is so common in society as to constitute the norm, the average, the way one expects it to be. Few people exist who know the depth of pleasure which is possible in sex. Recovery of this ability is a long trip and involves reidentification of oneself with sensations.

Giving and Receiving Sensual Attention

When you respect and admire your body, and when you transcend identification with the image you have of your body and perceive the body as sensation, you then are able to be conscious of the pleasure which always is present there. This is the condition of the body: pleasure.

However, that pleasure is not always experienced; in fact, it rarely is experienced. Alienation from the body is a result, first of identifying oneself as a body and nothing more, and then, to make matters worse, identifying oneself as the image of that body. When that happens, you live in a kind of cartoon as one of the cartoon characters. The way it feels to be alienated from the body is pleasureless, and in the extreme, it feels painful.

Body pain is a result of not living in the body but rather in an image of the body held in the mind. This is abandonment of the body. The way an abandoned body feels is painful. Real pleasure is no longer experienced, rather a caricature of pleasure is experienced.

When that caricature is all you have, you not only are separated from real pleasure, you are unaware that you are separated from pleasure.

This relates to the way people sex (and, yes, I mean that as a verb) with each other. When pleasure is experienced as a caricature of real pleasure, the senses are dulled. Normal touch does not feel pleasurable and therefore is largely abandoned in sex in favor of direct genital stimulation.

The genital organs have a large number of nerve endings compared to other parts of the body, so when they are stimulated the response is likely to be stronger. In extreme cases, however, when only a caricature of real pleasure is experienced, even direct genital stimulation produces little response. Carrying this approach to the extreme, one then buys some sort of artificial device; for example, a vibrating thing-a-ma-jig and then applies it directly to the genital organs in hopes of finally feeling something.

This is exactly the wrong approach if what you want is a return of your ability to experience real pleasure. The approach which works is to throw away all devices and abandon the fixation on direct stimulation of genitals.

Real pleasure begins with ordinary touching and being touched. One should stay with this until that touching and being touched is deeply pleasurable. Progression to genital stimulation should happen only when it can no longer be delayed or avoided. This progression should flow naturally without thinking, even without premeditation and without a distinct awareness of progressing from one sort of stimulation to another.

The first and most important sensory pleasure in lovemaking is visual. Seeing yourself and seeing your partner can be deeply pleasurable, and if it is not, back up and stay with that until it becomes pleasurable again. The second sensory pleasure in love making — and first for some people — is olfactory: smelling the other person and the other scents that may be present. That is why the perfume business will always be profitable.

Difficulties in lovemaking are encountered only in the presence of expectations. The presence of expectation creates the possibility of failure and, therefore, performance anxiety. In this circumstance, the approach to real pleasure is blocked, and what could be turn-on energy is diverted into the anxiety associated with the possibility of failure.

In an encounter, each person should approach the other with no expectations that anything in particular will happen. While merely looking at each other, looking is enough. Nothing else needs to happen. If this progresses to touching, touching is enough. Nothing else needs to happen. If this progresses, whatever happens is enough and need not progress to another stage. Satisfaction is available at each stage, and often the encounter will stop with looking or with touch or with kissing and satisfaction will be the condition of both people, if expectations are not present. When satisfaction is present, the experience of the encounter will feel good. If some feels good, more feels better, and progression is almost certain.

When the encounter does progress, sexual energy flows freely. This energy, in the absence of expectations, begins to flow with merely looking at your partner. The orgasm is "coming" from the first glance. The way I use the word "coming" means that the orgasm is on the way, whether or not it ever arrives. Coming can last a long time before orgasm, and for a long time after orgasm, as the energy continues to flow, although I suppose this would best be termed "going." Coming can last for hours, because it is the flow of energy between people who choose to love each other, sensually. Sensuality and sex are not different, but rather two expressions of the same energy flowing back and forth, one to the other.

OPINION

OPINION

After the last few years of researching the medical literature to discern the proper way to maximum health and vitality, I have come to realize how very obscured is my vision by the barriers set forth by vested capitalist interests in the health field. After all, the name of the game in business is to make money, and in order to make money in the health field it is necessary for people to be sick. If people lead healthy, vital lives with minimum sickness until their times to die come, then die quickly and easily, the shareholders in the various health-impact industries are not going to be happy — and they are going to take their money elsewhere.

Remember our example in the beginning of the book about a plant which grows anywhere, is nonpatentable and, when eaten, cures cancer, vascular disease and all other major diseases known to man. What happens when the discovery of this plant is made public? The medical establishment flexes its considerable public relations muscle, goes on television, gets into national news magazines and local newspapers and assures the public that this "cockamamie" new plant is a hoax. The public, unaccustomed to examining evidence and thinking for itself, automatically believes the medical establishment, and laws are passed to outlaw and eradicate this plant.

Meanwhile, a few doctors and other people who think for themselves grow this new plant, try it out for themselves, and find it to be as effective as advertised. Some of these doctors use it for themselves and their families and say nothing to their patients for fear or losing their licenses to practice medicine. Other doctors risk everything to offer this new treatment to their patients. Many of them lose their licenses, because they will not back down from their medical boards.

If you are going to live your life out in maximum health and vitality, it is essential that you understand this process and resolve to think for yourself regarding your medical treatment. Here is the essential truth: the desire for profits distorts the truth. Few people, including physicians, are able to see through these distortions.

At the beginning of the twentieth century, heart disease was almost unknown. Now heart disease is rampant, and the medical establishment is telling us that fat is the cause. If we would only cut our fat intake, our health would return, they say. However, fat intake in 1900 was greater than it is now. Where was heart disease then? Around that time, hydrogenated, trans fatty acids began to make their way into the American diet. This was a tragic instance of messing with nature, and plays a large part in the causation of heart disease. It is not fat, *per se*, which causes the problem, it is the type of fat. Saturated fats and hydrogenated (trans) fatty acids are key players in heart disease, along with vitamin C deficiency. The monounsaturated fats, such as virgin olive oil, have been shown over and over to protect the heart from atherosclerosis.

Since 1955, when fat phobia got its start, Americans have cut their fat intake by more than five percent, yet more people are obese and more people have vascular disease and cancer, both supposedly associated with eating fat. Does this make sense to you? What kind of health system are we living in if it does not encourage us to distinguish the different types of fat? Are we supposed to be too stupid to grasp the notion that not all fats are the same?

Average life expectancy at birth is greater now than at the turn of the century. The medical establishment tells us, "Oh, of course people live longer now, and therefore they live long enough to develop vascular disease." However, an examination of the facts reveals that if you reached age fifty in the year 1900, you could expect to live (on average) another 25 years. Now, in the 1990s, if you live to age fifty, you can expect to live another 26 years. Big difference, huh? So this line of reasoning explains nothing about why so much vascular disease is now present.

Since the year 1900, the industrial revolution has come to full fruition. People flocked to cities to work in factories in great numbers, leaving the countryside to be farmed by fewer people, using more efficient equipment. Large farm cooperatives, and later incredibly large food production companies, were created to fill the vacuum left by millions of farmers who had migrated to cities to participate in the industrialization process.

The desire for profits on the part of these food companies dovetailed nicely with the busy life of city folks, and the fast food revolution was born. Now you could go to the store and buy "food" to which you only needed to add water and/or heat, and the meal was ready. To achieve this, food was "processed," a term which covers a multitude of sins, including the addition of preservatives to increase the shelf life of this "food."

The processing of food sacrifices its nutritional value. Adding chemical preservatives to food throws another joker into the deck, because no one knows the exact results these chemicals have on the human body over a lifetime.

Of course, it is in the farmer's best economic interest to produce the highest yield of food, so he takes advantage of herbicides and pesticides to eliminate the competition of weeds and critters. There are standards set to tell the consumer the safe levels of these things in their food, when no one knows if any level is safe, over a lifetime.

As the modernization of farming technology took place, food for farm animals began to be manufactured rather than grown directly on the farm. "Animal feed," which the farmer could buy cheaper than he could grow animal food, was invented. Meat, eggs and milk products began to contain even higher levels of herbicides and pesticides than vegetables and fruits, thus contaminating the food supply on the other side of the plate. And guess where in their bodies animals store toxins? Same place you do: in the fatty tissues. Most herbicides, pesticides and preservatives are fat soluble, so they naturally end up in the fat tissues.

It's not the fat, folks **its the type of fat, and it's what is in the fat** that accounts for the three-fold increase in the incidence of cancer since the turn of the century. The real culprit behind vascular heart disease is the increased intake of carbohydrates in proportion to proteins since the medical establishment came out with that recommendation in 1955, and the increased intake of processed foods containing, among other things, hydrogenated, trans-fatty acids, and the continued intake of animal (saturated) fat.

It is true that you are better off to eat a low-fat diet, but you would be just as well off to eat a balance of fats, carbs, and proteins, as long as you can be sure they are produced without the aid of herbicides and pesticides, and that they are not stored in preservatives.

Perhaps it is not necessary be a vegetarian to enjoy maximal health and vitality. This begs the question of the moral and spiritual consideration of eating meat, which necessitates the taking of sentient life. The homocentric point of view is that it doesn't matter, and that God gave us the power to enslave, raise and slaughter animals — so it is right to do it. A more cosmic point of view would have something else to say about the morality of killing animals, particularly in face of the fact that we can obtain all necessary nutrients from plants.

Now, let us take a look at the problem of obesity. It is just amazing to me to go into public (a mall or supermarket) and see the sheer number of fat people — not just a little fat, but grossly fat — beached whale fat. One-third of Americans are obese! If you go to family albums and newspapers from the turn of the century, you see that people were not obese then, and they are now. Why?

To get the answer, let us take a look at what people try to do to handle the fat, namely diet and exercise. It is now well recognized, even among lay people, that diets do not work. Many people have tried dieting for years, and it just does not work to lose weight and keep it off. Stories abound of people, exemplified by certain celebrities such as Oprah Winfrey, who diet the pounds off only to have them return with friends in a few weeks or months. Exercise offers a bit more hope as long as you continue regular exercise, but if you quit — same story — the fat comes back, sometimes multiplied.

Many people are discouraged, and many have given up on diets and exercise and resolved to readjust their self image to allow themselves to be fat without regret. That is a good move, psychologically speaking, but it begs the question: why are people so fat these days?

I believe the problem is twofold. On one hand, herbicides, pesticides and preservatives, even in low concentrations, damage the hormonal regulatory systems of the body, particularly the adrenal gland, but also the thyroid, parathyroid, thymus, pancreas and the pineal gland itself. Not only is the production of hormones altered but so is the receptivity of the body's cells to these hormones. Add to that the fact that farm animals are fed hormones and antibiotics to increase production of meat, milk and eggs, and that many of these hormones and antibiotics find their way into the body of the consumer of these products, and you have a prescription for metabolic imbalance.

Then, when you consider the imbalanced diet the typical person eats, heavy on carbs, light on protein, you can begin to understand the amount of blubber folks are carrying around. The hormonal regulatory systems of the body are deeply disturbed, and all the complex carbs pass through digestion to simple carbs and storage as fat.

If you could imagine the exquisite process of life, in the normal state, as a kind of biochemical symphony, and imagine that the members of the orchestra playing this symphony all become high on drugs, each playing his or her own melody, you would have some kind of analogy to what happens in the human body after years of eating and drinking food laced with herbicides, pesticides, preservatives and hormones. If we test the performance of any one member of this orchestra we may find that the music produced is acceptable; however, it is not in sync with the rest of the orchestra.

Thus, we may measure the blood biochemistry of an obese person, or a person with immune deficiency, and find almost all the studies to be normal. So, the doctor says, "Your studies are normal. There is nothing I can do for you. You have to learn to live with yourself the way you are."

That response would be a relatively enlightened one for most doctors. What you are more likely to get is a prescription for an appetite suppressant and some incorrect, parent-like advice about diet and exercise. Meanwhile, you may notice that the doctor also is a little round and not looking like the picture of vitality.

In my opinion, allopathic doctors are doing far more harm than good, in the long run. Why do I say that? Let us look at the allopathic model of medicine. The allopathic paradigm is that the body is perfectly normal until symptoms of a distinct disease appear. The cause of that disease is thought to be one thing, and all you have to do is identify that one thing and give the one best antidote to return the patient to perfect health.

So, if there is an infection, the task is to identify the bacteria or other organism causing the infection and kill it with a chemical, usually an antibiotic. Or, if the problem is with the immune system, the cause must be one thing, perhaps a virus. So kill the virus or, if that is not possible, develop a vaccine to the virus and protect people who do not yet have the virus. If the offending agent is one of the patient's own organs — the stomach, colon, or gallbladder, for example — pour a chemical on it. If that doesn't work, cut it out, throw it away and pronounce the patient cured.

It may be that biology is a bit more complex than the allopathic, one cause, one cure paradigm would have it. It may be that the causes of today's illnesses, especially the ones which are epidemic (vascular disease, cancer and immune dysfunction), are multi-factorial: coming from many different insults to body metabolism.

The average person in America is exposed to 500 foreign chemicals each day. Each *day*! This is an assault on the human body without precedent in history. I am not amazed that so many people are sick, I am amazed that so many people are well.

Nevertheless, the dominant medical model today is the allopathic model, so even though the supposed single causes of most diseases have not been discovered, there still is the assumption that there is one cause, and there should therefore be one cure. But, what if the cause is multiple?

Let us say that you have been exposed to 500 chemicals each day for years, your immune system is somewhat depressed by having been insulted by molecules foreign to the human body, and you develop bronchitis. Then your doc gives you a prescription for an antibiotic — another foreign chemical. The antibiotic kills the bacteria causing your bronchitis. Success, right? Maybe not. Maybe the antibiotic to which you have just been exposed — in an amount larger than the amount of all the other foreign chemicals to which you have been exposed in the last two months combined — while having killed the bacteria, also has insulted your immune system even more, making it more likely for you to develop another infection, perhaps in a different part of your body. So you solve this problem with another antibiotic — with the same result.

A similar situation exists with the cancer patient. Perhaps the cancer is the result of multiple insults to the body, but then the doctor says "Here take this stuff; it will kill your cancer, if it doesn't kill you first."

Picture the heart patient with cardiovascular disease from who-knows-what-they-put-in-it, which he or she has been eating for years, and the doctor says, "Take some of this stuff. If you survive the side effects, your heart may work better." What kind of solution is that?

Or, picture the AIDS patient. Diagnosis made. Patient assured of the single cause of AIDS: the HIV-1 virus. Here, take this AZT. Patient looks at the package insert, which comes with his AZT and sees that the possible side effects of AZT look like a description of autoimmune deficiency. How much sense does it make to take a medicine which can produce the disease it is supposed to treat?

Contrary to popular opinion, cancer and AIDS survival rates are no better with chemical treatments than they are without. They are different, however: the doctor has something to do and the pharmaceutical industry is getting rich.

The best hounds barking up the wrong tree will never catch the cat. Can it be that we are barking up the wrong tree? What if all diseases have multiple causes and predisposing factors. How wise are we to ignore those factors and take another chemical? Is it possible that we are producing more, rather than less, disease — in the long run?

If I were living a typical American life — eating processed foods, occasionally visiting a fast-food restaurant, drinking soft drinks, as well as unfiltered water from the city water supply (full of chlorine and fluoride), eating meat, not exercising so much — and I turned up with cancer or AIDS, here is what I would do if I wanted my best chance of living a long and vital life.

I would clean up my act. I would move to the countryside, as far away from traffic and industrial pollution as possible. I would either grow my own food or eat certified organically grown food. I would stop taking all drugs, including nonprescription drugs. I would drink only distilled or filtered, reverse osmosis water. I would never smoke another cigarette or drink another alcoholic drink. I would take a full range of vitamin supplements. I would exercise — vigorous aerobic exercise — 30 minutes every day. I would meditate several hours each day. All my medicines would be derived from herbs and other plants. I would juice fast three days of each week. I would find a colon therapist and maintain a perfectly clean colon. I would find a progressive physician and request chelox therapy (a combination of chelation therapy and hydrogen peroxide therapy). I would read and learn new things to do for my health, and I would do them. I would think and act for myself.

On the other hand, why wait? Why not do these things now? This is the way I live my life, except I do not meditate hours each day. When you learn I have cancer, or any other degenerative disease, that is the day you can throw this book away and forget about it. It will not happen. It does not have to happen to you either. *Your health is in your hands*.

NETWORKING

The Alternative Medicine Network

In the New Age — and this *is* the New Age — things work by networking. An ideal network consists of almost infinite channels of communication in which every person in the network has access to every other person in the network. The world is rapidly becoming a vast network, thanks to a convergence of technology and spiritual transformation. Organizations and businesses which do not understand this will soon learn and change, or they will pass into history.

The Referral Network

In the ideal medical network, you would have access to the physicians who render the kind of therapy in which you are interested. To play my responsible part in the creation of such a network, **I offer you a referral service to those doctors who are in substantial agreement with the principles outlined in this book.** Naturally, this is quite an effort on my part and the part of my staff. Any donation you send along with your request for a referral will be appreciated. We suggest $20. Simply send a stamped, self-addressed envelope, along with your check, to:

Ron Kennedy, M.D.
P.O. Box 2909
Rohnert Park, CA 94927
U.S.A.

You will receive a list of the 5-10 doctors nearest you who offer the therapy in which you are interested, provided that therapy is mentioned in this book. Please do not call, as we are not prepared to deal with phone requests.

If you are a physician (M.D., D.O., or N.D.) and want to be part of the network, list the alternative services you offer and forward that information to me with a request to be included on the referral list.

Networking this Book

This book is not advertised in the conventional sense. The only way it will live in the market place is by word of mouth — when one person tells another of its value. If you find value in this book, I encourage you to share it with others, *because it is the right thing to do.*

You can order this book through Context Publications. On page 383 there is an order form for your convenience.

Ron Kennedy, M.D.

Major subjects covered are in bold.

BONUS SECTION

A Sample Copy of

The Kennedy Newsletter

The Kennedy Quarterly Newsletter

An individual by the name of Matthias Rath, M.D. has come up with a comprehensive explanation of the cause, prevention, and treatment of vascular disease which I find rational and compelling. Dr. Rath has done seminal research at the University of Hamburg and has published twelve papers in respected research journals on the subject of vascular disease. He now lives in the U.S. and was a friend and colleague of the only double Noble prize winner, the late Dr. Linus Pauling. Dr. Rath has established a company called Health Now to educate the public about the prevention and treatment of vascular disease. In his public presentations and in his book *Eradicating Heart Disease*, Dr. Rath explains the known facts from his research on vascular disease and provides proof at each critical turn in his reasoning. I have reviewed his work and concluded that what he has to say is critically important. Therefore, I choose to throw what weight I have behind the effort to bring Dr. Rath's information to your attention.

The best part of Dr. Rath's discoveries is that they provide effective action anyone can take to both prevent and treat vascular disease in a powerful way by natural means without relying on Draconian changes in diet and lifestyle or dangerous drugs which lower cholesterol but do nothing to decrease overall mortality. Let us go to the beginning of this story.

Our distant ancestors lost the ability to produce vitamin C.

It long has been known that human beings do not produce ascorbic acid (vitamin C). Because vitamin C — which I shall refer to as "ascorbate" from here on out — is essential to life and because we cannot produce it, it is known as a vitamin in human metabolism. We are rare among species, because almost all \mammals can make abundant supplies of ascorbate. There are only four species of mammals which do not make their own ascorbate. These are (1) humans, (2) gorillas, (3) guinea pigs and (4) fruit bats.

All these species, except humans, are vegetarian by nature. Humans probably were vegetarians with rare exception, until the invention of animal husbandry. Gorillas are constantly foraging for plant food rich in vitamin C. Guinea pigs do the same, and fruit bats, well, why do you suppose we them call them fruit bats? These three animals know, by instinct, they must ingest large quantities of ascorbate to stay healthy.

In the body of an ascorbate-making mammal, the ascorbate molecule is made from a few small modifications of the glucose molecule. Glucose is in abundant supply in humans and animals at all times. There are four enzymes required to convert glucose into vitamin C. Humans have the first three enzymes, having lost the fourth enzyme somewhere in evolution.

In mammals which retained the ability to make ascorbic acid, it is made in response to all sorts of stress, especially the stress of infection. The normal everyday nonstress production of ascorbate, when proportioned up to represent the amount made on a weight basis corrected to the size of the average man (seventy kilograms), is from five to ten grams (5,000-10,000 mg.) per day. Under stress, that amount can be quadrupled.

Compare this to the official federal government recommendation (RDA or recommended deficiency allowance) of 60 mg. (six one-hundredths of one gram or six one-thousands of five grams). The increased production of ascorbate under stress in animals goes a long way toward explaining why we do not see anything like the rate of infection among animals which we see in human beings. When was the last time you saw an animal with a cold?

Why did these four mammals — humans, gorillas, guinea pigs and fruit bats — lose the ability to make ascorbate? Probably, because they could. I suspect that these four animals had abundant sources of ascorbate in their diets, and loss of ability to produce their own ascorbate did not put them at excess risk of being weeded out by natural selection. Only the human being has changed his dietary preferences since then. Humans are the only species to both eat meat and be unable to produce ascorbate. There are no other carnivores which cannot make ascorbate.

This explanation dovetails nicely with research in genetics which suggests that we all had a common mother and a common father who lived sometime between 100,000 to 200,000 years ago, all other branches of the human family since having died out. This would explain why all, and not just some, humans are deficient in this fourth enzyme. These common ancestors are thought to have lived in tropical regions of Africa where ascorbate-containing food was abundant.

Ice ages, scurvy, and natural selection

However, our common ancestors did not stay in Africa. They migrated to cover the entire earth. Then came the Ices Ages, one after another, each lasting around 10,000 years. We know from the archeological evidence that human beings lived through these ice ages in northern climates. They somehow toughed it out. Ascorbate, because it is made by plant food, is not easy to come by in an ice age. The old vegetable garden does not do so well under a thick layer of ice. These ancestors suffered from ascorbate deficiency, a disease called scurvy, a fact borne out by examination of their remains.

Scurvy is marked by the breakdown of collagen tissue throughout the body and frequent infections. Collagen is the protein with which strong connective tissue is made throughout the body. Sailors were known to have had scurvy on long voyages, until someone discovered that a little citrus fruit intake avoided the disease. The way those "scorbutic" (the term we apply to a person with scurvy) sailors died was by leakage of blood out of their blood vessels. Their blood vessels literally cracked open and they bled to death.

The same sort of thing happened to many of our ancestors who lived through the ice ages. Many of them bled to death because they had little or no ascorbate, and without ascorbate there is no collagen production or repair throughout the body. The wall of a blood vessel is made of collagen. Therefore, when you run out of ascorbate, it is only a matter of time until that wall of collagen breaks down, is not repaired, cracks open and you bleed to death.

Risk factors: lipoprotein(a), LDL, lipids, and oxidized cholesterol.

However, not all our Ice Ages ancestors died of cracked open blood vessels. Many did, but some had the ability to repair leaky blood vessel walls without the assistance of ascorbate.

These people, as a group, lived long enough to have children, and we are the descendants of those children. Therefore, we have inherited this ability to repair our blood vessel walls without much ascorbate.

When a crack develops in a blood vessel wall due to a shortage of ascorbate, certain fat packages in the blood have the ability to plug the leak by forming a kind of plaster cast. These packages of fat are known as cholesterol, lipids, low density lipoproteins (LDL), and one especially effective leak plugger, lipoprotein(a), a special type of LDL.

LDL is a bag of several thousand cholesterol and other fat molecules with the bag itself made of protein. In itself, despite all the hype in the media, ordinary LDL is no problem. However, there is one type of LDL, namely lipoprotein(a) which has an extra protein cover on the outside of the usual protein cover. Lipoprotein(a) is a double bag of fat. This outer bag is called apoprotein(a) or apo(a). The "a" could well stand for *adhesive*, because it is a very sticky substance. When a crack develops in the wall of a blood vessel, this sticky double-bagged fat sack finds its way through the crack. Once there, the apo(a) adhesive outer bag glues it down and begins the process of plugging the leak. This both avoids death by scurvy and sets the stage for blood vessel disease.

Once having plugged the leak the apo(a) outer bag sticks to whatever other bags of cholesterol (i.e. LDL) float by and glues them down as well. The process looks like the following:

1. The scorbutic (ascorbate deficient) crack in the blood vessel wall is the first step in atherosclerosis.

2. The plugging of the leak with lipoprotein(a) is the second step.

3. The gluing down of other LDL (single layer bags of cholesterol and lipids which are not sticky in themselves) is the third step.

4. The fourth step is the stimulation, by lipoprotein(a), of the muscle cells in the artery wall to multiply, thus forming a tumor (swelling).

5. Then the cleanup crew arrives, also known as macrophages, and they try to eat the whole mess and carry it away. However, many of them overeat, get fat, and become part of the problem by dying and being glued down into the plaque. Because they contain so much fat, they appear under the microscope to be full of foam, and they are therefore known as "foam cells."

The tumor, i.e., the proliferation of excess smooth muscle cells is not cancerous. Nevertheless, it can cause death by pushing this mass of plaque into the lumen (passage way) of the blood vessel in which this process is happening. This narrows the passage way through which blood passes and can eventually lead to heart attack, stroke and other problems, depending on where in the body it develops.

Here are all the known actions of ascorbate:

1. Increases HDL (high density lipoprotein) production. (HDL is able to help resorb fat located in plaque. In the process it changes from a disc shape to a globular form of HDL, and takes this fat to the liver to be burned.)

2. Decreases the production of lipoprotein(a). (Somehow the liver knows when there is plenty of ascorbate on board, and therefore no need for high levels of lipoprotein(a) which is, after all, a repair factor for the cracks in blood vessel walls which come up in the absence of sufficient ascorbate.)

3. Down-regulates cholesterol and triglyceride production in the liver. (These are secondary repair factors in that they are glued into the plaque by lipoprotein(a).)

4. Lowers blood sugar and insulin requirements.

5. By relaxing the blood vessel walls, lowers blood pressure when hypertension is present. (This is not the total answer to a case of hypertension, but it can help.)

6. Inhibits inappropriate intravascular clot formation (the final and sometimes deadly event in cases of heart attacks and strokes).

Lipoprotein(a) is the real risk factor for vascular disease.

The bottom line is that lipoprotein(a) is the real risk factor in cardiovascular disease and that ascorbate and niacin are the only major lines of defense against high levels of lipoprotein(a). Cholesterol, even LDL cholesterol, can serve as a statistical risk factor only to the degree that it is correlated with the level of the real problem: the special type of LDL called lipoprotein(a).

The best test, by far, for risk of cardiovascular disease is the direct measurement of this special type of LDL, namely a lipoprotein(a) level. A lipoprotein(a) level is ten times more accurate and specific for prediction of vascular disease.

You may have to educate your doctor.

By the way, this is new information, right out of the research journals. It will be many years before the average doctor knows about it and many more years before it is generally accepted and then a few more years before this test is routinely ordered in the evaluation for vascular disease. Medicine is dominated by a conservative inertia in which, for what they conceive of as medical-legal safety, 95% of the entire pack moves forward slowly, and together, to incorporate advances in science.

If you want this test now, you will probably have to educate your doctor about it and then insist on it. Also, you can be sure the anticholesterol industry is not going give up their position easily and adopt lipoprotein(a) as the new standard, regardless of the scientific truth behind the matter. If they do, they lose big money!

The presently accepted levels of lipoprotein(a) are the following.

0 - 20 mg./dl		low risk
20 - 40 mg./dl.		moderate risk
>40 mg./dl.		high risk

Here are the startling facts about lipoprotein(a).

1.   Lipoprotein(a) levels are largely determined by inheritance.

2.   Special diet does not influence lipoprotein(a) levels.

3.   None of the available cholesterol lowering drugs lower lipoprotein(a) blood levels.

4.   Ascorbate and niacin both lower lipoprotein(a) blood levels.

5.   L-lysine and L-proline, two natural amino acids, can prevent the apo(a) adhesive from sticking, serving as a kind of Teflon coating. Of these, L-proline is several times more powerful than L-lysine. These aminos also assist to shrink the plaque which is already present.

6.   Lipoprotein(a) blood level is the single greatest risk factor predicting the restenosis of vessels used in bypass surgery.

Animals in the wild do not get heart attacks.

The process of atherosclerosis is limited to humans. Animals in the wild do not develop atherosclerosis, therefore no heart attacks and no strokes occur among these citizens of nature. To induce an animal to have atherosclerosis you have to put it in captivity and feed it the kind of diet which humans use to cause the problem. The guinea pig and fruit bat make good models, if this is what you want to do. The gorilla would make a good model, but who wants fifty gorillas lined up in a laboratory?

Animals in the wild do not get heart attacks because they make their own ascorbate, and therefore the process of atherosclerosis does not begin. We humans could take the hint, load up on vitamin C and a few other vitamins twice each day for life and eradicate heart disease. This is already happening in the U.S. where ascorbate consumption has skyrocketed over the past 25 years, and heart disease has dropped by one third. The war against smoking may also have something to do with this, yet in countries where smoking has declined in the absence of increased ascorbate consumption, there has been no equivalent change in heart disease rates.

The cost in lives

Nevertheless, there is still a long way to go. In the U.S., every other person will die of vascular heart disease. Many more will die of stroke, another complication of vascular disease. Every year 1.5 million Americans die of heart attack, one fifth of them suddenly, before reaching the hospital or medical attention. Death is the first symptom of heart disease for forty percent of those who learn they have it. More than seven million Americans are living with vascular heart disease right now, and 2.5 million have cerebrovascular disease. Eight million Americans have arrythmias: irregular heartbeat related to vascular disease.

The cost in dollars

One hundred billion dollars are spent on vascular heart disease every year, $200,000 every minute of every day. Coronary bypass, an extremely inappropriate procedure for the great majority of heart patients — considering the alternatives — sucks ten billion dollars out of American pockets every year.

The only people gaining from this situation are the drug companies, the hospital industry, vascular surgeons and cardiologists. Do you think any of these folks are going to tell you what I am telling you about ascorbate and heart disease? Would you cut off your income, given the opportunity. No you would not. If you were even sufficiently up-to-date with the current scientific literature to know these things, you would develop doubts and rationalizations about the research demonstrating the relationship between heart disease and anything which the public could control on its own. You would then believe your own doubts and rationalizations. In your own private life, you would load up on ascorbate everyday, just in case.

Program for the reversal of heart disease

If you have vascular disease, and if you want not to have it, there is a plan for you.

1. Get yourself into chelation therapy and stay the course. This is the fastest, most proven method of dealing with this life-threatening condition. The literature proving this is extensive, despite what uninformed doctors may tell you. Then, in consultation with a doctor who practices nutritional medicine, take the following steps:

    (All the following dosages may be adjusted by your doctor, based on his or her experience and medical opinion.)

2. Vitamin C to bowel tolerance — as much as you can take without diarrhea. For most people this will be in the range of five to ten grams (5,000-10,000 mg.) each day. Spread this amount into two equal doses 12 hours apart. (Vitamin C prevents further cracking of the blood vessel wall — the beginning of the disease.)

3. Co-enzyme Q10 90-180 mg. twice each day (strengthens the heart muscle).

4. L-carnitine 3 grams twice each day (also strengthens the heart muscle).

5. L-lysine 3 grams twice each day (acts to release lipoprotein(a) from plaque formation and prevent further deposition of same).

6. L-proline 3 grams twice each day (acts to release lipoprotein(a) from plaque formation and prevent further deposition of same).

7. Niacin decreases the production of lipoprotein(a) in the liver. Inositol nicotinate is a form of naicin which gives less of a problem with flushing and therefore allows for larger therapeutic doses. Begin with 250 mg. at lunch, 500 mg. at dinner and 500 mg. at bedtime the first day; then increase gradually over a few days until you reach four grams per day, or the highest dose under four grams you can tolerate. Be sure to aks your doctor for liver enzyme level tests every two months or less to be sure your liver is able to handle the dose you are taking.

8. Vitamin E (as Unique E) 800-2400 IU per day. (This inhibits the proliferation of smooth muscle cells in the walls of arteries undergoing the atherosclerotic changes.)

9. Stop smoking. (This decreases the free radical load on your body.)

10. Adopt a sensible diet with plenty of veggies and not so much fat. (The metabolism of fat decreases your body vitamin pool dramatically.)

11. Ask your doctor for a comprehensive stool analysis (Great Smokies Lab) to see if you are digesting well all that good food. Your diet does not matter much if it is not getting into your body.

12. Lower stress in your life however you can.

13. Adopt a sensible exercise program in collaboration with your doctor.

  The Kennedy Quarterly Newsletter comes out Spring, Summer,

Fall and Winter. Its purpose is to provide life-saving, life-extending information.

How to order the Kennedy Newsletter

Follow the instruction of the Order Form on page 383 of this book.

Sources

Rath M, Niendorf A, Reblin T, Dietel M, Krebber H-J, and Beisiegel U   Detection and quantification of lipoprotein(a) of the atertial wall of 107 coronary bypass patients. Arteriosclerosis 9:579-92 (1989)

Rath M and Pauling L   Hypothesis: Lipoprotein(a) is a surrogate for ascorbate Proceedings of the National Acad of Sciences USA 87:6204-07 (1990a)

Rath M and Pauling L   Immunological evidence for the accumulation of lipoprotein(a) in the atherosclerotic lesion of the hypoascorbemic guinea pig   Proceeding of the National Academy of Sciences USA 87:9388-90 (1990b)

Rath M and Pauling L   Solution to the puzzle of human cardiovascular disease: its primary cause is ascorbate deficiency leading to the deposition of lipoprotein (a) and fibrinogen/fibrin in the vascular wall. J of Orthomolecular Med 6:125-34(1991a)

Rath M and Pauling L   Apoprotein(a) is an adhesive protein   J of Orthomolecular Med 6:139-43(1991b)

Rath M and Pauling L   A unified theory of human cardiovascular disease leading the way to abolition of this disease as a cause for human mortality   J of Orthomolecular Med 7:5-15(1992a)

Rath M and Pauling L   Plasma induced proteolysis and the role of lipoprotein(a), lysine and synthetic lysine analogs   J of Orthomolecular Med 7:17-23(1992b)

Rath M   Lipoprotein(a) reduction by ascorbate   J of Orthomolecular Med 7:81-2(1992c)

Rath M   Solution to the puzzle of human evolution   J of Orthomolecular Med 7:73-80(1992d)

Rath M   Reducing the risk for cardiovascular disease with nutritional supplements   J of Orthomolecular Med 7:153-62(1992e)

Rath M   Cationic-anionic and anionic-cationic oligopeptides in apoprotein(a) and other proteins as modulators of protein action and of biological communication   J of Applied Nutrition 44:62-9(1992f)

Rath M   Discovery of new elements of biological communication leading the way to the abolition of infectious diseases, cancer and other diseases as causes of human mortality J of Orthomolecular Med 8:11-20(1993)

We invite
you to visit our
World Wide Web site,

The Alternative Medicine Network
at:
http://www.sonic.net/~nexus

You can order copies of
this and other books by internet.
Simply fill out the order form at:
http://www.sonic.net/~nexus/order.html

Educational
consultations with
Dr. Kennedy are available.
Fill out the application form at
http://www.sonic.net/~nexus/kennedy.html

ORDER FORM

(Permission to photocopy this order form is granted.)

Write the number of books you are ordering in the box below.

☐ **THE THINKING PERSON'S GUIDE TO PERFECT HEALTH,**
Ron Kennedy, M.D. **Prices per book include shipping and handling.**

$ 25.^{00} in U.S., outside California
26.^{50} in California (includes sales tax)
31.^{00} (USD) Canada or Mexico
36.^{00} (USD) outside No. America, **surface mail**
44.^{00} (USD) outside No. America, **airmail**

Please check this next box if you want to order:

☐ **Dr. Kennedy's Quarterly Newsletter** for one (1) year!
I have enclosed $30 for my subscription ($36 outside U.S.)

ORDERING INSTRUCTIONS

Multiply the number of books ordered by the price per book, and choose your preferred method of payment. *Your check must be drawn on a U.S. bank. Any bank outside the U.S. can sell you a bank check drawn on one of their U.S. bank accounts. Make checks payable to: Context Publications.*

Method of Payment : ☐ Check   ☐ Money order   ☐ Visa   ☐ MasterCard

_____   _____

Your credit card number↗   Expiration date↗

_____   _____

Your name as it appears on card↗   Your authorized signature↗

Ship book(s) to:

↘

_____   _____
name   phone number

_____   _____
street address   suite or apartment number

_____   _____
city   state   zip or postal code

_____
country

Mail order form to:

Context Publications
P.O. Box 2909
Rohnert Park, CA 94927
U.S.A.

Or, you may phone, fax, or internet your order:

Tel. **(707) 576-1700** ✦ Fax **(707) 575-6830**
Telephone credit card orders only: **(800) 963-2633**
By internet: *http://www.sonic.net /~nexus/order.html*

A Final Word

Life can become unimaginably diffucult, and some of those difficulties appear as illness in the body. Ill health can be heard as a wake up call for the spirit, if you stop to listen. In this sense, every illness represents the possibility of spiritual transformation as incredible as the illness is troublesome, right up to, and including, the final event of life.

Writing this book was a labor of love. If you saw only the information and missed the love, you did not read between the lines. I wish for you, and for those people you love, long and healthy lives in which you live out the purposes for which you came into this world. And at the end, I wish for you the peace only God can bring.

Ron Kennedy

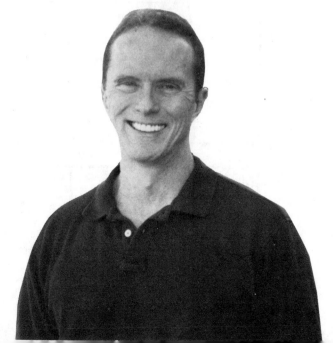